MR in the Emergency Room

Editor

JORGE A. SOTO

MAGNETIC RESONANCE IMAGING CLINICS OF NORTH AMERICA

www.mri.theclinics.com

Consulting Editors
SURESH K. MUKHERJI
LYNNE S. STEINBACH

May 2016 • Volume 24 • Number 2

ELSEVIER

1600 John F. Kennedy Boulevard • Suite 1800 • Philadelphia, Pennsylvania, 19103-2899

http://www.mri.theclinics.com

MRI CLINICS OF NORTH AMERICA Volume 24, Number 2
May 2016 ISSN 1064-9689, ISBN 13: 978-0-323-44469-9

Editor: John Vassallo (j.vassallo@elsevier.com)
Developmental Editor: Meredith Clinton

© **2016 Elsevier Inc. All rights reserved.**

This periodical and the individual contributions contained in it are protected under copyright by Elsevier, and the following terms and conditions apply to their use:

Photocopying
Single photocopies of single articles may be made for personal use as allowed by national copyright laws. Permission of the Publisher and payment of a fee is required for all other photocopying, including multiple or systematic copying, copying for advertising or promotional purposes, resale, and all forms of document delivery. Special rates are available for educational institutions that wish to make photocopies for non-profit educational classroom use. For information on how to seek permission visit www.elsevier.com/permissions or call: (+44) 1865 843830 (UK)/ (+1) 215 239 3804 (USA).

Derivative Works
Subscribers may reproduce tables of contents or prepare lists of articles including abstracts for internal circulation within their institutions. Permission of the Publisher is required for resale or distribution outside the institution. Permission of the Publisher is required for all other derivative works, including compilations and translations (please consult www.elsevier.com/permissions).

Electronic Storage or Usage
Permission of the Publisher is required to store or use electronically any material contained in this periodical, including any article or part of an article (please consult www.elsevier.com/permissions). Except as outlined above, no part of this publication may be reproduced, stored in a retrieval system or transmitted in any form or by any means, electronic, mechanical, photocopying, recording or otherwise, without prior written permission of the Publisher.

Notice
No responsibility is assumed by the Publisher for any injury and/or damage to persons or property as a matter of products liability, negligence or otherwise, or from any use or operation of any methods, products, instructions or ideas contained in the material herein. Because of rapid advances in the medical sciences, in particular, independent verification of diagnoses and drug dosages should be made.

Although all advertising material is expected to conform to ethical (medical) standards, inclusion in this publication does not constitute a guarantee or endorsement of the quality or value of such product or of the claims made of it by its manufacturer.

Magnetic Resonance Imaging Clinics of North America (ISSN 1064-9689) is published quarterly by Elsevier Inc., 360 Park Avenue South, New York, NY 10010-1710. Months of issue are February, May, August, and November. Business and Editorial Offices: 1600 John F. Kennedy Blvd., Ste. 1800, Philadelphia, PA 19103-2899. Customer Service Office: 3251 Riverport Lane, Maryland Heights, MO 63043. Periodicals postage paid at New York, NY and additional mailing offices. Subscription prices are $380.00 per year (domestic individuals), $636.00 per year (domestic institutions), $100.00 per year (domestic students/residents), $420.00 per year (Canadian individuals), $828.00 per year (Canadian institutions), $545.00 per year (international individuals), $828.00 per year (international institutions), and $275.00 per year (international and Canadian students/residents). International air speed delivery is included in all *Clinics* subscription prices. All prices are subject to change without notice. **POSTMASTER:** Send address changes to *Magnetic Resonance Imaging Clinics*, Elsevier Health Sciences Division, Subscription Customer Service, 3251 Riverport Lane, Maryland Heights, MO 63043. Customer Service (orders, claims, online, change of address): Elsevier Health Sciences Division, Subscription **Customer Service, 3251 Riverport Lane, Maryland Heights, MO 63043. Tel:1-800-654-2452 (U.S. and Canada); 314-447-8871 (outside U.S. and Canada). Fax: 314-447-8029. E-mail: journalscustomer** service-usa@elsevier.com **(for print support);** journalsonlinesupport-usa@elsevier.com **(for online support).**

Reprints. For copies of 100 or more of articles in this publication, please contact the Commercial Reprints Department, Elsevier Inc., 360 Park Avenue South, New York, NY 10010-1710. Tel.: 212-633-3874; Fax: 212-633-3820; E-mail: reprints@elsevier.com.

Magnetic Resonance Imaging Clinics of North America is covered in the *RSNA Index of Imaging Literature, MEDLINE/PubMed (Index Medicus),* and *EMBASE/Excerpta Medica.*

Printed in the United States of America.

Contributors

CONSULTING EDITORS

SURESH K. MUKHERJI, MD, MBA, FACR
Department of Radiology, Michigan State
University, East Lansing, Michigan

LYNNE S. STEINBACH, MD, FACR
Professor of Radiology and Orthopaedic
Surgery, Department of Radiology and
Biomedical Imaging, University of California
San Francisco, San Francisco, California

EDITOR

JORGE A. SOTO, MD
Professor, Department of Radiology, Boston
Medical Center, Boston University School of
Medicine, Boston, Massachusetts

AUTHORS

HANI H. ABUJUDEH, MD
Department of Radiology, Massachusetts
General Hospital, Boston, Massachusetts

WILSON ALTMEYER, MD
Assistant Professor of Radiology;
Neuroradiology Fellowship Director, University
of Texas Health Science Center at San Antonio,
San Antonio, Texas

AKSHAY D. BAHETI, MD, DO
Department of Radiology, University of
Washington, Seattle, Washington

DAVID D.B. BATES, MD
Radiology Resident, Department of Radiology,
Boston Medical Center, Boston University
School of Medicine, Boston, Massachusetts

GENEVIEVE L. BENNETT, MD
Department of Radiology, New York University
School of Medicine, New York, New York

PUNEET BHARGAVA, MD
Department of Radiology, University of
Washington, Seattle, Washington

RITU BORDIA, MBBS, MPH
Section of Neuroradiology, Department of
Radiology, Winthrop-University Hospital,
Mineola, New York

PATRICIA T. CHANG, MD
Department of Radiology, Boston Children's
Hospital, Harvard Medical School, Boston,
Massachusetts

MARGARET N. CHAPMAN, MD
Assistant Professor of Radiology,
Department of Radiology, Boston
Medical Center, Boston University School
of Medicine, Boston, Massachusetts;
Radiology Service, VA Boston
Healthcare System, West Roxbury,
Massachusetts

MATTHEW DATTWYLER, MD
Department of Radiology, Massachusetts
General Hospital, Boston, Massachusetts

AKIFUMI FUJITA, MD, PhD
Associate Professor of Radiology,
Department of Radiology, Jichi Medical
University School of Medicine, Tochigi,
Japan

ALI GUERMAZI, MD, PhD
Professor of Radiology, Section Head, Section of Musculoskeletal Imaging, Department of Radiology, Boston Medical Center, Boston University School of Medicine, Boston, Massachusetts

AVNEESH GUPTA, MD
Clinical Associate Professor, Department of Radiology, Boston Medical Center, Boston University School of Medicine, Boston, Massachusetts

JUAN GUTIERREZ, MD
Director of Neuroradiology Division, Medico Neuroradiologo, Centro Avanzado de Diagnóstico Médico CEDIMED, Medellin, Colombia

RATHACHAI KAEWLAI, MD
Radiologist, Department of Diagnostic and Therapeutic Radiology, Faculty of Medicine, Ramathibodi Hospital, Mahidol University, Bangkok, Thailand

DOUGLAS S. KATZ, MD
Department of Radiology, Winthrop-University Hospital, Mineola, New York

DANIEL KAWAKYU-O'CONNOR, MD
Assistant Professor, Division of Emergency Imaging, Department of Imaging Sciences, University of Rochester Medical Center, Rochester, New York

ANDREW KOMPEL, MD
Assistant Professor of Radiology, Section of Musculoskeletal Imaging, Department of Radiology, Boston Medical Center, Boston University School of Medicine, Boston, Massachusetts

WAYNE KUBAL, MD
Professor of Radiology, Department of Medical Imaging, University of Arizona, Tucson, Arizona

MANICKAM KUMARAVEL, MD
Associate Professor, Director Musculoskeletal Imaging Division, Department of Diagnostic and Interventional Imaging, University of Texas Health Science Center at Houston, Houston, Texas

CHRISTINA A. LeBEDIS, MD
Assistant Professor of Radiology, Department of Radiology, Boston Medical Center, Boston University School of Medicine, Boston, Massachusetts

EDWARD Y. LEE, MD, MPH
Chief, Division of Thoracic Imaging, Department of Radiology, Boston Children's Hospital, Harvard Medical School, Boston, Massachusetts

MARIAM MOSHIRI, MD
Department of Radiology, University of Washington, Seattle, Washington

AKIRA MURAKAMI, MD
Assistant Professor of Radiology, Section of Musculoskeletal Imaging, Department of Radiology, Boston Medical Center, Boston University School of Medicine, Boston, Massachusetts

KAMBIZ NAEL, MD
Assistant Professor of Radiology, Director of Neuro MRI, CT and Advanced Imaging, Department of Radiology, Icahn School of Medicine at Mount Sinai, New York, New York; Department of Medical Imaging, University of Arizona, Tucson, Arizona

REFKY NICOLA, MS, DO
Division of Emergency Imaging, Department of Imaging Sciences; Department of Radiology, University of Rochester Medical Center, Rochester, New York

NAOKO SAITO, MD, PhD
Assistant Professor of Radiology, Department of Radiology, Saitama International Medical Center, Saitama Medical University, Saitama, Japan

OSAMU SAKAI, MD, PhD
Professor of Radiology, Otolaryngology – Head and Neck Surgery, and Radiation Oncology; Chief of Neuroradiology, Department of Radiology, Boston Medical Center, Boston University School of Medicine, Boston, Massachusetts

AJAY K. SINGH, MD
Department of Radiology, Massachusetts
General Hospital, Boston, Massachusetts

JORGE A. SOTO, MD
Professor, Department of Radiology, Boston
Medical Center, Boston University School of
Medicine, Boston, Massachusetts

ANDREW STEVEN, MD
Assistant Professor of Radiology, University of
Maryland Medical System, Baltimore,
Maryland

DAVID W. SWENSON, MD
Department of Radiology, Boston Children's
Hospital, Harvard Medical School, Boston,
Massachusetts

NEIL THAYIL, MD
Department of Radiology, Boston Medical
Center, Boston University School of Medicine,
Boston, Massachusetts

WILLIAM M. WEATHERS, MD
Department of Radiology, University of Texas
Health Science Center at Houston, Houston,
Texas

SIROTE WONGWAISAYAWAN, MD
Radiologist, Department of Diagnostic and
Therapeutic Radiology, Faculty of Medicine,
Ramathibodi Hospital, Mahidol University,
Bangkok, Thailand

EDWARD YANG, MD, PhD
Department of Radiology, Boston Children's
Hospital, Harvard Medical School, Boston,
Massachusetts

Contents

> Neuroimaging plays a critical role in the management of patients with acute stroke syndrome, with diagnostic, therapeutic, and prognostic implications. A multiparametric magnetic resonance (MR) imaging protocol in the emergency setting can address both primary goals of neuroimaging (ie, detection of infarction and exclusion of hemorrhage) and secondary goals of neuroimaging (ie, identifying the site of arterial occlusion, tissue characterization for defining infarct core and penumbra, and determining stroke cause/mechanism). MR imaging provides accurate diagnosis of acute ischemic stroke (AIS) and can differentiate AIS from other potential differential diagnoses.

> Magnetic resonance (MR) imaging is an extremely useful tool in the evaluation of traumatic brain injury in the emergency department. Although Computed tomography (CT) still plays the dominant role in urgent patient triage, MR imaging's impact on traumatic brain injury imaging continues to expand. MR imaging has shown superiority to CT for certain traumatic processes, such as diffuse axonal injury, cerebral contusion, and infarction. Magnetic resonance angiography and magnetic resonance venography allow emergent vascular imaging for patients that should avoid ionizing radiation or intravenous contrast.

> Magnetic resonance (MR) imaging of the spine is increasingly being used in the evaluation of spinal emergencies because it is highly sensitive and specific in the diagnosis of acute conditions of the spine. The prompt and accurate recognition allows for appropriate medical and surgical intervention. This article reviews the MR imaging features of common emergent conditions, such as spinal trauma, acute disc herniation, infection, and tumors. In addition, we describe common MR imaging sequences, discuss challenges encountered in emergency imaging of the spine, and illustrate multiple mimics of acute conditions.

> This article discusses the use of magnetic resonance (MR) imaging in various acute infectious diseases of the head and neck, with particular emphasis on situations

where MR imaging provides additional information that can significantly impact treatment decisions and outcomes. MR imaging findings of various disease processes are discussed, based on the head and neck compartments from which they originate. Specifically, infectious entities of the orbit, paranasal sinuses, pharynx, oral cavity (including periodontal disease), salivary glands, temporal bone, and lymph nodes are described in detail.

Many pathologies of the musculoskeletal system involve nontraumatic causes. Magnetic resonance (MR) imaging is used in the diagnosis because of its high sensitivity and specificity compared with other modalities. Osteomyelitis, osteonecrosis of the femoral head, and stress fractures are pathologies of bone where early diagnosis and intervention usually lead to an improved outcome. Joint aspiration and culture is the standard for diagnosing septic arthritis. MR imaging can support the diagnosis and allows evaluation for adjacent abscess and osteomyelitis. Early in the disease process, necrotizing fasciitis may not be clinically suspected and imaging may provide the first indication of the presence of this potentially deadly infection.

Musculoskeletal (MSK) trauma is commonly encountered in the emergency department. Computed tomography and radiography are the main forms of imaging assessment, but the use of magnetic resonance (MR) imaging has become more common in the emergency room (ER) setting for evaluation of low-velocity/sports-related injury and high-velocity injury. The superior soft tissue contrast and detail provided by MR imaging gives clinicians a powerful tool in the management of acute MSK injury in the ER. This article provides an overview of techniques and considerations when using MR imaging in the evaluation of some of the common injuries seen in the ER setting.

The utility of magnetic resonance (MR) imaging in evaluating abdominal and pelvic pain in the pregnant patient is discussed. Details regarding the indications, technical aspects, and imaging findings of various common abdominal and pelvic abnormalities in pregnancy are reviewed.

Magnetic resonance (MR) imaging is gaining increased acceptance in the emergency setting despite the continued dominance of computed tomography. MR has the advantages of more precise tissue characterization, superior soft tissue contrast, and a lack of ionizing radiation. Traditional barriers to emergent MR are being overcome by streamlined imaging protocols and newer rapid-acquisition sequences. As the utilization of MR imaging in the emergency department increases, a strong working knowledge of the MR appearance of the most commonly encountered abdominopelvic pathologies is essential. In this article, MR imaging protocols and findings of acute pelvic, scrotal, and gastrointestinal pathologies are discussed.

MAGNETIC RESONANCE IMAGING CLINICS OF NORTH AMERICA

VISIT THE CLINICS ONLINE!
Access your subscription at:
www.theclinics.com

PROGRAM OBJECTIVE
The goal of *Magnetic Resonance Imaging Clinics of North America* is to keep practicing physicians up to date with current clinical practice by providing timely articles reviewing the state of the art in patient care.

TARGET AUDIENCE
All practicing physicians and healthcare professionals who provide patient care utilizing findings from Magnetic Resonance Imaging.

LEARNING OBJECTIVES
Upon completion of this activity, participants will be able to:
1. Review the use of MR in musculoskeletal emergencies.
2. Discuss the use of MR in pelvic, gastrointestinal, and obstetric emergencies.
3. Recognize the use of MR in head traumas and infections.

ACCREDITATION
The Elsevier Office of Continuing Medical Education (EOCME) is accredited by the Accreditation Council for Continuing Medical Education (ACCME) to provide continuing medical education for physicians.

The EOCME designates this enduring material for a maximum of 15 *AMA PRA Category 1 Credit*(s)™. Physicians should claim only the credit commensurate with the extent of their participation in the activity.

All other health care professionals requesting continuing education credit for this enduring material will be issued a certificate of participation.

DISCLOSURE OF CONFLICTS OF INTEREST
The EOCME assesses conflict of interest with its instructors, faculty, planners, and other individuals who are in a position to control the content of CME activities. All relevant conflicts of interest that are identified are thoroughly vetted by EOCME for fair balance, scientific objectivity, and patient care recommendations. EOCME is committed to providing its learners with CME activities that promote improvements or quality in healthcare and not a specific proprietary business or a commercial interest.

The planning committee, staff, authors and editors listed below have identified no financial relationships or relationships to products or devices they or their spouse/life partner have with commercial interest related to the content of this CME activity:
Wilson Altmeyer, MD; David D.B. Bates, MD; Genevieve L. Bennett, MD; Puneet Bhargava, MD; Ritu Bordia, MBBS, MPH; Patricia T. Chang, MD; Margaret N. Chapman, MD; Akshay D. Baheti, MD, DO; Anjali Fortna; Akifumi Fujita, MD, PhD; Ali Guermazi, MD, PhD; Avneesh Gupta, MD; Juan Gutierrez, MD; Rathachai Kaewlai, MD; Douglas S. Katz, MD; Daniel Kawakyu O'Connor, MD; Andrew Kompel, MD; Wayne Kubal, MD; Manickam Kumaravel, MD; Christina A. LeBedis, MD; Edward Y. Lee, MD, MPH; Mariam Moshiri, MD; Suresh K. Mukherji, MD, MBA, FACR; Akira Murakami, MD; Kambiz Nael, MD; Refky Nicola, MS, DO; Naoko Saito, MD, PhD; Osamu Sakai, MD, PhD; Erin Scheckenbach; Jorge A. Soto, MD; Andrew Steven, MD; Karthik Subramaniam; David W. Swenson, MD; Neil Thayii, MD; John Vassallo; William M. Weathers, MD; Sirote Wongwaisayawan, MD; Edward Yang, MD.

UNAPPROVED/OFF-LABEL USE DISCLOSURE
The EOCME requires CME faculty to disclose to the participants:
1. When products or procedures being discussed are off-label, unlabelled, experimental, and/or investigational (not US Food and Drug Administration [FDA] approved); and
2. Any limitations on the information presented, such as data that are preliminary or that represent ongoing research, interim analyses, and/or unsupported opinions. Faculty may discuss information about pharmaceutical agents that is outside of FDA-approved labelling. This information is intended solely for CME and is not intended to promote off-label use of these medications. If you have any questions, contact the medical affairs department of the manufacturer for the most recent prescribing information.

TO ENROLL
To enroll in the *Magnetic Resonance Imaging Clinics of North America* Continuing Medical Education program, call customer service at 1-800-654-2452 or sign up online at http://www.theclinics.com/home/cme. The CME program is available to subscribers for an additional annual fee of USD 250.

METHOD OF PARTICIPATION
In order to claim credit, participants must complete the following:
1. Complete enrolment as indicated above.
2. Read the activity.
3. Complete the CME Test and Evaluation. Participants must achieve a score of 70% on the test. All CME Tests and Evaluations must be completed online.

CME INQUIRIES/SPECIAL NEEDS
For all CME inquiries or special needs, please contact elsevierCME@elsevier.com.

Foreword

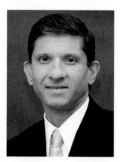

Suresh K. Mukherji, MD, MBA, FACR
Consulting Editor

The largest growing segment, and some would argue specialty, is emergency radiology. The cause of the growth is very complicated and due to multiple factors, including access, payments, and our "on-demand" culture. With the continuing growth of this specialty, the challenge of utilization and appropriateness must be addressed. MR is being increasingly considered the first-line test in a variety of clinical conditions that require immediate imaging evaluation in the emergency room. But what is the real value of MR in the emergency setting?

This issue of the *Magnetic Resonance Imaging Clinics* focuses on the proper use of MR in the emergency setting. Dr Jorge Soto has done a masterful job assembling world-renowned experts to write articles on MR of acute stroke, cranial trauma, spinal emergencies, head and neck infections, musculoskeletal emergencies, and acute conditions of the abdomen and pelvis. He also has included articles pertaining to the emergency MR imaging performed in children and in pregnancy. I want to personally thank Dr Soto for his willingness to take on this challenging topic and congratulate him and his colleagues for creating such an outstanding issue of *Magnetic Resonance Imaging Clinics*.

Suresh K. Mukherji, MD, MBA, FACR
Department of Radiology
Michigan State University
846 Service Road
East Lansing, MI 48824, USA

E-mail address:
mukherji@rad.msu.edu

Magn Reson Imaging Clin N Am 24 (2016) xiii
http://dx.doi.org/10.1016/j.mric.2016.02.002
1064-9689/16/$ – see front matter © 2016 Published by Elsevier Inc.

Foreword

Preface
MR in the Emergency Room

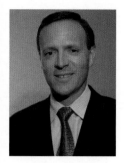

Jorge A. Soto, MD
Editor

The practice of Emergency Radiology continues to undergo rapid and substantial changes. The number and complexity of imaging tests performed on acutely ill patients have expanded rapidly. So has the need for near real-time interpretations of these examinations, which has resulted in an exponential growth in the number of emergency centers that provide around-the-clock coverage by onsite radiologists. Almost simultaneously, there has been a growing concern among health care providers and the public in general about the harmful consequences of the indiscriminate use of ionizing radiation (mostly delivered with computed tomography [CT]). Although the numerous benefits of the proper use of CT in the emergency setting are unquestionable, it is also true that alternative imaging tests are desirable in certain patient populations that are particularly prone to the potentially negative effects of the excessive use of this modality, such as children, young adults, and pregnant patients. Thus, it is not surprising that MR is being increasingly considered as the first-line test in a variety of clinical conditions that require immediate imaging evaluation in the emergency room. MR is also the "go to" modality when results of other examinations (CT, ultrasound) are inconclusive or nondiagnostic. The number of MR scanners installed in, or adjacent to, the emergency room of tertiary care centers has increased considerably, and this trend will only continue.

This issue of *Magnetic Resonance Imaging Clinics of North America* focuses on the proper use of MR in the emergency setting. Some articles address conditions that have been traditionally evaluated with MR, such as suspected stroke, spinal emergencies, and abdominal/pelvic pain in the pregnant patient. Other articles focus on the use of MR as a problem-solver or second-line modality, such as cranial trauma, head and neck infections, pancreaticobiliary emergencies, and musculoskeletal emergencies (traumatic and nontraumatic). Finally, the common theme in the remaining two articles is the use of MR in clinical situations, where this modality is a good alternative for diagnosis without the use of ionizing radiation: pediatric emergencies and a subgroup of acute pelvic and gastrointestinal emergencies. I am indebted to the contributing authors, who understood the importance of the topics and ensured that every article delivers a clear message about the appropriateness of the use of MR in specific circumstances. I also want to thank Suresh Mukherji, MD, for trusting me with the responsibility of editing this issue of *Magnetic Resonance Imaging Clinics of North America*, and Meredith Clinton and the Elsevier staff, for their continuous help.

Jorge A. Soto, MD
Department of Radiology
Boston Medical Center
Boston University School of Medicine
FGH Building, 3rd Floor
820 Harrison Avenue
Boston, MA 02118, USA

E-mail address:
jorge.soto@bmc.org

Magn Reson Imaging Clin N Am 24 (2016) xv
http://dx.doi.org/10.1016/j.mric.2016.02.001
1064-9689/16/$ – see front matter © 2016 Published by Elsevier Inc.

Magnetic Resonance Imaging of Acute Stroke

Kambiz Nael, MD[a,b,*], Wayne Kubal, MD[b]

KEYWORDS

- MR imaging • Stroke • Emergency imaging • MR perfusion • MR angiography

KEY POINTS

- Neuroimaging plays a critical role in the management of patients with acute stroke syndrome, with diagnostic, therapeutic, and prognostic implications.
- A multiparametric magnetic resonance (MR) imaging protocol in the emergency setting can address both primary goals of neuroimaging (ie, detection of infarction and exclusion of hemorrhage) and secondary goals of neuroimaging (ie, identifying the site of arterial occlusion, tissue characterization for defining infarct core and penumbra, and determining stroke cause/mechanism).
- MR imaging provides accurate diagnosis of acute ischemic stroke (AIS) and can differentiate AIS from other potential differential diagnoses.

INTRODUCTION

Stroke is a common and serious disorder, with an annual incidence of approximately 795,000 in the United States, of which approximately 85% are ischemic and 15% are hemorrhagic.[1] Neuroimaging plays a critical role in the diagnosis and management of patients with acute stroke. The neuroimaging evaluation of patients with suspected acute stroke has significantly evolved over the past few decades from a simple noncontrast computed tomography (CT) to now frequently including multiparametric data, including vascular and perfusion imaging.

Although the time window of 3.0 to 4.5 hours still applies for intravenous–thrombolytic treatment, recent clinical trials with encouraging results on the potential role of endovascular treatment[2–4] have created new possibilities for advanced stroke treatment, with the potential for treatment of many more patients beyond the 4.5 hours time window. This possibility makes the role of advanced imaging even more crucial, with the potential for

expanding the treatment window for patients with acute stroke if carefully screened and selected based on appropriate imaging criteria. The paradigm is changing from "time is brain" to "imaging is brain."

This article reviews the role of magnetic resonance (MR) imaging and multiparametric MR imaging for the evaluation of patients presenting with acute stroke syndrome, such as acute ischemic stroke (AIS), intracranial hemorrhage (ICH), and transient ischemic attack (TIA), and some of the potential challenging differential diagnoses in the acute emergency setting. It also reviews our institutional technical and clinical experience in MR imaging of patients with acute stroke and provides some clinical examples.

ROLE OF MAGNETIC RESONANCE IMAGING IN STROKE IMAGING

The primary goals of neuroimaging are to determine the presence of infarction and to distinguish between hemorrhagic and ischemic stroke. The

Disclosure: The authors have nothing to disclose.
[a] Department of Radiology, Icahn School of Medicine at Mount Sinai, One Gustave L. Levy Place, Box 1234, New York, NY 10029, USA; [b] Department of Medical Imaging, University of Arizona, PO Box 245067, 1501 N Campbell Ave, Room 1365, Tucson, AZ 85724-5067, USA
* Corresponding author.
E-mail address: Kambiznael@gmail.com

Magn Reson Imaging Clin N Am 24 (2016) 293–304
http://dx.doi.org/10.1016/j.mric.2015.11.002
1064-9689/16/$ – see front matter © 2016 Elsevier Inc. All rights reserved.

secondary goals of stroke imaging, largely applied to ischemic strokes, are to identify the location and extent of intravascular clot as well as the presence and extent of penumbra (hypoperfused tissue at risk for infarction).[5,6] To be effective, comprehensive stroke protocols should be able to address the aforementioned primary and secondary goals in a timely manner.

Although CT is the most commonly used modality for stroke imaging, partly because of its wide availability and faster acquisition time, some comprehensive stroke centers choose MR imaging rather than CT for 2 major reasons. First, higher sensitivity and specificity of MR imaging for delineation of hyperacute ischemia. Diffusion-weighted imaging (DWI) provides the most specific way to image acute infarction and perfusion imaging can help in delineation of ischemic penumbra. The advent of MR imaging has redefined stroke syndromes such as acute ischemic infarction and TIA from an all-or-none process to a dynamic and evolving process, providing meaningful physiologic and functional information. Second, the absence of radiation. A comprehensive CT stroke protocol delivers a mean effective dose of 16.4 mSv,[7] which is approximately 6 times the dose of an unenhanced CT head. This difference is particularly important for patients who need repeat examinations following treatment or have a change in their neurologic examination, in whom the repeated CT scans can be prohibitive because of the accumulated radiation dose.

HOW I DO IT?
Image Acquisition (Technical Aspects)

At our institution, if there is no contraindication, MR is the default imaging modality for patients presenting with suspicion of AIS. After activation of the stroke code and the patient's arrival at the emergency department, an MR safety questionnaire is administered and MR-compatible electrocardiogram leads are placed as the patient is being evaluated by the neurology team. The patient is then placed on an MR-compatible table and wheeled to the MR magnet for imaging.

We have 2 stroke MR protocols in place: (1) a fast stroke protocol that takes approximately 6 minutes to acquire,[8] and (2) a routine stroke protocol that takes about 20 to 25 minutes. Although many factors contribute to the decision of which protocol to perform, the fast MR protocol is mainly used for patients who are considered strong candidates for an interventional procedure, such as mechanical embolectomy, to minimize the imaging time without delaying treatment. The routine stroke protocol encompasses other imaging

components that allow for further detailed evaluation of the brain, taking into account other differential diagnoses and stroke mimics.

Improvements in MR imaging hardware technology, including the introduction of multicoil technology for better signal reception and higher magnetic fields (≥3 T), which afford higher signal/noise ratio, have increased the efficiency with which fast imaging tools can be applied. In addition, fast sequence design such as echo planar imaging (EPI) and rapid imaging tools such as parallel acquisition algorithms[9] have resulted in significant improvements in the efficiency of MR imaging in terms of both spatial and temporal resolution. Taking advantage of these combinations, we have designed and are effectively using a fast MR imaging protocol with total acquisition time of approximately 6 minutes, a 4-fold reduction in scan time compared with conventional MR stroke imaging.[10,11] For comprehensive stroke centers that choose MR imaging as their imaging modality, the described protocol allows a comparable acquisition time and efficiency to that of multimodal CT protocols, and takes advantage of the superior tissue resolution, the higher sensitivity, and the higher specificity for delineation of infarction afforded by MR imaging.[12]

IMAGING COMPONENTS

Comprehensive MR stroke protocols used routinely in major stroke centers have 3 essential components: (1) parenchymal imaging, which identifies the presence and size of an irreversible infarcted core, determines presence of hemorrhage, and helps to age the ischemic event; (2) MR angiogram to determine the location of arterial occlusion and presence of an intravascular thrombus that can be treated with thrombolysis or thrombectomy; (3) perfusion imaging to determine the presence of hypoperfused tissue at risk for subsequent infarction if adequate perfusion is not restored.

Each of these components and their potential clinical applications are reviewed here.

Parenchymal Imaging

Parenchymal imaging usually encompasses 3 components:

Diffusion-weighted imaging
Diffusion-weighted imaging (DWI) can detect ischemic tissue within minutes of ictus and has emerged as the most sensitive and specific imaging technique for acute ischemia (**Fig. 1**), far beyond nonenhanced CT or any other type of MR imaging sequences.[12] In addition, the pattern of

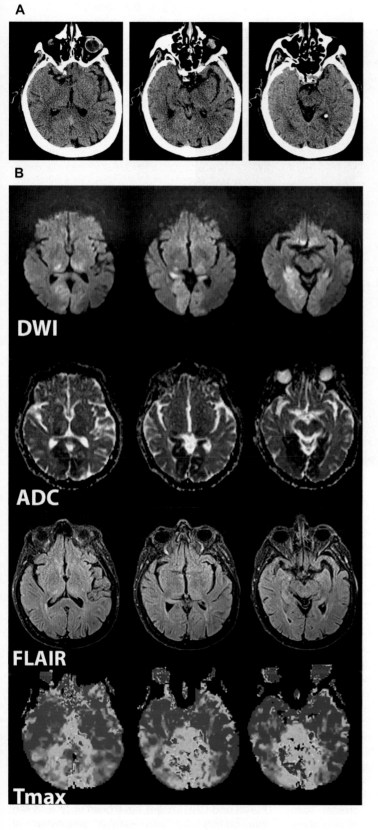

Fig. 1. A 91-year-old woman with history of diabetes, atrial fibrillation, and hypertension presented with acute onset of severe headache and then became unresponsive. Baseline National Institutes of Health Stroke Scale (NIHSS): 26. Time from onset to imaging was approximately 2 hours. Sequential aligned noncontrast CT (*A*) and MR imaging DWI, apparent diffusion coefficient (ADC), fluid-attenuated inversion recovery (FLAIR), and dynamic susceptibility contrast (DSC) time to maximum (T_{max}) (*B*) and a coronal and sagittal maximum intensity projection from the contrast-enhanced magnetic resonance angiography (CE-MRA) image (*C*) are shown. There is a hyperacute infarction seen on DWI-ADC images involving bilateral posterior cerebral artery (PCA) territories, including bilateral thalami and occipital lobes. Note that the infarction is not seen on CT or FLAIR, which is suggestive of hyperacuity. There is matched perfusion deficit on DSC-T_{max}. CE-MRA images show an absence of flow within the left vertebral artery, diminutive flow within the intradural segment of the right vertebral artery and proximal basilar artery, with occlusion and absence of flow within the distal basilar and proximal PCA arteries caused by acute basilar artery thrombosis.

C

Fig. 1. (*continued*)
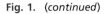

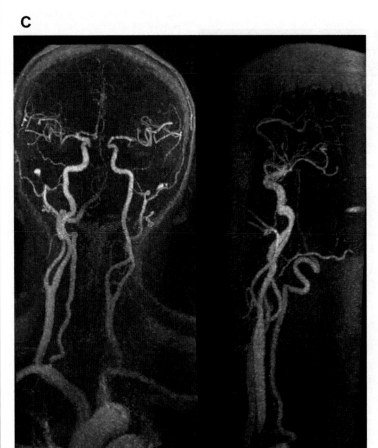

the DWI abnormalities provides insight into the underlying cause and stroke subtype. For example, visualization of multiple small bright lesions on DWI sequences within different vascular territories may indicate an embolic stroke mechanism.

Fluid-attenuated inversion recovery

Fluid-attenuated inversion recovery (FLAIR) helps to determine the age of the infarction,[13,14] permits detection of subtle cerebral subarachnoid hemorrhage, and can add diagnostic value to gradient-echo (GRE) images for detecting intra-arterial clot.[15–17] The most important use of FLAIR imaging in the setting of acute stroke is to identify acute ischemic infarcts that lie within the thrombolytic time window in patients with symptoms first noted on awakening (wake-up stroke),[18] or patients with unwitnessed onset who are unable to provide an accurate history. As a rule, lesion visibility on FLAIR increases as time passes from the stroke onset and up to 93% of acute stroke lesions can have positive FLAIR findings at greater than 6 hours.[13,18,19] FLAIR sequences may also show

hyperintense vessels following a proximal occlusion even in the absence of parenchymal signal changes. These findings may indicate slow flow in the collateral circulation. In our 6-minute stroke protocol we have replaced conventional FLAIR with EPI-FLAIR.[8] We have shown that EPI-FLAIR has similar diagnostic performance and quantitative and qualitative results to conventional FLAIR (**Fig. 2**), but only requires one-third of the acquisition time.[20] Because of the shorter acquisition time, EPI-FLAIR may provide better image quality with less motion artifact, particularly in uncooperative patients (**Fig. 3**).

Gradient-echo imaging

GRE imaging is used to detect intracranial hemorrhage and intraluminal thrombus formation (**Fig. 4**). Although CT is the standard method used to rule out intracranial hemorrhage, GRE has been shown to be at least as accurate as CT for the detection of acute intraparenchymal hemorrhage.[21] Both FLAIR and GRE images have been used to detect intra-arterial clot with variable sensitivity and

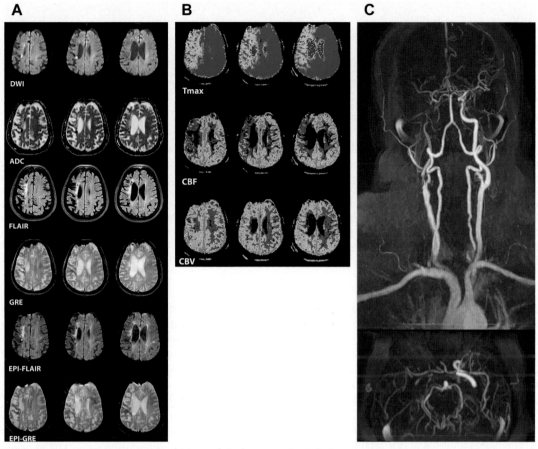

Fig. 2. A 68-year-old woman with a history of stroke approximately 1 year earlier that left her with residual left-sided deficits now presents with a new onset of left-sided weakness. NIHSS: 7. Sequentially aligned DWI, ADC, FLAIR, GRE, EPI-FLAIR, and EPI-GRE (*A*) are shown. There is a small acute infarction in the right posterior centrum semiovale on the background of chronic infarction in the right cerebral deep white matter seen on FLAIR images. There are chronic blood products and hemosiderin staining within the chronic infarction seen on GRE images. EPI-FLAIR and EPI-GRE, used in our 6-minute stroke protocol, are acquired in a fraction (one-third) of the time compared with conventional FLAIR and GRE, but with identical image quality and diagnostic information. CE-MRA (*C*) shows diminutive flow signal in the high cervical segment and occlusion of the petrous segment of the right internal carotid artery. There is reconstitution of flow signal in the cavernous and supraclinoid segment and proximal anterior cerebral artery and middle cerebral artery branches with less signal intensity compared with the normal left side, likely through collateral flow. On DSC-T_{max} and CBF (*B*), there is a large perfusion deficit that indicates delayed perfusion and hypoperfusion respectively. In contrast, CBV has significantly increased, suggesting collateralization in this patient with a history of chronic infraction.

specificity.[15,16] Again, in our 6-minute stroke protocol, EPI-GRE has replaced conventional GRE with similar diagnostic performance but only a fraction of the acquisition time[8] (see **Fig. 2**).

GRE is significantly more sensitive for detection of chronic intracerebral microhemorrhages, which may be the sequelae of amyloid angiopathy or chronic hypertension. The clinical importance of these microbleeds is unknown. At present, there is no statistically significant increased risk of ICH when patients with a small number of chronic microhemorrhages (<5) are treated with thrombolysis.[22,23]

However, the risk of hemorrhage in patients with more than 5 chronic microhemorrhages is unknown.[24]

Hemorrhagic transformation (HT) of an ischemic infarction is a common occurrence, and can be seen in 30% to 74% of patients, particularly in patients with embolic strokes and those treated with thrombolytic or mechanical revascularization therapies. Although CT is equally sensitive for detection of parenchymal hematomas, petechial hemorrhages on the more subtle spectrum of HT are detected by GRE with significantly higher

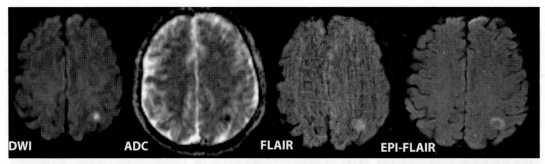

Fig. 3. A 28-year-old man with past medical history of intravenous drug abuse and infective endocarditis presented with right-sided weakness 6 hours before imaging. Baseline NIHSS: 5. The patient was uncooperative and could not hold still. There is an acute infarction in the left postcentral gyrus with associated FLAIR hyperintensity, presumably caused by septic embolism in this patient who had positive blood culture (methicillin-resistant *Staphylococcus aureus*) and positive echocardiography with vegetations. Note the significantly better image quality on EPI-FLAIR image compared with conventional FLAIR, which is degraded by motion artifact. This difference is a clear advantage of the EPI-FLAIR technique used in our 6-minute MR stroke protocol because of the shorter acquisition time (52 seconds in EPI-FLAIR compared with 3 minutes in conventional FLAIR), in particular in uncooperative patients.

sensitivity. The clinical significance of petechial hemorrhage is unknown.

Magnetic Resonance Angiogram

An important aspect of the work-up of patients with AIS or TIA is the imaging of both the intracranial and extracranial vasculature. Intravenous thrombolysis has been shown to be more effective in reperfusing small distal vessels than larger proximal vessels.[25] Larger vessel occlusion may be more effectively treated with intra-arterial thrombolysis or mechanical thrombectomy, which are associated with fewer complications.[26,27] Precise imaging of the vascular tree is required during the initial assessment of patients with acute stroke, not only to accurately detect the site of the arterial disease but also to identify the underlying stroke cause, such as carotid atherosclerotic disease; vascular dissection with or without intraluminal thrombosis (see **Fig. 1**); vasculopathy, such as fibromuscular dysplasia; and other treatable structural causes.

The magnetic resonance angiography (MRA) techniques often used in stroke imaging include the noncontrast time-of-flight (TOF) technique and contrast-enhanced MRA (CE-MRA). Limitations of TOF-MRA include long acquisition times and overestimation of arterial stenosis caused by spin saturation and phase dispersion secondary to slow, in-plane, turbulent, or complex flow.[28,29] An improved CE-MRA technique with higher spatial resolution and faster acquisition time afforded by advances in technology such as multicoil technology and parallel imaging can now be used in acute stroke imaging for complete evaluation of both the extracranial and intracranial (see **Figs. 2 and 4**) supra-aortic arteries,[30,31] resulting in significant improvement in the performance of stroke protocols in terms of image quality and speed.[8,32]

Magnetic Resonance Perfusion

Bolus dynamic susceptibility contrast (DSC) and arterial spin labeling are two methods of measuring cerebral perfusion using MR imaging, each with different strengths and limitations.[33–35] Faster image acquisition and the ability to generate perfusion maps in a few minutes have made DSC a more robust and widely accepted technique to measure cerebral perfusion in patients with acute stroke. The gadolinium contrast dose is approximately 0.1 mmol/kg. Perfusion imaging in patients with presentation of acute stroke syndromes can be used in the following scenarios:

Defining ischemic penumbra

Following a cerebral arterial occlusion, there is a developing infarction core and surrounding hypoperfused brain tissue that is potentially at risk of infarction if blood flow is not restored in a timely manner. This potentially salvageable tissue is called the ischemic penumbra. The rate of change in the extent of infarction core and penumbra is a dynamic process that depends on the recanalization of the occlusion and presence of collateral flow. In the absence of effective revascularization, the infarction core is likely to grow and progressively replace the penumbra (**Fig. 5**). In the case of early revascularization, either spontaneously or resulting from thrombolysis, the penumbra may be salvaged from infarction.[36]

A

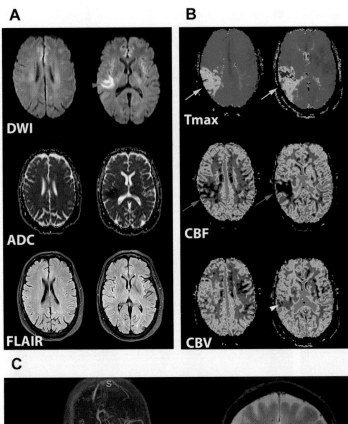

B

Fig. 4. A 71-year-old woman with past medical history of hypertension and coronary artery disease with cardiomyopathy presented with sudden onset of left-sided facial, upper extremity, and lower extremity weakness. Baseline NIHSS: 4. Time from onset to imaging: 110 minutes. Sequentially aligned DWI, ADC, FLAIR, DSC-T_{max}, CBF, and CBV (*A*) and a coronal and axial maximum intensity projection from CE-MRA in addition to coronal GRE image (*B*) are shown. There is an acute infarction involving the right opercular region (*arrowhead on DWI*). Note that there is no corresponding FLAIR hyperintensity, which indicates the hyperacute nature of the infarction (time from onset to imaging was 110 minutes). On perfusion images (*B*), the T_{max} lesion (delayed perfusion) (*white arrows*) and CBF lesion (hypoperfusion) (*red arrows*) are both larger than acute infarcted tissue seen on DWI (*arrowhead in A*), a representation of ischemic penumbra (so called diffusion-perfusion mismatch). The CBV lesion (*white arrowhead*) is significantly smaller, closely mimicking the infarction core, as expected. CE-MRA (*C*) shows normal appearance of the cervical arteries. There is occlusion of the right M2 posterior division (*arrowhead*). GRE (*C*) shows increased blooming, indicating a thrombus (*arrow*).

C

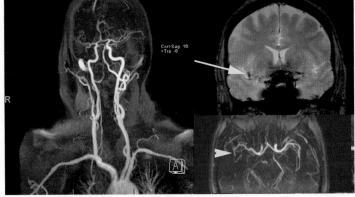

Perfusion imaging can be used to determine the extent of ischemic penumbra. Although the clinical utility of ischemic penumbra defined by perfusion imaging and its effect on patient outcomes remains controversial,[37,38] it has been used with some success to identify patients who may respond favorably to revascularization therapies and in the identification of potentially salvageable tissue.[3,10,11,39]

DSC perfusion can provide various maps showing regions of hemodynamic compromise. These maps often include a measure of time such as mean transit time (MTT) or time to maximum (T_{max}), cerebral blood flow (CBF), and cerebral blood volume (CBV). Following an arterial occlusion, regions of irreversible infarction show low CBV, low CBF, and increased MTT/T_{max}. The ischemic penumbra is expected to have CBV within normal ranges, moderate reduction in CBF, and moderately increased MTT/T_{max}. Modest changes in these values can be seen in regions of benign oligemia: tissue with modest hemodynamic compromise that does not reach the level of being at risk of infarction, regardless of reperfusion status. Differentiation of penumbra and benign oligemia remains a diagnostic challenge because absolute thresholds have not been fully validated.

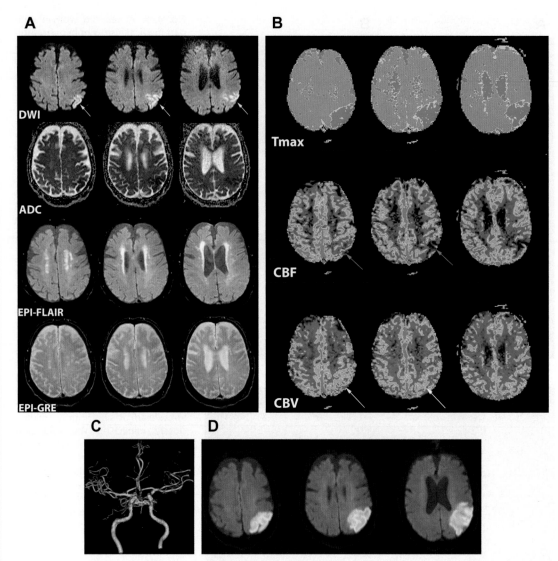

Fig. 5. A 58-year-old man with past medical history of atrial fibrillation hypertension, presents with right-sided weakness. Baseline NIHSS: 6. Time of onset to first MR imaging was approximately 90 minutes. Using the 6-minute MR stroke protocol, there is a hyperacute infarction involving left posterior frontal and parietal lobes (*A*) (*white arrows on DWI images*). Note the absence of FLAIR hyperintense signal, which is suggestive of hyperacuity. There is no hemorrhage on EPI-GRE images. There is a larger perfusion deficit (so-called diffusion-perfusion mismatch) best seen on DSC-T_{max} greater than 6 seconds (*B*), which is suggestive of critical delayed perfusion. There is regional increased CBV (*white arrows*) caused by increased autoregulation, which seems inadequate because there is decreased CBF (*red arrows*). MRA (*C*) shows no proximal arterial stenosis. On follow-up MR imaging (*D*) obtained 12 hours later, there is progression and growth of infarction now encompassing the entire hypoperfused region detected on the initial MR imaging.

Collateral flow status

Perfusion imaging can provide an indirect measure of collateral flow.[10,40,41]

Several investigators have shown reverse correlation between the degree of collateral flow and the extent and severity of hypoperfusion defined on MR perfusion data.[39,42–44]

Collateral flow is often directly evaluated with vascular imaging such as catheter angiography,

CT angiography (CTA), or MRA. Because of inherent limited spatial and temporal resolution of cross-sectional vascular imaging such as CTA or MRA to evaluate the full extent of collateral flow, catheter angiography remains the gold standard method for imaging collateral vasculature. Because multivessel conventional angiography is impractical for all patients in routine practice, the development of noninvasive approaches that combine angiographic information with perfusion data can significantly enhance understanding of the collateral circulation.

Perfusion deficit noted on MR perfusion time maps (such as T_{max}) encompasses both delayed perfusion caused by underlying arterial occlusion and delayed flow through collateral circulation, without the ability to distinguish antegrade from collateral flow. In contrast, CBF and CBV maps provide information regarding the amount of blood flow to specific regions of the brain, although the arterial source of sustained perfusion may not be evident, some of which may be from collateral flow. Therefore a mismatch between the volume of brain with time delay on T_{max} and the volume of brain with hypoperfusion on CBF/CBV may in part be a good representation of collateral flow (see **Figs. 2** and **4**).

Furthermore, MR perfusion data, as an indirect measure of collateral flow, have been used as a marker of successful recanalization, which in turn can improve therapeutic decision making, tailoring patient selection and enrollment to those who will most benefit from recanalization procedures.[3,42,45] A further imaging-driven collateral flow index has been developed, enabling risk stratification for

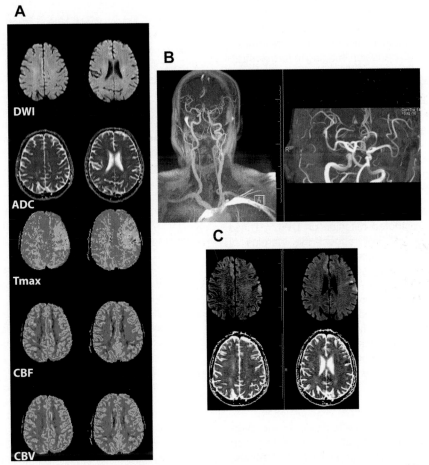

Fig. 6. A 67-year-old man with past medical history of atrial fibrillation and prior TIAs presents with complaints of garbled speech for 10 minutes before it resolved. Time of onset to first MR imaging was approximately 2 hours. On initial MR images (*A*), there is no acute infarction on the DWI-ADC images. Perfusion imaging (*A*) reveals a regional perfusion deficit evident by increased T_{max} involving the left operculum and Broca area. Note compensatory increased in CBV suggestive of autoregulation and luxury perfusion to maintain the CBF. MRA (*B*) shows a normal proximal arterial tree without evidence of hemodynamically significant stenosis. The patient was discharged from the emergency department with the diagnosis of TIA; however, 14 hours later his garbled speech returned and was noted to be persistent. He also complained of a patch of right-sided upper lip numbness. He was able to follow commands and communicate by writing, but was noted to have a severe expressive aphasia. Second MR imaging (*C*) reveals restricted diffusion and acute infarction involving the frontal operculum and Broca area, in the region of previously identified delayed perfusion.

individual treatment decision making, expanding treatment options for patients with AIS.

Differential diagnosis: transient ischemic attack, seizure

Transient ischemic attack With the introduction of DWI into routine clinical practice, studies have shown that up to 40% of patients with clinically defined TIA have evidence of restricted diffusion that indicates ischemic infarction. This finding has led to a recent American Stroke Association–endorsed proposal to revise the definition of TIA from time-based to tissue-based criteria.[46] However, DWI-negative patients remain a source of uncertainty and a great clinical challenge. Many of these patients may have transient cerebral ischemia in which the degree of hemodynamic compromise did not reach the threshold for tissue injury. Acknowledging this challenge, several investigators used perfusion imaging to further stratify patients with TIA.[47–50] In our experience, perfusion imaging, when incorporating both T_{max} and CBF parametric maps, has added diagnostic value to the detection of regions of hypoperfusion or postischemic hyperperfusion in approximately one-quarter of patients with DWI-negative TIA (**Fig. 6**), thus providing additional evidence to confirm a footprint of ischemia that would otherwise go undetected.[51]

Seizure Prolonged seizures or status epilepticus can lead to restricted diffusion on DWI.[52] These changes often do not respect the margins of vascular territories and are associated with increased, not decreased, perfusion.[53] Another helpful imaging finding to differentiate seizure from AIS is the pulvinar sign, which is restricted diffusion and increased CBF in the ipsilateral thalamic pulvinar. This finding may be caused by extensive neuronal connections between the thalamus and parietotemporal regions, which are often involved in seizure activity.[53]

SUMMARY

MR imaging can be used effectively for the diagnosis and evaluation of patients presenting with acute stroke syndrome in emergency settings. Recent advances in MR imaging technology have allowed fast and efficient multimodal MR imaging, such as the described 6-minute MR stroke protocol that can be used for the evaluation of patients with AIS, with resultant significant reduction in scan times, rivaling those multimodal CT protocols.

Because recent clinical trials have established endovascular procedures as effective treatment strategies for patients with acute stroke, multimodal neuroimaging will continue to play an increasingly important role in the evaluation and management of patients with stroke. Advanced imaging techniques provide important insights into individual patient pathophysiology, stroke cause, and prognosis. This information may be used by clinicians to make treatment decisions for both acute therapies and long-term secondary prevention approaches.

REFERENCES

1. Lloyd-Jones D, Adams RJ, Brown TM, et al. Heart disease and stroke statistics–2010 update: a report from the American Heart Association. Circulation 2010;121:e46–215.
2. Goyal M, Demchuk AM, Menon BK, et al. Randomized assessment of rapid endovascular treatment of ischemic stroke. N Engl J Med 2015;372:1019–30.
3. Campbell BCV, Mitchell PJ, Kleinig TJ, et al. Endovascular therapy for ischemic stroke with perfusion-imaging selection. N Engl J Med 2015; 372:1009–18.
4. Berkhemer OA, Fransen PSS, Beumer D, et al. A randomized trial of intraarterial treatment for acute ischemic stroke. N Engl J Med 2015;372:11–20.
5. Schellinger PD. The evolving role of advanced MR imaging as a management tool for adult ischemic stroke: a western-European perspective. Neuroimaging Clin North Am 2005;15:245–58, ix.
6. Rowley HA. Extending the time window for thrombolysis: evidence from acute stroke trials. Neuroimaging Clin North Am 2005;15:575–87, x.
7. Mnyusiwalla A, Aviv RI, Symons SP. Radiation dose from multidetector row ct imaging for acute stroke. Neuroradiology 2009;51:635–40.
8. Nael K, Khan R, Choudhary G, et al. Six-minute magnetic resonance imaging protocol for evaluation of acute ischemic stroke: pushing the boundaries. Stroke 2014;45:1985–91.
9. Griswold MA, Jakob PM, Heidemann RM, et al. Generalized autocalibrating partially parallel acquisitions (GRAPPA). Magn Reson Med 2002;47: 1202–10.
10. Albers GW, Thijs VN, Wechsler L, et al. Magnetic resonance imaging profiles predict clinical response to early reperfusion: the Diffusion and Perfusion Imaging Evaluation for Understanding Stroke Evolution (DEFUSE) study. Ann Neurol 2006;60:508–17.
11. Davis SM, Donnan GA, Parsons MW, et al. Effects of alteplase beyond 3 h after stroke in the echoplanar imaging thrombolytic evaluation trial (epithet): a placebo-controlled randomised trial. Lancet Neurol 2008;7:299–309.
12. Fiebach JB, Schellinger PD, Jansen O, et al. CT and diffusion-weighted MR imaging in randomized order: diffusion-weighted imaging results in higher

accuracy and lower interrater variability in the diagnosis of hyperacute ischemic stroke. Stroke 2002; 33:2206–10.

13. Thomalla G, Cheng B, Ebinger M, et al. DWI-FLAIR mismatch for the identification of patients with acute ischaemic stroke within 4.5 h of symptom onset (pre-FLAIR): a multicentre observational study. Lancet Neurol 2011;10:978–86.

14. Aoki J, Kimura K, Iguchi Y, et al. FLAIR can estimate the onset time in acute ischemic stroke patients. J Neurol Sci 2010;293:39–44.

15. Flacke S, Urbach H, Keller E, et al. Middle cerebral artery (MCA) susceptibility sign at susceptibility-based perfusion MR imaging: clinical importance and comparison with hyperdense MCA sign at CT. Radiology 2000;215:476–82.

16. Assouline E, Benziane K, Reizine D, et al. Intra-arterial thrombus visualized on T2* gradient echo imaging in acute ischemic stroke. Cerebrovasc Dis 2005; 20:6–11.

17. Noguchi K, Ogawa T, Seto H, et al. Subacute and chronic subarachnoid hemorrhage: diagnosis with fluid-attenuated inversion-recovery MR imaging. Radiology 1997;203:257–62.

18. Thomalla G, Rossbach P, Rosenkranz M, et al. Negative fluid-attenuated inversion recovery imaging identifies acute ischemic stroke at 3 hours or less. Ann Neurol 2009;65:724–32.

19. Petkova M, Rodrigo S, Lamy C, et al. MR imaging helps predict time from symptom onset in patients with acute stroke: implications for patients with unknown onset time. Radiology 2010;257:782–92.

20. Meshksar A, Villablanca JP, Khan R, et al. Role of EPI-FLAIR in patients with acute stroke: a comparative analysis with FLAIR. AJNR Am J Neuroradiol 2014;35(5):878–83.

21. Kidwell CS, Chalela JA, Saver JL, et al. Comparison of MRI and CT for detection of acute intracerebral hemorrhage. JAMA 2004;292:1823–30.

22. Kakuda W, Thijs VN, Lansberg MG, et al. Clinical importance of microbleeds in patients receiving IV thrombolysis. Neurology 2005;65:1175–8.

23. Lee SH, Kang BS, Kim N, et al. Does microbleed predict haemorrhagic transformation after acute atherothrombotic or cardioembolic stroke? J Neurol Neurosurg Psychiatry 2008;79:913–6.

24. Wintermark M, Sanelli PC, Albers GW, et al. Imaging recommendations for acute stroke and transient ischemic attack patients: a joint statement by the American Society of Neuroradiology, the American College of Radiology and the Society of Neurointerventional Surgery. J Am Coll Radiol 2013;10:828–32.

25. del Zoppo GJ, Poeck K, Pessin MS, et al. Recombinant tissue plasminogen activator in acute thrombotic and embolic stroke. Ann Neurol 1992;32:78–86.

26. Furlan A, Higashida R, Wechsler L, et al. Intra-arterial prourokinase for acute ischemic stroke. The PROACT II study: a randomized controlled trial. Prolyse in Acute Cerebral Thromboembolism. JAMA 1999;282:2003–11.

27. Becker KJ, Brott TG. Approval of the MERCI clot retriever: a critical view. Stroke 2005;36:400–3.

28. Lin W, Tkach JA, Haacke EM, et al. Intracranial MR angiography: application of magnetization transfer contrast and fat saturation to short gradient-echo, velocity-compensated sequences. Radiology 1993; 186:753–61.

29. Isoda H, Takehara Y, Isogai S, et al. MRA of intracranial aneurysm models: a comparison of contrast-enhanced three-dimensional MRA with time-of-flight MRA. J Comput Assist Tomogr 2000;24:308–15.

30. Nael K, Villablanca JP, Pope WB, et al. Supraaortic arteries: contrast-enhanced MR angiography at 3.0 T–highly accelerated parallel acquisition for improved spatial resolution over an extended field of view. Radiology 2007;242:600–9.

31. Phan T, Huston J 3rd, Bernstein MA, et al. Contrast-enhanced magnetic resonance angiography of the cervical vessels: experience with 422 patients. Stroke 2001;32:2282–6.

32. Nael K, Meshksar A, Ellingson B, et al. Combined low-dose contrast-enhanced MR angiography and perfusion for acute ischemic stroke at 3T: a more efficient stroke protocol. AJNR Am J Neuroradiol 2014;35:1078–84.

33. Detre JA, Leigh JS, Williams DS, et al. Perfusion imaging. Magn Reson Med 1992;23:37–45.

34. Wolf RL, Alsop DC, McGarvey ML, et al. Susceptibility contrast and arterial spin labeled perfusion MRI in cerebrovascular disease. J Neuroimaging 2003;13: 17–27.

35. Smith AM, Grandin CB, Duprez T, et al. Whole brain quantitative CBF and CBV measurements using MRI bolus tracking: comparison of methodologies. Magn Reson Med 2000;43:559–64.

36. Read SJ, Hirano T, Abbott DF, et al. The fate of hypoxic tissue on 18F-fluoromisonidazole positron emission tomography after ischemic stroke. Ann Neurol 2000;48:228–35.

37. Hacke W, Furlan AJ, Al-Rawi Y, et al. Intravenous desmoteplase in patients with acute ischaemic stroke selected by MRI perfusion-diffusion weighted imaging or perfusion CT (DIAS-2): a prospective, randomised, double-blind, placebo-controlled study. Lancet Neurol 2009;8:141–50.

38. Kidwell CS, Jahan R, Gornbein J, et al. A trial of imaging selection and endovascular treatment for ischemic stroke. N Engl J Med 2013;368:914–23.

39. Lansberg MG, Straka M, Kemp S, et al. MRI profile and response to endovascular reperfusion after stroke (DEFUSE 2): a prospective cohort study. Lancet Neurol 2012;11:860–7.

40. Olivot JM, Mlynash M, Thijs VN, et al. Geography, structure, and evolution of diffusion and perfusion

lesions in Diffusion and Perfusion Imaging Evaluation for Understanding Stroke Evolution (DEFUSE). Stroke 2009;40:3245–51.

41. Soares BP, Tong E, Hom J, et al. Reperfusion is a more accurate predictor of follow-up infarct volume than recanalization: a proof of concept using CT in acute ischemic stroke patients. Stroke 2010;41: e34–40.

42. Nicoli F, Lafaye de Micheaux P, Girard N. Perfusion-weighted imaging-derived collateral flow index is a predictor of MCA M1 recanalization after I.V. thrombolysis. AJNR Am J Neuroradiol 2013;34:107–14.

43. Bang OY, Saver JL, Alger JR, et al. Determinants of the distribution and severity of hypoperfusion in patients with ischemic stroke. Neurology 2008;71: 1804–11.

44. Olivot JM, Mlynash M, Inoue M, et al. Hypoperfusion intensity ratio predicts infarct progression and functional outcome in the DEFUSE 2 cohort. Stroke 2014; 45:1018–23.

45. Nicoli F, Scalzo F, Saver JL, et al. The combination of baseline magnetic resonance perfusion-weighted imaging-derived tissue volume with severely prolonged arterial-tissue delay and diffusion-weighted imaging lesion volume is predictive of MCA-M1 recanalization in patients treated with endovascular thrombectomy. Neuroradiology 2014;56:117–27.

46. Easton JD, Saver JL, Albers GW, et al. Definition and evaluation of transient ischemic attack: a scientific statement for healthcare professionals from the American Heart Association/American Stroke Association Stroke Council; Council on Cardiovascular Surgery and Anesthesia; Council on Cardiovascular Radiology and Intervention; Council on Cardiovascular Nursing; and the Interdisciplinary Council on Peripheral Vascular Disease. The American Academy of Neurology affirms the value of this statement as an educational tool for neurologists. Stroke 2009; 40:2276–93.

47. Restrepo L, Jacobs MA, Barker PB, et al. Assessment of transient ischemic attack with diffusion- and perfusion-weighted imaging. AJNR Am J Neuroradiol 2004;25:1645–52.

48. Krol AL, Coutts SB, Simon JE, et al. Perfusion MRI abnormalities in speech or motor transient ischemic attack patients. Stroke 2005;36:2487–9.

49. Mlynash M, Olivot JM, Tong DC, et al. Yield of combined perfusion and diffusion MR imaging in hemispheric TIA. Neurology 2009;72:1127–33.

50. Kleinman JT, Zaharchuk G, Mlynash M, et al. Automated perfusion imaging for the evaluation of transient ischemic attack. Stroke 2012;43:1556–60.

51. Grams R, Kidwell C, Shroff S, et al. Tissue negative-transient ischemic attack: is there a role for MR perfusion? Paper presented at the ASNR 52nd Annual Meeting. Montréal, Canada, May 22, 2014.

52. Londono A, Castillo M, Lee YZ, et al. Apparent diffusion coefficient measurements in the hippocampi in patients with temporal lobe seizures. AJNR Am J Neuroradiol 2003;24:1582–6.

53. Szabo K, Poepel A, Pohlmann-Eden B, et al. Diffusion-weighted and perfusion MRI demonstrates parenchymal changes in complex partial status epilepticus. Brain 2005;128:1369–76.

Use of Magnetic Resonance in the Evaluation of Cranial Trauma

Wilson Altmeyer, MD[a],*, Andrew Steven, MD[b],
Juan Gutierrez, MD[c]

KEYWORDS

- Cranial trauma • Diffuse axonal injury • Contusion • Hematoma • MR imaging

KEY POINTS

- MR imaging is commonly performed as an adjunct imaging modality after initial trauma evaluation with CT.
- MR imaging is the most sensitive imaging modality for diagnosis of diffuse axonal injury (DAI), parenchymal contusion, and traumatic cerebral infarction.
- MR imaging is just as sensitive as CT for the detection of acute subarachnoid hemorrhage (SAH) and is more sensitive in detection of subacute to chronic SAH.
- Magnetic resonance angiography (MRA) is a useful tool for interrogating the intracranial vasculature in children, pregnant patients, and patients with renal insufficiency or acute kidney injury.

INTRODUCTION

Approximately 1.7 million Americans present to emergency departments (EDs) each year with head trauma.[1] Of these patients, 52,000 die and 275,000 require hospitalization. Traumatic brain injury (TBI) is a contributing factor in one-third of all traumatic deaths in the United States, with motor vehicle accidents comprising the leading cause of TBI-related mortality.[1]

CT traditionally serves as the initial imaging modality of choice in the evaluation of TBI secondary to its widespread availability, speed, cost, and sensitivity for both acute intracranial hemorrhage and fractures. There has been a steady increase, however, in the use of MR imaging by EDs over the past decade.[2-4] Factors contributing to the increased rate of MR imaging use include improved availability, reduced cost, faster acquisition times, and lack of ionizing radiation.[3] MR imaging also offers improved soft tissue contrast with increased sensitivity for detection for a wide variety of traumatic pathologies, such as DAI and cerebral contusions.[5,6] This increased sensitivity for TBI is particularly useful in the setting of mild head trauma where initial imaging CT may be negative[7] (Fig. 1).

The brain and spine are the most common anatomic locations to be imaged with MR imaging by the ED. The most common indications for emergent MR imaging of the brain are stroke, headache, and trauma.[3,8] This article provides a succinct review of the MR imaging appearance of the common traumatic intracranial pathologies that are encountered in an ED setting.

INTRA-AXIAL TRAUMA
Contusions

Cerebral contusions are parenchymal bruises that occur when the brain has an impact on the surface

The authors have nothing to disclose.
[a] Department of Radiology, University of Texas Health Science Center at San Antonio, 7703 Floyd Curl Drive, San Antonio, TX 78229-3900, USA; [b] Department of Radiology, University of Maryland Medical System, 22 South Green Street, Baltimore, MD 21201, USA; [c] Centro Avanzado de Diagnóstico Médico CEDIMED, Calle 18 AA sur # 29 c 340, Medellín, Colombia
* Corresponding author.
E-mail address: altmeyer@uthscsa.edu

Magn Reson Imaging Clin N Am 24 (2016) 305–323
http://dx.doi.org/10.1016/j.mric.2015.11.011
1064-9689/16/$ – see front matter © 2016 Elsevier Inc. All rights reserved.

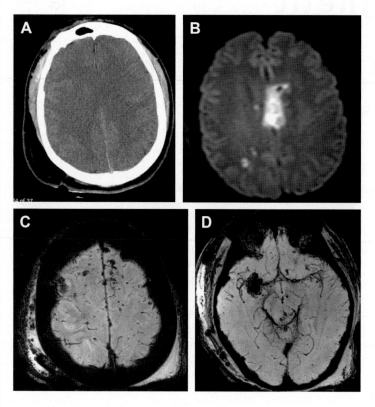

Fig. 1. (*A*) Axial noncontrast CT fails to reveal TBI after motor vehicle collision. MR imaging clearly depicts restricted diffusion in the (*B*) body of the corpus callosum, (*C*) small foci of hemorrhage at the frontal gray-white junction, and (*D*) punctate midbrain hemorrhages on axial SWI sequences, consistent with the final diagnosis of DAI.

of the skull, falx cerebri, or tentorium. Blunt, closed head injury is the most frequent cause of brain contusions. The inferior frontal and anterior temporal lobes are the most common locations for cerebral contusion because the adjacent anterior and middle cranial fossae of the skull base have a relatively sharp, irregular contour.[9] The occipital lobes are almost always spared from contusion because the bordering occipital bone exhibits a smooth inner table. A contusion at the site of trauma is referred to as a *coup contusion*. When the contusion is 180° opposite the site of direct impact, the contusion is termed, *contrecoup* (**Fig. 2**). Contusion may be difficult to visualize on initial CT examination in an ED. Contusions, however, have a tendency to enlarge and become more apparent on follow-up imaging.

Contusion by definition must involve the cortical surface of the brain, a feature that helps differentiate from subcortical DAI. The imaging appearance of cerebral contusion may vary from subtle petechial hemorrhage to multiple large parenchymal hematomas with severe mass effect. A CT examination classically demonstrates foci of hyperattenuating hemorrhage within a wedge-shaped region of hypodense cerebral edema. MR imaging is more sensitive than CT for the detection of cerebral contusion.[6,7,10] The fluid-attenuated

inversion recovery (FLAIR) sequence is superior to T1-weighted and T2-weighted sequences for detection of cerebral edema in the setting of a brain contusion (**Fig. 3**). The appearance of hemorrhagic contusions change on T1-weighted and T2-weighted sequences along a predictable pattern based on the age of blood products (**Table 1**). Hemorrhagic contusions often contain blood products in various stages of degradation within the hematoma, with the evolution progressing in a centripetal fashion. Subacute blood products are one of only a few pathologic processes that are hyperintense on T1-weighted sequences.

Gradient-recalled echo (GRE) and susceptibility-weighted images (SWIs) are the most sensitive sequences for detection of hemorrhagic contusion. Hemorrhage appears as black "blooming" artifact on these sequences. There is growing evidence in the literature confirming SWI's superiority to GRE for the detection of intracranial hemorrhage.[11–13] Foci of DWI hyperintensity within a cerebral contusion may reflect either blood products or regions of cytotoxic edema and neuronal death.[9]

Penetrating Injury

Penetrating injuries are characterized by a projectile piercing the skull, dura, and brain. The

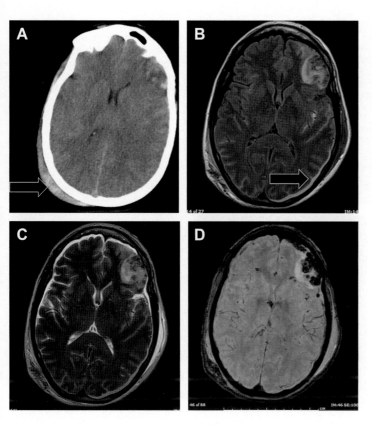

Fig. 2. (A) Axial noncontrast CT demonstrates a wedge shaped hypoattenuating left frontal contusion with internal small hemorrhagic foci. Notice the subcutaneous swelling is 180° opposite of brain injury, confirming contrecoup contusion (arrow). The exact margins of the contusion are better delineated on (B) FLAIR and (C) T2-weighted sequences. A small SDH is also more evident on the FLAIR sequence ([B] arrow). (D) Gradient susceptibility on the axial SWI sequence confirms the presence of blood.

projectile leaves a trail of destruction with damaged brain parenchyma and torn vasculature. When the cerebral defect is linear in morphology, the term, cerebral laceration, is often used (Fig. 4). Gunshot and stabbing assaults are the most common sources of penetrating injury.[14]

CT imaging can show metallic density ballistic fragments, comminuted skull fractures, macerated brain parenchyma, cerebral contusion, and liner lacerations. MR imaging is not often performed in the ED on patients with penetrating cerebral injuries to avoid the potential harm that may be caused by displacement of intracranial metallic bullet fragments and the high rate of patient mortality shortly after admission. When performed, MR imaging can further characterize the primary penetrating injury as well as detect superimposed DAI and cerebral infarctions.

Diffuse Axonal Injury

Severe rotational acceleration/deceleration stress on the brain results in DAI. The cerebral gray matter and white matter have different density and stiffness and, therefore, accelerate and decelerate at different speeds. This differential movement results in stretching or shearing injury centered at the junction between the cerebral gray and white matter. Motor vehicle collisions are the most common causes of DAI. DAI has a strong predilection for the gray-white junction of the frontotemporal lobes, corpus callosum, brainstem, and internal capsule. Adams and colleagues[15] introduced a staging system for DAI in 1989. The stage of DAI is determined by lesion location and helps predict patient prognosis (Table 2).

There is often a significant discordance between the dismal clinical appearance of the DAI patient and the surprisingly normal-appearing head CT.[16] Noncontrast head CT performed in an ED is often normal in the setting of mild to moderate DAI.[17] A majority (80%) of DAI lesions are nonhemorrhagic[18] and these foci are particularly difficult to diagnose with CT. CT may demonstrate a few punctate, hyperattenuating foci of hemorrhage. These foci represent the tip of the iceberg, with additional nonvisualized brain injury highly likely. CT in an ED also allows fast triage and exclusion of concurrent injuries, such as skull fractures, cerebral herniations, contusions, and parenchymal hematomas.

MR imaging has a much higher sensitivity than CT for DAI, particularly for the more common nonhemorrhagic variety.[17] Paterakis and colleagues[5] examined more than 1000 trauma cases over a

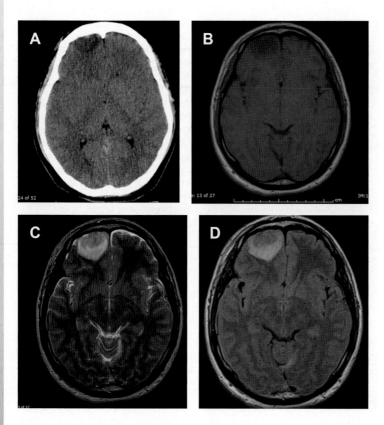

Fig. 3. The right frontal cerebral contusion is more apparent on (*C*) axial T2-weighted and (*D*) FLAIR sequences compared with (*A*) non-contrast CT and (*B*) T1-weighted sequences.

2-year period. They isolated 33 patients who had normal admission head CT examinations but clinical evidence of TBI. Follow-up MR imaging performed with 48 hours confirmed DAI in 24 of the 33 patients (73%). MR imaging shows small, ovoid foci of restricted diffusion and T2 hyperintensity in the setting of acute DAI (**Figs. 5** and **6**). The long axis of the ovoid DAI lesion is aligned in the direction of the regional white matter fibers. In the setting of hemorrhagic DAI, MR imaging demonstrates oval foci of gradient susceptibility.

It is imperative that a trauma MR imaging protocol includes a heme-sensitive sequence. Spitz and colleagues[19] have shown SWI more sensitive than FLAIR imaging for detection of lesions in the setting of hemorrhagic DAI. SWI is more sensitive than traditional T2* GRE imaging for the detection of intracranial blood products in a variety of pathologic conditions.[11–13] Beauchamp and colleagues[20] reported that SWI can reveal up to 30% more lesions than CT or conventional MR imaging in the setting of TBI. In another study, Tong and colleagues[21] concluded that SWI depicts significantly more hemorrhagic DAI lesions than does conventional T2* GRE imaging.

Traumatic Cranial Nerve Injury

Cranial nerve injury is not uncommon in the setting of head trauma.[22,23] In general, cranial nerves I

Table 1
MR imaging appearance of intracranial hematoma

	Time	Blood Product	T1	T2	T2*
Hyperacute	<24 h	Oxy-Hgb	Iso	Bright	Dark rim
Acute	1–3 d	Deoxy-Hgb	Iso	Dark	Dark
Early subacute	3 d to 1 wk	Intracellular met-Hgb	Bright	Dark	Very dark
Late subacute	>1 wk	Extracellular met-Hgb	Bright	Bright	Variable signal intensity
Chronic	Months	Hemosiderin	Dark	Dark	Very Dark

Abbreviations: Deoxy, deoxygenated; Hgb, hemoglobin; Met, methemoglobin; Oxy, oxygenated.

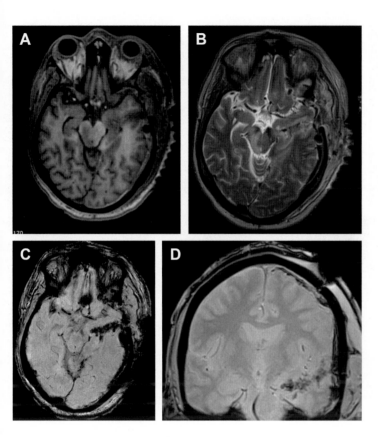

Fig. 4. A linear parenchymal defect courses through the left temporal lobe status post–motor vehicle collision, consistent with penetrating injury. (*A*) T1-weighted axial, (*B*) axial T2-weighted, (*C*) axial SWI, and (*D*) coronal T2* GRE sequences.

through VII are most frequently injured.[18] Blunt trauma is associated with injury of the olfactory, facial, and vestibulocochlear nerves.[23] Penetrating orbital trauma or fractures through the optic canal may result in optic nerve injury. The oculomotor, trochlear, and abducens nerves are commonly injured or even avulsed in the setting of trauma (**Fig. 7**). Transverse temporal bone fractures have a high incidence of facial nerve injury at the level of the geniculate ganglion. MR imaging is the

modality of choice in evaluating the cranial nerves and may reveal irregularity or discontinuity of the nerve fibers. Dedicated high-resolution, thin MR imaging sequences are required for interrogation of the cranial nerves. Heavily T2-weighted 3-D sequences, such as constructive interference in steady state (CISS) and fast imaging employing steady-state acquisition (FIESTA), are typically selected because they provide the needed special resolution to delineate these small structures. Hemorrhage and edema may be evident on routine MR imaging sequences at the root entry zone of the brainstem.

EXTRA-AXIAL TRAUMA
Subarachnoid Hemorrhage

Bleeding into the space between the arachnoid membrane and the pia results in SAH. Trauma is the most common cause of SAH. Additional nontraumatic causes of SAH include aneurysm rupture, arteriovenous malformation, vasculopathy, and coagulopathy, among other entities. SAH is exceedingly common in the setting of moderate to severe head injury and is associated with both blunt and penetrating head trauma. SAH can often be

Table 2
Adams and Gennarelli staging of diffuse axonal injury

Grade	Anatomic Region of Injury
1	Gray-white matter junction (most common in frontal and temporal lobes)
2	Grade 1 with additional lesions in corpus callosum (most common in splenium)
3	Grade 2 with additional lesions in brainstem

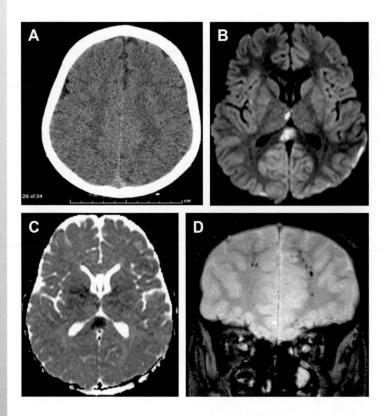

Fig. 5. (A) CT is largely without abnormality. (B) DWI and (C) ADC map reveal restricted diffusion in the splenium of the corpus callosum. (D) Coronal T2* GRE depicts multiple hemorrhagic foci at the gray-white junction of the corpus callosum, overall consistent with Adams and Gennarelli grade II DAI.

found in isolation or adjacent to subdural hematomas (SDHs) and parenchymal contusions.

On CT, acute SAH manifests as curvilinear hyperattenuation that insinuates along the surface of the brain parenchyma and fills the cerebral sulci, slyvian fissures, and basilar cisterns. MR imaging has been shown to be just as good as CT in detection of acute SAH and superior to CT in detection of subacute to chronic SAH.[24–26] Verma and colleagues[27] examined 25 consecutive patients that presented to the ED with acute SAH. They found that the SWI and FLAIR MR imaging sequences yielded a distinctly higher detection rate for SAH than CT. The SWI and FLAIR sequences played complementary roles in SAH detection (Figs. 8 and 9). SWI was superior for detection of central SAH (interheispheric and intraventricular) and FLAIR was superior for detection of peripheral

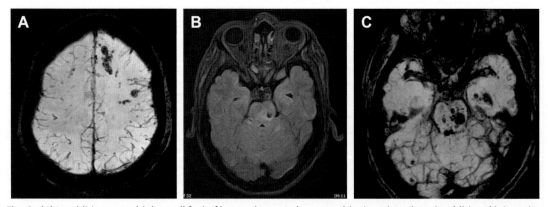

Fig. 6. (A) In addition to multiple small foci of hemorrhage at the gray-white junction, there is additional injury visualized in the dorsolateral brainstem on (B) FLAIR and (C) SWI, consistent with Adams and Gennarelli grade III DAI.

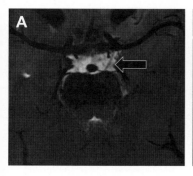
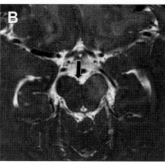

Fig. 7. (B) 3-D, heavily T2-weighted sequence with (A) minimal intensity projection reformatted image reveal disrupted right oculomotor nerve (A arrow) with severed proximal nerve fibers at the root entry zone of the interpeduncular fossa (B arrow).

SAH over the convexities. The high sensitivity of FLAIR for SAH is confounded by a high false-positive rate. Cerebrospinal fluid (CSF) pulsation can result in flow-related artifacts in the basilar cisterns that may be confused for SAH on the FLAIR sequences (**Fig. 10**). FLAIR hyperintensity in this anatomic region should alert the radiologist to examine the CT or additional MR imaging sequences (SWI, T2*, and T1) to exclude SAH. FLAIR hyperintensity in the cerebral sulci is also not specific for SAH. The differential diagnosis includes meningitis (**Fig. 11**), leptomeningeal carcinomatosis, melanosis, artifact from poor CSF suppression (**Fig. 12**), and hyperoxygenation in the setting of anesthesia.

Epidural Hematoma

Epidural hematomas result from bleeding into the potential space between the dura mater and the inner table of the skull. Epidural hematomas are highly associated with skull fracture, in particular the flat, thin pterion. Pterion fractures may result in laceration of a branch of the middle meningeal artery with subsequent hemorrhage into the epidural space. Approximately 10% to 30 % of epidural hematomas are venous in etiology.[9,28] The major venous sinuses lie within the dura mater and tearing of the peripheral wall result in venous epidural hematomas (**Fig. 13**). Epidural hematomas are typically lentiform in shape because

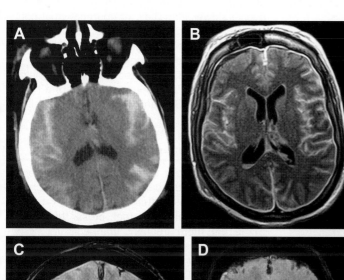

Fig. 8. (A) CT, (B) fast-acquisition axial FLAIR, (C) coronal T2* GRE, and (D) axial SWI demonstrate SAH insinuating into the sulci over the convexities. Intraventricular hemorrhage layers in trigones of the lateral ventricles on the FLAIR sequence.

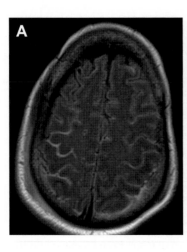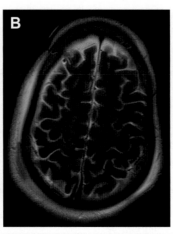

Fig. 9. CSF saturation on the (*A*) FLAIR sequence increases the ability to detect SAH compared with (*B*) standard T2.

the dura is firmly attached to the skull and cranial sutures. These hematomas classically do not cross the cranial suture lines unless the fracture transgresses the suture or there is associated sutural diastasis.[29] Epidural hematomas are most likely to occur at the site of direct impact, so-called coup epidural hematoma.

CT density evolves over time based on the acuity of blood. Epidural hematomas are hyper-attenuating in the acute phase and then slowly fade in density over time. A swirled or mixed attenuation within the hematoma raises concern for a hyperacute epidural hematoma with active hemorrhage and increased risk for enlargement.[30] CT remains the preeminent imaging modality in evaluating acute traumatic injury and suspected epidural hematoma, because it is vastly superior for the exclusion of fracture. MR imaging can help interrogate for concurrent TBI, such as DAI or infarction. The MR imaging appearance of epidural hematomas vary based on age (see **Table 1**). Extra-axial hematomas evolve slower than their intraparenchymal counterparts.[31] The vascular nature of the dura results in a high regional oxygen tension with subsequent slowing of hemoglobin degradation. T1-weighted and T2-weighted images are helpful for determining the approximate age of a hematoma, whereas SWI and T2* GRE add sensitivity for detection.

Subdural Hematoma

SDHs result from bleeding into the potential space between the dura mater and the arachnoid membrane, most often due to laceration of bridging cortical veins that cross this space. SDHs are more frequent than epidural hematomas, are rarely associated with skull fractures, and may occur on the coup or contrecoup side of the impact. SDHs readily cross sutures but not dural reflections (falx and tentorium cerebri). They are linear or crescentic in shape and, when large, may extend over an entire hemisphere (**Figs. 14** and **15**). Bilateral SDHs are present in 15% of cases.[9] SDHs can occur in patients of any age but are much more common in the elderly secondary to the increased prevalence of cerebral atrophy and the increased likelihood of cortical vein laceration. In contrast,

Fig. 10. The FLAIR sequence is susceptible to flow-related artifacts, particularly near the basilar artery (*arrow*) and foramen of Monro. No prepontine abnormality could be identified on the other MR imaging sequences.

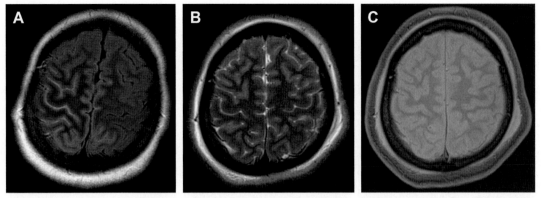

Fig. 11. Many different pathologies may result in hyperintense FLAIR signal in the subarachoid space. This patient, who was diagnosed with N-methyl-D-aspartate receptor antibody-related meningoencephalitis, demonstrates hyperintense signal in the subarachnoid space (A, B). (C) Notice the lack of susceptibility on axial T2* GRE.

epidural hematomas are more common in adolescents and young adults. Recurrent or mixed-attenuation SDHs should raise suspicion for nonaccidental trauma in children.

Acute SDHs appear as hyperattenuating, crescentic extra-axial masses on CT examinations. Mixed attenuation can be seen in SDH with hyperacute bleeding, acute-on-chronic hematoma, coagulopathy, or mixed SDH/hygroma in the setting of arachnoid membrane laceration. The hematoma should decrease by approximately 1.5 Hounsfield units per day and become isoattenuating to adjacent brain parenchyma at approximately days 5 to 7. SDHs have a variable appearance on MR imaging dependent on their age. Like epidural hematomas, SDHs evolve slower than intraparenchymal hematomas secondary to the high regional oxygen tension. The FLAIR, T2* GRE, and SWI sequences are particularly useful in detecting SDH. As with epidural

hematoma, MR imaging is most helpful in evaluation of concurrent TBI, such as DAI, infarction, and contusion.

Subdural Hygromas

A subdural hygroma is an abnormal accumulation of CSF within the subdural space. These CSF collections are likely secondary to either small tears in the arachnoid membrane or traumatic separation of the arachnoid-dura mater interface.[32] Subdural hygromas are highly associated with trauma and may appear immediately or within the first few days of injury.[32,33] Hygromas are typically found along the cerebral convexities, with an infratentorial location uncommon.[32,34] As with SDHs, traumatic subdural hygromas are typically crescentic in shape, cross sutures, and respect the midline (**Fig. 16**). Subdural hygromas are most likely bilateral. A hygroma should be isoattenuating to CSF

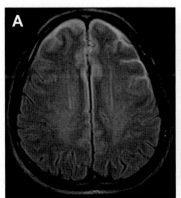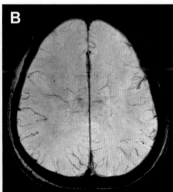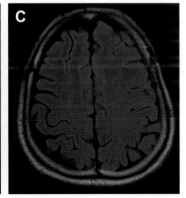

Fig. 12. (A) Incomplete fluid suppression can mimic SAH on FLAIR sequence. (B) No hemorrhage was identified on axial SWI. (C) Immediate repeat FLAIR excluded SAH.

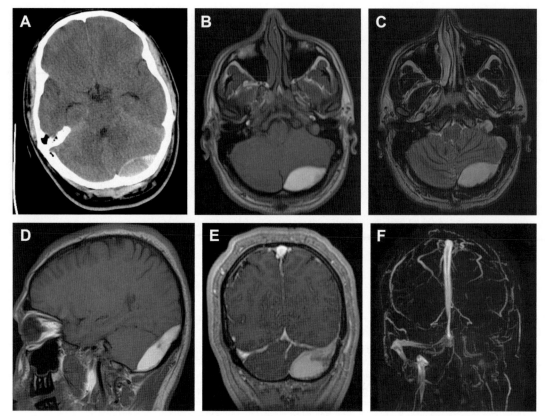

Fig. 13. (*A*) CT reveals a lens-shaped blood collection in the posterior fossa. Follow-up MR imaging demonstrates a hyperintense epidural hematoma on (*B*) T1-weighted and (*C*) T2-weighted sequences. (*D*) The sagittal T1 sequences shows the blood collection crossing the tentorium, content with epidural hematoma. (*E*) Coronal postcontrast T1 image confirms that the hematoma arises from the left transverse venous sinus. (*F*) This sinus is occluded on MRV.

on CT examination and isointense to CSF on all MR imaging sequences. Careful examination of the FLAIR and T2* sequences allows distinction between SDHs and hygromas. Cerebral atrophy with enlargement of the subarachnoid space may mimic bilateral, traumatic subdural hygromas. In these cases, inspection of the cortical veins is helpful. Cortical veins course through the enlarged subarachnoid spaces in the setting of atrophy (**Fig. 17**), whereas in subdural hygromas the veins are displaced centrally and are not seen coursing through subdural hygromas.[35]

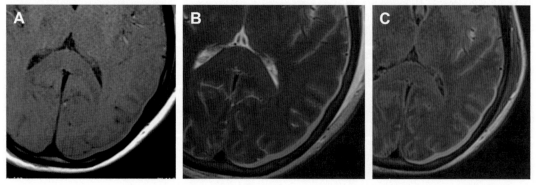

Fig. 14. (*A*) T1, (*B*) T2, and (*C*) FLAIR images show a small crescentic, extra-axial hematoma overlying the left hemisphere, consistent with SDH. SAH is also visualized in the left sylvian fissure on the FLAIR sequence.

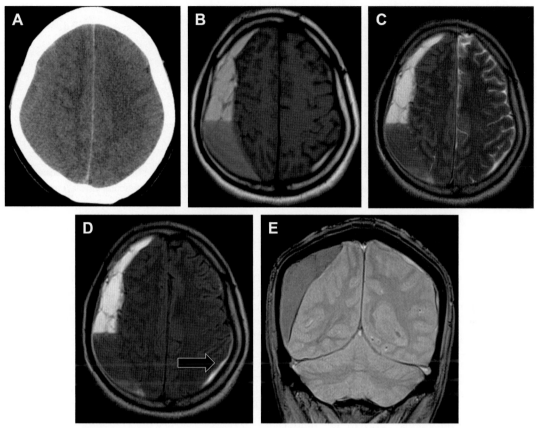

Fig. 15. Patient presents to the ED for "headache after minor trauma 2 weeks ago." (*A*) CT reveals a subtle isoattenuating SDH over the right convexity. (*B–E*) MR imaging confirms a mixed signal intensity SDH. The anterior component of the SDH has an appearance consistent with extracellular met-hemoglobin (T1 and T2 hyperintense). (*D*) FLAIR demonstrates a small contralateral SDH (*arrow*).

SECONDARY BRAIN INJURY

Secondary brain injuries (SBIs) are defined those that occur after the initial traumatic event. SBIs may take days to develop and can be even more devastating than the primary injury. Examples of SBI include cerebral edema, herniation, infarction, and CSF leak.

Posttraumatic Cerebral Edema

Posttraumatic brain edema can cause severe morbidity and mortality because it results in increasing intracranial pressure with subsequent impairment of cerebral blood flow. Traumatic cerebral edema is thought to comprise components of both vasogenic and cytotoxic

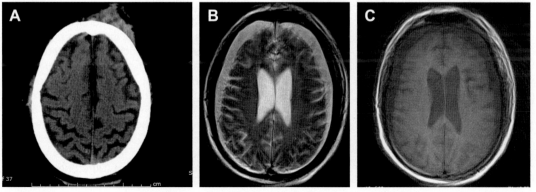

Fig. 16. Initial head CT after (*A*) MVC is unremarkable. (*B, C*) Follow-up MR imaging with fast-acquisition technique reveals development of subdural hygromas that are isointense to CSF on all sequences.

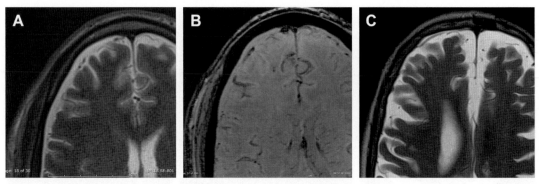

Fig. 17. (*A, B*) Subdural hygromas medially displace the cortical vessels. (*C*) No such vascular displacement is seen in the setting of atrophy.

edema,[36] with cytotoxic edema playing the predominant role in morbidity.[37] Although the exact etiology of brain swelling is unknown, the leading hypotheses are increased intracranial fluid from blood-brain barrier breakdown and cerebral hyperemia from disrupted autoregulation. Traumatic cerebral edema preferentially affects children and young adults and classically takes 24 to 48 hours to develop.[9] Posttraumatic delayed cerebral edema manifests as diffuse or focal loss of the normal gray-whiter matter distinction, sulcal effacement, and ventricular compression. MR imaging demonstrates T1 hypointensity, T2 hyperintensity, and restricted diffusion in the affected brain. As with hypoxic-ischemic injury, traumatic brain edema may preferentially involve the cerebrum with sparing of the brainstem or cerebellum.

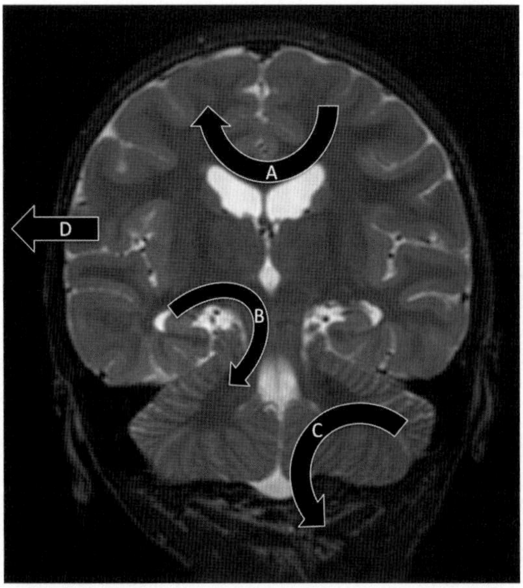

Cerebral Herniations

The intracranial vault has a defined volume. Therefore, any traumatic injury that produces mass effect may displace the brain into a contiguous compartment, a process termed *cerebral herniation* (**Fig. 18**). Examples of traumatic intracranial mass lesions include extra-axial hematomas, brain contusions, and cerebral edema. Subfalcine herniation is the most common cerebral herniation and results when a unilateral hemispheric lesion, such as an SDH, displaces the ipsilateral cingulate gyrus under the free edge of the falx. This midline shift can cause contralateral ventricular trapping from obstruction of the foramen of Monro and infarction of the anterior cerebral artery territory secondary to vascular compression on the falx. Downward transtenorial, or uncal, herniation is the second most frequent herniation syndrome and occurs when mass effect shifts the cerebrum caudally through the tentorial incisura. Unilateral supratentorial mass effect results in downward transtenorial herniation of the ipsilateral uncus and surrounding temporal lobe. Bilateral supratentorial mass effect can result in herniation of both medial temporal lobes, so-called central descending herniation. Complications of downward transtentorial herniation include oculomotor cranial nerve palsy, brainstem (Duret) hemorrhages, and posterior cerebral artery infarcts from vascular compression on the tentorium. Less commonly, mass effect in the posterior fossa

Fig. 18. A, subfalcine; B, downward transtenorial/uncal; C, tonsilar; and D, transcranial cerebral herniations.

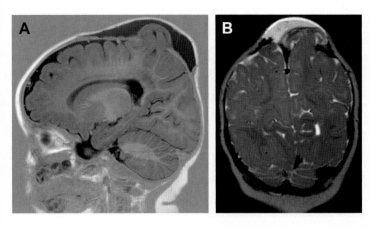

Fig. 19. A 1-year-old patient presented to the ED with seizures after craniosynostosis surgery 1 week prior. (A, B) MR imaging confirmed transcranial cerebral herniation.

may result in upwards transtentorial herniation or tonsilar herniation through the foramen magnum. Rarely, transcranial herniation occurs when the brain protrudes through a traumatic defect in the skull (Fig. 19).

Posttraumatic Infarction

Although acute brain ischemia and infarction are covered in depth (see Kambiz Nael, Wayne Kubal: MR Imaging of Acute Stroke, in this issue), it is important to stress the strong association

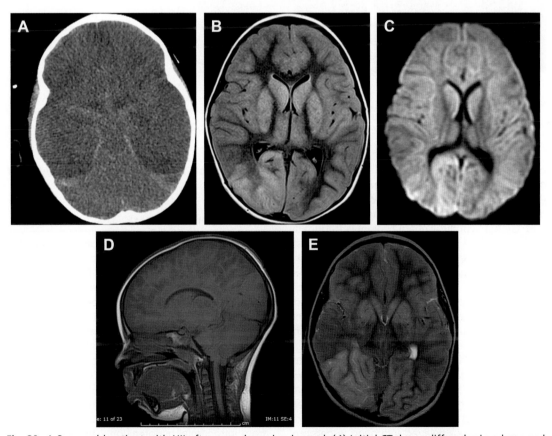

Fig. 20. A 3-year-old patient with HII after near-drowning in pool. (A) Initial CT shows diffuse brain edema and severe HII. Notice the preferential involvement of the supratentorial structures, the so-called white cerebellar sign. (B, C) Diffuse cortical and basil ganglia Hypoxic Ischemic Injury (HII) with restricted diffuse are present on MR imaging. Mass effect results in (D) tonsilar and (E) downward tentorial cerebral herniations. (E) Notice the lack of a suprasellar cistern.

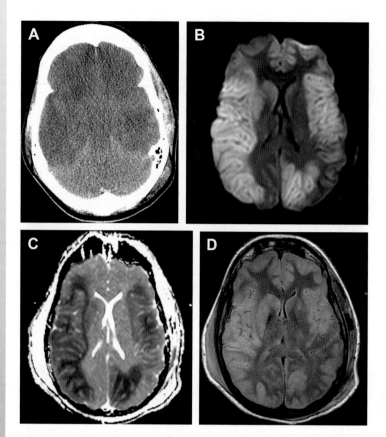

Fig. 21. (*A*) CT examination after strangulation accident demonstrates the white cerebellar sign due to preferential supratentorial HII. (*B–D*) MR imaging reveals cortical and right basal ganglia restricted diffusion and edema consistent with severe HII.

between trauma and infarction. The initial traumatic event may result in cerebral infarction through either global hypoxic-ischemic injury or damage/compression of the intracranial vasculature. Global hypoxic-ischemic injury is frequently encountered in the setting of cardiac arrest, strangulation, and drowning (**Figs. 20** and **21**). Penetrating injury to the circle of Willis can generate large vascular territory infarctions. Embolic and hypoperfusion infarctions are associated with dissection of the arteries of the neck and other vascular injuries (**Fig. 22**). Secondary brain infarcts occur days to weeks after the initial injury and may be even more devastating than the precipitating traumatic event (**Fig. 23**). Tawil and colleagues[38] examined 384 consecutive patients with severe TBI and found that 8% developed infarctions on follow-up imaging. The most common cause of delayed infarction is cerebral herniation, as discussed previously. Arterial vasospasm and venous congestion also play a role in delayed posttraumatic cerebral infarction. MR imaging is more sensitive than CT for

detection of acute infarction, regardless of cause.[39]

Cerebrospinal Fluid Leak

CSF leaks occur when head or spine injuries lacerate the dura. CSF leaks occur in 1% to 3% of close head injuries.[40] Friedman and colleagues[41] studied 51 consecutive patients who developed CSF leaks after head trauma. They found that 84% of the CSF leaks were associated with a definable skull base fracture. The frontal sinuses and cribriform plate are the most frequent locations of traumatic CSF leak.[40,41] The leaking CSF may manifest clinically as rhinorrhea (80%) or otorrhea (20%) and increases the likelihood of posttraumatic meningitis.[40] The patient may also develop postural headaches from intracranial hypotension. The precise location of the leak may be identified with CT or nuclear medicine cisternography. MR imaging may demonstrate the classic triad of intracranial hypotension: pachymeningeal enhancement,

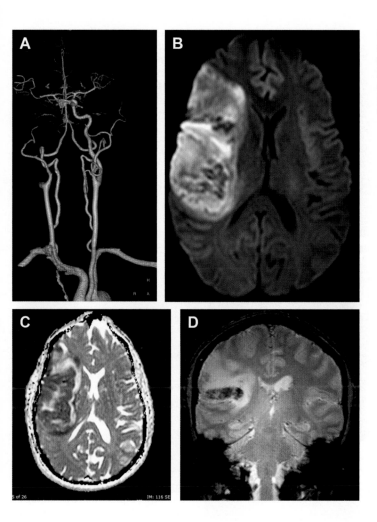

Fig. 22. Traumatic right ICA dissection after motor vehicle accident is demonstrated nicely on (*A*) CTA. Associated right MCA infarction is depicted on (*B*) DWI and (*C*) ADC sequences. (*D*) Hemorrhagic transformation is detected on coronal T2* GRE.

brainstem slumping, and SDHs/hygromas (**Fig. 24**). The classic triad is only present in approximately 50% of cases.[42] Additional signs of intracranial hypotension include distension of the dural venous sinuses, engorged pituitary gland, and downward descent of the cerebellar tonsils.[42–44]

VASCULAR IMAGING

Historically, the role of noninvasive cerebrovascular imaging in the ED was confined to CT angiography. Although this modality still plays a dominant role, MRA is extremely useful in certain urgent situations. For instance, a test that does not deliver ionizing radiation is preferred in certain patient populations, such as pregnant patients and children. MRA can be used to screen the cervical and intracranial vasculature in these patients. Iodinated contrast should be avoided in patients with chronic renal insufficiency or acute kidney injury to mitigate the risks of contrast-induced nephropathy. Noncontrast MRA techniques provide an alternative way to image both the arterial and venous vasculature in these patients, avoiding concerns for contrast-related renal damage.

A detailed discussion of the various MRA sequences and underlying physics extends beyond the scope of this issue. MRA of the head or neck, however, can be performed either with or without intravenous gadolinium contrast. Noncontrast time-of-flight MRA is frequently the sequence of choice for imaging the circle of Willis. Time-of-flight capitalizes on flowing blood's lack of saturation following a suppression pulse, so-called flow-related enhancement. Contrast-enhanced MRA is useful for evaluating the neck

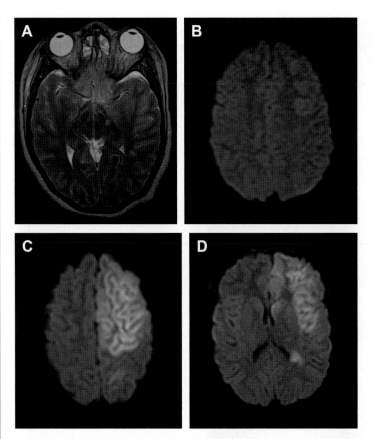

Fig. 23. (*A*, *B*) Initial MR imaging after head trauma reveals only bifrontal contusions. (*C*, *D*) Repeat MR imaging on day 4 of hospitalization show the development of secondary brain infarctions.

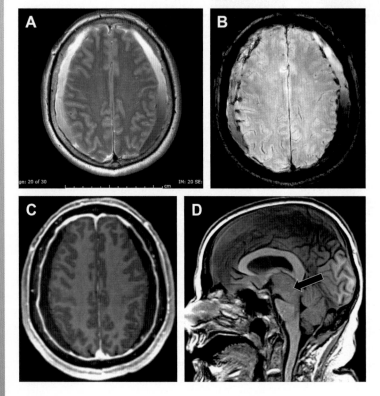

Fig. 24. Classic triad of MR imaging findings in posttraumatic intracranial hypotension include (*A*, *B*) bilateral SDHs, (*C*) pachymeningeal enhancement, and (*D*) midbrain slumping (*arrow*).

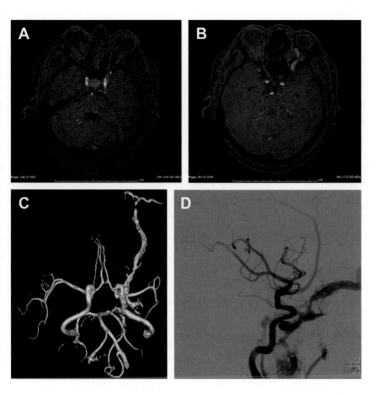

Fig. 25. An industrial explosion resulted in clinical left carotid cavernous fistula. MRA-confirmed arterialized blood flow in (A) the left cavernous sinus and (B, C) superior ophthalmic vein. (D) Lateral projection angiogram confirms diagnosis.

vessels because it allows imaging a larger field of view. Contrast-enhanced MRA relies on the T1 shortening effects of intravascular gadolinium contrast. Although CTA is the dominant imaging modality in the ED, MRA has proved a viable tool for radiologists in diagnosing traumatic carotid-cavernous fistula (Fig. 25), internal carotid artery dissection, dural arteriovenous fistula, arterial occlusion, and secondary delayed vasospasm.[45–47]

Noncontrast axial T1 fat-saturated images are particularly helpful for detecting subacute dissection, because the intramural clot appears hyperintense relative to the surrounding structures (Fig. 26).[48] MR venography (MRV) can help isolate posttraumatic venous sinus occlusion, sinus laceration (see Fig. 13), or cortical vein injury, particularly in cases where intravenous iodinated contrast is contraindicated.[49–51]

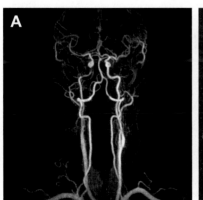
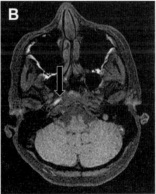

Fig. 26. (A) 3-D reformatted image from Contrast-enhanced MRA reveals a subacute right ICA dissection. (B) The axial fat saturated noncontrast T1 sequence shows a hyperintense subacute clot within the dissected petrous ICA (arrow).

SUMMARY

MR imaging is an extremely valuable tool in the evaluation of TBI in the ED. CT still plays the dominant role in urgent patient triage due to its speed, cost, and sensitivity for detecting fractures and intracranial hemorrhage. The role of MR imaging in the imaging of TBI in the emergency setting, however, continues to expand. MR imaging has shown superiority to CT for depicting multiple traumatic processes, such as DAI, cerebral contusion, and infarction. MRA and MRV allow emergent vascular imaging for patients in whom ionizing radiation and/or iodinated contrast agents should be avoided.

REFERENCES

1. Faul M, Xu L, Wald M, et al. Traumatic brain injury in the United States: emergency department visits, hospitalizations and deaths 2002-2006. Cent Dis Control Prev Natl Cent Inj Prev Control; 2010. Available at: http://www.cdc.gov/traumaticbrain injury/pdf/blue_book.pdf.
2. Ahn S, Kim WY, Lim KS, et al. Advanced radiology utilization in a tertiary care emergency department from 2001 to 2010. PLoS One 2014;9(11):e112650.
3. Rankey D, Leach JL, Leach SD. Emergency MRI utilization trends at a tertiary care academic medical center: baseline data. Acad Radiol 2008;15(4):438–43.
4. Agarwal R, Bergey M, Sonnad S, et al. Inpatient CT and MRI utilization: trends in the academic hospital setting. J Am Coll Radiol 2010;7(12):949–55.
5. Paterakis K, Karantanas AH, Komnos A, et al. Outcome of patients with diffuse axonal injury: the significance and prognostic value of MRI in the acute phase. J Trauma 2000;49:1071–5.
6. Yokota H, Kurokawa A, Otsuka T, et al. Significance of magnetic resonance imaging in acute head injury. J Trauma 1991;31(3):351–7.
7. Lee H, Wintermark M, Gean AD, et al. Focal Lesions in Acute Mild Traumatic Brain Injury and Neurocognitive Outcome: CT versus 3T MRI. J Neurotrauma 2008;25(9):1049–56.
8. Quaday KA, Salzman JG, Gordon BD. Magnetic resonance imaging and computed tomography utilization trends in an academic ED. Am J Emerg Med 2014;32(6):524–8.
9. Osborn A. Osborn's brain: imaging, pathology, and anatomy. 1st edition. Manitoba (Canada): Amirsys Publishing Inc; 2013.
10. Orrison WW, Gentry LR, Stimac GK, et al. Blinded comparison of cranial CT and MR in closed head injury evaluation. AJNR Am J Neuroradiol 1994; 15(2):351–6.
11. de Souza JM, Domingues RC, Cruz LCH, et al. Susceptibility-weighted imaging for the evaluation of patients with familial cerebral cavernous malformations: a comparison with T2-weighted fast spin-echo and gradient-echo sequences. AJNR Am J Neuroradiol 2008;291:154–8.
12. Cheng A-L, Batool S, McCreary CR, et al. Susceptibility-weighted imaging is more reliable than T2*-weighted gradient-recalled echo MRI for detecting microbleeds. Stroke 2013;44(10):2782–6.
13. Shams S, Martola J, Cavallin L, et al. SWI or T2*: which MRI sequence to use in the detection of cerebral microbleeds? The Karolinska imaging dementia study. AJNR Am J Neuroradiol 2015;36(6): 1089–95.
14. Jandial R, Reichwage B, Levy M, et al. Ballistics for the neurosurgeon. Neurosurgery 2008;62(2):472–80 [discussion: 480].
15. Adams JH, Doyle D, Ford I, et al. Diffuse axonal injury in head injury: definition, diagnosis and grading. Histopathology 1989;15(1):49–59.
16. Davis PC, Expert Panel on Neurologic Imaging. Head trauma. AJNR Am J Neuroradiol 2007;28(8): 1619–21.
17. Mittl RL, Grossman RI, Hiehle JF, et al. Prevalence of MR evidence of diffuse axonal injury in patients with mild head injury and normal head CT findings. AJNR Am J Neuroradiol 1994;15(8):1583–9.
18. Yousem D, Grossman R. Neuroradiology: the requisites. 3rd edition. Philadelphia: Elsevier Health Sciences; 2010.
19. Spitz G, Maller JJ, Ng A, et al. Detecting lesions after traumatic brain injury using susceptibility weighted imaging: a comparison with fluid-attenuated inversion recovery and correlation with clinical outcome. J Neurotrauma 2013;3024:2038–50.
20. Beauchamp MH, Ditchfield M, Babl FE, et al. Detecting traumatic brain lesions in children: CT versus MRI versus susceptibility weighted imaging (SWI). J Neurotrauma 2011;28(6):915–27.
21. Tong KA, Ashwal S, Holshouser BA, et al. Hemorrhagic shearing lesions in children and adolescents with posttraumatic diffuse axonal injury: improved detection and initial results. Radiology 2003;227(2):332–9.
22. Coello AF, Canals AG, Gonzalez JM, et al. Cranial nerve injury after minor head trauma. J Neurosurg 2010;113(3):547–55.
23. Evans RW. Neurology and trauma. New York: Oxford University Press; 2006.
24. Da Rocha AJ, da Silva CJ, Gama HPP, et al. Comparison of magnetic resonance imaging sequences with computed tomography to detect low-grade subarachnoid hemorrhage: role of fluid-attenuated inversion recovery sequence. J Comput Assist Tomogr 2006;302:295–303.
25. Mitchell P, Wilkinson ID, Hoggard N, et al. Detection of subarachnoid haemorrhage with magnetic resonance imaging. J Neurol Neurosurg Psychiatry 2001;70(2):205–11.

26. Yuan M-K, Lai P-H, Chen J-Y, et al. Detection of subarachnoid hemorrhage at acute and sub-acute/chronic stages: comparison of four magnetic resonance imaging pulse sequences and computed tomography. J Chin Med Assoc 2005; 68(3):131–7.

27. Verma RK, Kottke R, Andereggen L, et al. Detecting subarachnoid hemorrhage: comparison of combined FLAIR/SWI versus CT. Eur J Radiol 2013; 82(9):1539–45.

28. Zimmerman RA, Bilaniuk LT. Computed tomographic staging of traumatic epidural bleeding. Radiology 1982;144(4):809–12.

29. Huisman TA, Tschirch FT. Epidural hematoma in children: do cranial sutures act as a barrier? J Neuroradiol 2009;36(2):93–7.

30. Al-Nakshabandi NA. The swirl sign. Radiology 2001; 218(2):433.

31. Siddiqui FM, Bekker SV, Qureshi AI. Neuroimaging of hemorrhage and vascular defects. Neurotherapeutics 2011;8(1):28–38.

32. Lee KS. The pathogenesis and clinical significance of traumatic subdural hygroma. Brain Inj 1998; 12(7):595–603.

33. Zanini MA, de Lima Resende LA, de Souza Faleiros AT, et al. Traumatic subdural hygromas: proposed pathogenesis based classification. J Trauma 2008;643:705–13.

34. Kabir SMR, Jennings SJ, Makris D. Posterior fossa subdural hygroma with supratentorial chronic subdural haematoma. Br J Neurosurg 2004;18(3): 297–300.

35. McCluney KW, Yeakley JW, Fenstermacher MJ, et al. Subdural hygroma versus atrophy on MR brain scans: "the cortical vein sign". AJNR Am J Neuroradiol 1992;13(5):1335–9.

36. Unterberg AW, Stover J, Kress B, et al. Edema and brain trauma. Neuroscience 2004;129(4): 1021–9.

37. Ito J, Marmarou A, Barz Kress B, et al. Edema and brain trauma. J Neurosurg 1996;841: 97–103.

38. Tawil I, Stein DM, Mirvis SE, et al. Posttraumatic cerebral infarction: incidence, outcome, and risk factors. J Trauma 2008;64(4):849–53.

39. Srinivasan A, Goyal M, Azri FA, et al. State-of-the-Art imaging of acute stroke. Radiographics 2006; 26(Suppl 1):S75–95.

40. Lloyd KM, DelGaudio JM, Hudgins PA. Imaging of skull base cerebrospinal fluid leaks in adults. Radiology 2008;248(3):725–36.

41. Friedman JA, Ebersold MJ, Quast LM. Post-traumatic cerebrospinal fluid leakage. World J Surg 2001;25(8):1062–6.

42. Shah LM, McLean LA, Heilbrun ME, et al. Intracranial hypotension: improved MRI detection with diagnostic intracranial angles. AJR Am J Roentgenol 2013;200(2):400–7.

43. Farb RI, Forghani R, Lee SK, et al. The venous distension sign: a diagnostic sign of intracranial hypotension at mr imaging of the brain. AJNR Am J Neuroradiol 2007;28(8):1489–93.

44. Pannullo SC, Reich JB, Krol G, et al. MRI changes in intracranial hypotension. Neurology 1993;43(5):919.

45. Vertinsky AT, Schwartz NE, Fischbein NJ, et al. Comparison of multidetector CT angiography and MR imaging of cervical artery dissection. AJNR Am J Neuroradiol 2008;29(9):1753–60.

46. Chen CC-C, Chang PC-T, Shy C-G, et al. CT angiography and mr angiography in the evaluation of carotid cavernous sinus fistula prior to embolization: a comparison of techniques. AJNR Am J Neuroradiol 2005;26(9):2349–56.

47. Grandin CB, Cosnard G, Hammer F, et al. Vasospasm after subarachnoid hemorrhage: diagnosis with MR angiography. AJNR Am J Neuroradiol 2000;21(9):1611–7.

48. Rodallec MH, Marteau V, Gerber S, et al. Craniocervical arterial dissection: spectrum of imaging findings and differential diagnosis. Radiographics 2008;286:1711–28.

49. Zhang Z, Long J, Li W. Cerebral venous sinus thrombosis: a clinical study of 23 cases. Chin Med J (Engl) 2000;113(11):1043–5.

50. Wasay M, Azeemuddin M. Neuroimaging of cerebral venous thrombosis. J Neuroimaging 2005;15(2): 118–28.

51. Choudhary AK, Bradford R, Dias MS, et al. Venous injury in abusive head trauma. Pediatr Radiol 2015; 45(12):1803–13.

Magnetic Resonance Imaging of Spinal Emergencies

Daniel Kawakyu-O'Connor, MD[a],*,
Ritu Bordia, MBBS, MPH[b], Refky Nicola, MS, DO[a]

KEYWORDS

- Emergency • MR imaging spine • Spinal cord • Protocols • Mimics • Trauma

KEY POINTS

- Magnetic resonance (MR) imaging of the spine is increasingly being performed for the evaluation of emergent conditions.
- MR imaging can readily differentiate between acute and chronic fractures identified by computed tomography (CT), and is sensitive and specific in detecting and describing ligament, disc, and spinal cord injury.
- MR imaging is preferred over CT in the evaluation of acute back pain in patients with history of malignancy or infection.
- MR imaging protocols should be tailored for a specific indication so as to increase the sensitivity and specificity of the examination, and decrease scan time.

INTRODUCTION

The role of MR imaging is expanding in the assessment of patients in the emergent setting. However, MR imaging has several limitations due to its longer scan times, higher expense, and the need for highly trained personnel. For this reason, the radiologist and referring clinicians should discuss the indication for the study before the MR examination.[1]

Also, the familiarization with appropriate MR imaging protocols for specific indications enables an appropriate utilization of MR imaging as a diagnostic tool, provides a higher degree of diagnostic certainty, and avoids unnecessary costs and delays to the patient and referring physician.[2]

PROTOCOLS AND SEQUENCES

A detailed patient's history is essential before the study is started. There are elements that are critically important, such as presence of devices or implants that are contraindicated for an MR examination (eg, electronic spine stimulator devices, cardiac pacers, defibrillators) or that may degrade examination quality (eg, spinal fusion hardware). Others include a history of malignancy or renal insufficiency, a documented history of reactions to gadolinium-based contrast agents, previous spine surgery, and clinical suspicion or risk factors for an infection (eg, current or recent central line use, suspected infections outside the spine, history or suspicion of intravenous drug use, and/or immunocompromised status).

The authors have nothing to disclose.
[a] Division of Emergency Imaging, Department of Imaging Sciences, University of Rochester Medical Center, 601 Elmwood Avenue, Box 648, Rochester, NY 14642, USA; [b] Section of Neuroradiology, Department of Radiology, Winthrop University Hospital, 259 1st Street, Mineola, NY 11501, USA
* Corresponding author.
E-mail address: Daniel_Oconnor@URMC.Rochester.edu

Magn Reson Imaging Clin N Am 24 (2016) 325–344
http://dx.doi.org/10.1016/j.mric.2015.11.004
1064-9689/16/$ – see front matter © 2016 Elsevier Inc. All rights reserved.

The MR imaging sequences that should be incorporated in the emergency MR imaging spine protocol are listed in **Table 1**.[3]

T1-weighted imaging (T1WI) is used to assess for any osseous abnormalities that may replace or infiltrate the normal fat-containing bone marrow, such as metastasis, edema, or infection. T1WI also provides information regarding the anatomy and signal characteristics of peri-spinal soft tissues.

T2-weighted imaging (T2WI) depicts spinal cord lesions that are hyperintense relative to the surrounding spinal cord and result in effacement of cerebrospinal fluid (CSF). Paraspinal soft tissue edema and fluid collections are best seen on T2WI sequences.

T2-weighted sequences with fat suppression (T2WI-FS) use lipid signal-specific fat suppression to provide accurate suppression of fat signal and excellent anatomic detail. T2WI-FS is sensitive to magnetic field inhomogeneity and may result in suboptimal fat suppression at the interface between air, fat, bone, or in the presence of metallic implants or foreign bodies.

Short tau/T1 inversion recovery (STIR) is a fat-suppression technique that is relatively insensitive to field inhomogeneity, although signal-to-noise ratio is typically decreased relative to T2WI-FS.

Signal suppression in STIR is not lipid specific and T1 signal associated with proteinaceous fluid (such as mucous or hemorrhage) also can be suppressed.

Proton density–weighted imaging (PDWI) is best for characterizing T2-hyperintense lesions of the spinal cord that are obscured on heavily T2-weighted acquisitions, and can be added or substituted if cord lesions are of primary clinical concern (eg, multiple sclerosis). PDWI is incorporated into protocols designed to identify disc herniation due to good anatomic detail and spatial resolution.

T2*-weighted gradient-recalled echo imaging (T2*WI or GRE) or newer *susceptibility-weighted imaging (SWI)* are commonly included in MR imaging spine trauma protocols to increase examination sensitivity for detection of hemosiderin-containing blood products within the spinal cord or epidural space.

Diffusion-weighted imaging (DWI) has a complementary role in the imaging of spinal cord neoplasms, epidural abscesses, and cord infarction, but is not included in the routine emergent spine MR imaging protocol.

Contrast-enhanced T1-weighted fat-suppressed imaging (T1WI-FS + Gd) is useful in

Table 1
Recommended magnetic resonance imaging sequences for the evaluation of spine

Sequence	Structures Evaluated	Disease Processes
T1WI	Bone marrow	Fractures, spine metastases, osteomyelitis
	Epidural space	Hematoma, abscess
T2WI	Spinal cord	Cord edema/inflammation or demyelination
T2WI with fat suppression	Bone marrow	Fractures, bone metastases, osteomyelitis
	Spinal cord	Cord edema/inflammation or demyelination
	Paraspinal soft tissues	Edema/fluid collections
STIR	Alternative to T2W fat suppression sequence	Similar to T2WI-FS
PDWI	Spinal cord	Demyelination
DWI	Bone marrow	Osteomyelitis/discitis
	Epidural space	Epidural abscess
	Spinal cord	Spinal cord infarction
	Anywhere	Neoplasm
T2*-GRE WI	Spinal cord	Hemorrhage (trauma cases)
T1WI with contrast and fat suppression	Bone marrow	Osteomyelitis/discitis
		Metastases
	Epidural space	Epidural phlegmon/abscess
	Spinal cord	Active inflammation/demyelination, leptomeningeal or dural metastases
	Paraspinal soft tissues	Abscess
	Anywhere	Neoplasm

Abbreviations: DWI, diffusion-weighted image; GRE, gradient-recalled echo imaging; PDWI, proton density–weighted image; STIR, short tau/T1 inversion recovery; T1WI, T1-weighted image; T2WI, T2-weighted image.

patients with history of tumor, infection, or recurrent disc herniation following surgery. Fat suppression is necessary to identify enhancement that would otherwise be obscured or equivocal due to high T1-weighted marrow or paraspinal soft tissue signal. In the spinal cord, T1WI-FS + Gd identifies regions of cord inflammation, active demyelination, or neoplasm.

Selection of a proper *field of view (FOV)* is a trade-off between scan time and spatial resolution. A *large FOV* allows evaluation of multiple spinal levels at a lower spatial resolution in a given time interval, and can be performed in multiple stages with a sagittal view extending from the skull base to the upper thoracic spine, and another from the lower thoracic spine to the lumbosacral junction. Large FOV protocols are indicated for unknown or multiple suspected noncontiguous levels of involvement (eg, metastatic disease to bone, suspected epidural abscess or disseminated osteomyelitis, or multiple age-indeterminate compression fractures). On the other hand, a *small FOV* is best for evaluating fewer spinal levels at greater spatial resolution in a given time interval.

Magnet field strength in emergent evaluation is less critical. Images acquired at 1.5 T are typically adequate for assessing fractures, cord lesions/hemorrhage, epidural fluid collections, and disc herniation. However, higher field-strength systems (eg, 3.0 T and higher) are increasingly becoming available.

SPINE TRAUMA

Trauma is the most common indication for spinal MR imaging. Most spinal injuries are caused by motor vehicle collisions (MVCs), with the remainder resulting from sports-related injuries, falls, and violent acts.[4] Young men are disproportionately commonly affected by spine trauma, although the average age is increasing in most developed countries because of the longer life expectancy of the population.[5]

The incidence of spinal injuries at different segments is related to the anatomic variability of the spinal column.[6] The cervical spine is the shortest in length; however, smaller bone and ligament structures, greater flexibility and articulation, and mass of the head predispose the cervical spine to injury, predominately at the C2 and C6-C7 levels.[7]

The thoracolumbar region (T11-T12 though L3-L4) represents the second most common region of traumatic injury within the spine.[8] Injury is less common at the upper thoracic levels due to the rigid and protective rib cage, and at the lumbosacral junction where osseous and supporting ligamentous structures are more robust. Uncommon patterns of spinal injuries are encountered in patients with predisposing conditions, such as osteopenia, ankylosing spondylitis, metastatic or primary bone lesions, and history of previous spine injury and/or surgery.[9]

UPPER CERVICAL SPINE TRAUMA

Injuries of the upper cervical spine (occiput through C2) may be considered separately from those below the level of C2 because of the unique anatomy of the spine at these levels and the distinct patterns of injury. Cervical spine fractures below the level of C2 (subaxial fractures) are described in terms similar to the thoracic and lumbar levels and are considered separately in the following paragraphs.

- *Atlanto-occipital and atlanto-axial dislocation-type injuries* result from flexion, flexion-distraction, or flexion-rotation mechanisms. This can be seen on multidetector CT (MDCT) or radiography directly or indirectly with the use of several metrics (eg, Powers ratio, basion-dental interval, the basion-posterior axial interval).[10,11]

However, MR imaging is important in assessing the integrity of the atlanto-occipital ligaments (anterior, posterior, and lateral), atlanto-axial ligaments (anterior and posterior), capsular ligaments, cruciate ligament of the atlas, and alar ligaments of the dens (**Fig. 1**).

- *C1 (Jefferson) burst fractures* are caused by axial loading of the cervical spine. This represents a fracture of the anterior and posterior arches of C1, as the wedge-shaped lateral masses of C1 are displaced laterally between the larger and more robust occipital condyles and the lateral masses of C2 (**Fig. 2**). Although the osseous injury is best detected on MDCT, MR imaging is critical for evaluating the involvement of the cruciate ligament of the atlas, which is important in assessing the stability of the injury.[12]
- *Odontoid fractures* are caused by flexion or extension injuries, often in conjunction with other injuries of the cervical spine.[13,14]

An isolated *type I odontoid fracture* is typically stable and involves the dens above the level of the transverse ligament. A *type II odontoid fracture* is considered unstable, commonly involves the base of the odontoid process at the junction of the body of C2, and is associated with a high rate of nonunion with conservative, nonoperative management (**Fig. 3**). A *type III odontoid fracture*

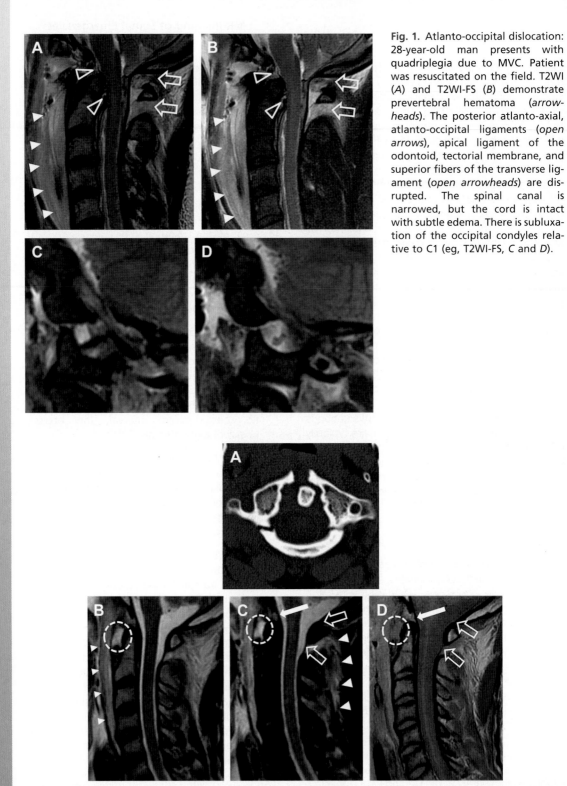

Fig. 1. Atlanto-occipital dislocation: 28-year-old man presents with quadriplegia due to MVC. Patient was resuscitated on the field. T2WI (A) and T2WI-FS (B) demonstrate prevertebral hematoma (arrowheads). The posterior atlanto-axial, atlanto-occipital ligaments (open arrows), apical ligament of the odontoid, tectorial membrane, and superior fibers of the transverse ligament (open arrowheads) are disrupted. The spinal canal is narrowed, but the cord is intact with subtle edema. There is subluxation of the occipital condyles relative to C1 (eg, T2WI-FS, C and D).

Fig. 2. C1 burst fracture (Jefferson): 40-year-old man presents neck pain after MVC. (A) Fractures of the anterior and posterior arches of C1 is seen in initial CT. (B) T2WI demonstrates large prevertebral fluid hematoma (white arrowheads). (C) T2WI -FS demonstrates increased signal in the deep soft tissue of the neck posteriorly consistent with interspinous ligament injury (arrowheads), and intact tectorial membrane (arrow) and posterior atlanto-occipital and atlanto-axial ligaments (open arrows). (D) PD sequences more clearly depict the intact tectorial membrane (arrow) and posterior atlanto-occipital and atlanto-axial ligaments (open arrows). The anterior arch of C1 is not seen on the sagittal images due to lateral displacement (dashed circle). The anterior arch of C1 is not seen on the sagittal images due to lateral displacement (dashed circle, B-D).

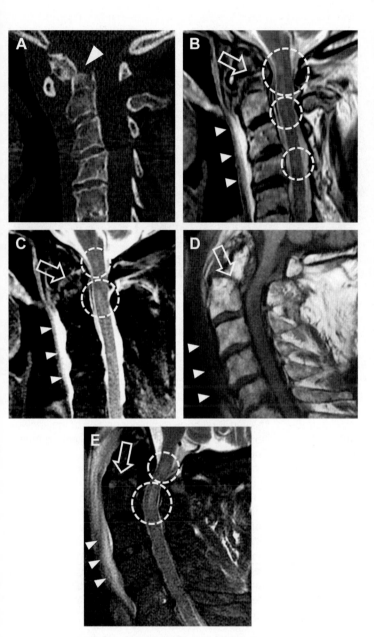

Fig. 3. Odontoid fracture, type 2: 80-year-old man has a history of recent fall and intermittent neuropathic pain. Sagittal CT image (*A*) demonstrates fracture of the dens at the level of the mid transverse ligament (*arrowhead*) with anterior translation of the anterior arch of C1. Post reduction T2WI (*B*) and T2WI-FS (*C*) demonstrate near-anatomic alignment of the dens, prevertebral hematoma (*arrowheads*), fracture line and marrow edema (*open arrow*), and increased T2 signal within the cord (*dashed white circles*) consistent with cord edema. An 82-year-old man presents with paraplegia. T1WI (*D*) demonstrates low signal at site of fracture (*open white arrow*) and prevertebral thickening (*white arrowheads*) and dorsal angulation of the dens. T2WI-FS (*E*) depicts edema (*dashed white circles*) and compression of the cord with paravertebral hematoma (*arrowheads*) and fracture with marrow edema (*open white arrow*).

extends from the base of the odontoid inferiorly into the body of C2 and is also considered unstable.

- *C2 (Hangman) fractures* (ie, traumatic spondylolisthesis of C2) are the result of sudden hyperextension and distraction of the head and upper neck with axial loading of the posterior elements of C2. MDCT readily detects pars interarticularis fractures, degree of anterolisthesis, and facet joint dislocation, and is sufficient for commonly used grading systems (ie, Effendi,

Levine).[15] Although the fracture is intrinsically unstable, spinal cord injury is uncommon except in high-grade fractures. MR imaging is used to assess injury of the cord, vertebral arteries, ligaments, and evidence of a prevertebral hematoma or marrow edema (**Fig. 4**).

Mimic: Chronic compression fractures due to remote trauma or osteopenia with adjacent marrow edema secondary to active disc arthropathy (ie, Modic changes) can mimic acute traumatic marrow edema.

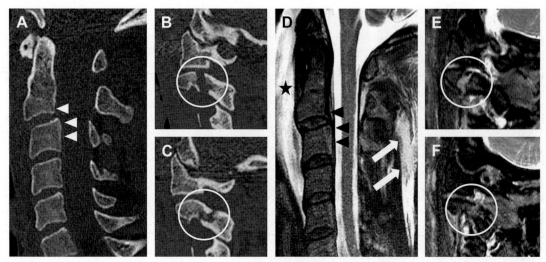

Fig. 4. Traumatic C2 spondylolysis ("Hangman fracture"): 38-year-old man status post MVC with steering wheel injury to mandible. CT images demonstrate anterior subluxation of C2 with (*A, arrowheads*) bilateral *spondylolisthesis* (*B, C, circles*) consistent with a "Hangman fracture." Sagittal MR imaging T2WI-FS (*D, arrowheads*) and spondylolisthesis of C2 (*E, F, circles*). Prevertebral hematoma (*D, black star*) and edema of the interspinous ligaments (*D, arrows*) is present.

- *Flexion teardrop* and *extension*-type injuries have similar radiographic and CT features. The primary role of MR imaging is to detect spinal cord injury. In flexion teardrop injuries, anterior compression and posterior distraction causes widening and dislocation of the posterior element and facet joints. The posterior translation of the major fracture fragment with respect to the cervical spine inferiorly, and loss of vertebral body height anteriorly is also seen (**Fig. 5**).

In extension injuries, anterior distraction and posterior compression forces result in widening of the disc with preserved vertebral body height (**Fig. 6**).

In equivocal cases, marrow edema involving the posterior elements or anterior longitudinal ligament disruption suggests an extension-type injury. Anterior vertebral body marrow edema or interspinous ligament injury suggests a flexion injury.

Mimic: Incompletely fused anterior endplate osteophytosis, or calcification of the anterior longitudinal ligament, can mimic a teardrop fracture.

SUBAXIAL CERVICAL, THORACIC, AND LUMBAR SPINE TRAUMA

Fractures and ligamentous injuries of the subaxial cervical spine are comparable to fractures of the thoracic and lumbar spine.[16] The "3-column" model divides the osseous and supporting ligamentous structures of the vertebral column into 3 adjacent columns: anterior, middle, and posterior.[8]

The anterior column includes the anterior half of the vertebral body, anterior portion of annulus fibrosis, and the anterior longitudinal ligament. The middle column includes the posterior half of the vertebral body, posterior portion of the annulus fibrosis, and the posterior longitudinal ligament. The posterior column includes the neural arch, facet joints and capsules, and the interspinous ligaments.

Other classification systems, such as the thoracolumbar injury classification severity score, also can be used.[17] This includes description of the morphology, mechanism of injury, and displacement of the spinal column (ie, compression, burst, translational/rotational, or distraction type injuries) and ligamentous injury with the neurologic assessment of injury are all combined to determine a conservative versus operative management.[18]

- *Compression fractures* result from an axial loading or flexion injury. The anterior portion of the vertebral body is most commonly involved resulting in a *wedge fracture*.

However, fractures may include the superior endplate, inferior endplate, or anterior cortex, and contiguous levels may be involved. Paraspinal hematoma may be present.

If the posterior column is not involved, compression fractures are typically stable and are not associated with acute spinal cord injury.[19] Marrow edema is characteristic, seen as decreased T1WI, increased T2WI-FS, and STIR signal relative to the adjacent marrow. The *burst fracture* is a more severe injury, involving all 3 columns, often

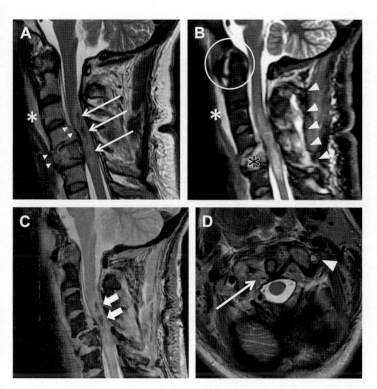

Fig. 5. Flexion teardrop fracture, C5 with cord contusion and hemorrhage in a 51-year-old woman following MVC, quadriplegia. Sagittal T2WI (*A*) demonstrates disruption of the cortex of C5 anteriorly and C6 posteriorly, teardrop fragment, disruption of the anterior and posterior longitudinal ligaments (*arrowheads*). There is evidence of cord contusion and hemorrhage (*arrows*) with a prevertebral hematoma from C1 to C5 (*asterisk*). Sagittal STIR (*B*) depicts marrow edema at C5 (black *asterisk*), prevertebral hematoma (white *asterisk*), interspinous ligament injury (*arrowheads*), and cord swelling with edema. Fluid in the predental space suggests additional injury at the C1-C2 level (*circle*). Sagittal GRE (*C*) confirms cord hemorrhage as central susceptibility within the cord (*white arrows*). Axial T2WI (*D*) at the level of the dens demonstrates disruption of the transverse ligament on the right (*arrow*) and absence of flow void with the left vertebral artery (*arrowhead*) consistent with occlusion.

with herniation of the nucleus pulposus into the adjoining endplates, comminuted vertebral body fractures, and loss of vertebral body height. Stability of the vertebral column at the level of injury is determined by the integrity of the anterior and posterior longitudinal ligaments and of the posterior elements, including the facet joints and neural arch and associated ligaments.[20] Posterior displacement of fracture fragments can result in stenosis of the spinal canal (**Fig. 7**).

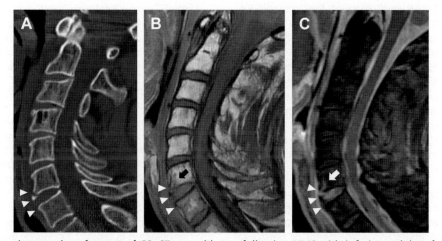

Fig. 6. Extension teardrop fracture of C6; 67 year-old man following MVC with inferior endplate fracture and widening of C6-C7 disc space in initial CT examination (*A, arrowheads*). Sagittal T1WI (*B*) confirms small fracture fragment from inferior endplate of C6 (*black arrow*), widening of C6-C7 disc space (*arrowheads*), and decreased marrow signal at fracture donor site consistent with edema. Uniform T1 marrow signal hyperintensity at the C1 through C6 levels is secondary to prior radiation therapy of head and neck cancer. Sagittal STIR (*C*) demonstrates both anterior longitudinal ligament injury and C6-C7 disc injury (*arrowheads*) and confirms marrow edema at C6 (*arrow*).

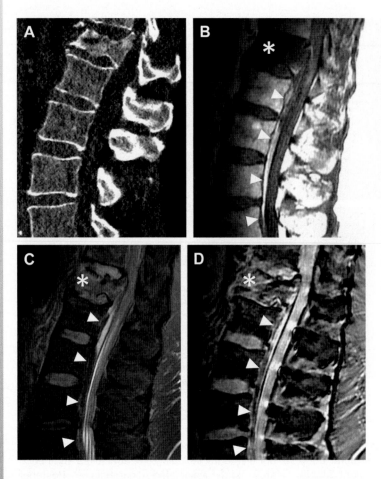

Fig. 7. Epidural hematoma, burst fracture of T12: 49 year-old man with spine pain and lower extremity paresthesia following MVC. Sagittal CT image (*A*) demonstrates T12 burst fracture and narrowing of the spinal canal. Sagittal T1WI (*B*) demonstrates decreased marrow signal (*white asterisk*) at the level of the burst fracture consistent with acute marrow edema and epidural thickening ventral to the thecal sac (*arrowheads*). Sagittal T2WI-FS (*C*) and GRE (*D*) demonstrate hyperintense signal within the fracture (*asterisks*); the epidural collection is hyperintense superiorly and hypointense inferiorly (*white arrowheads*) consistent with epidural hematoma with clot retraction.

- *Isolated spinous process fractures* are usually caused by a direct blow to the dorsal spine (**Fig. 8**). An evaluation of the interspinous, anterior longitudinal, and posterior longitudinal ligaments is necessary to confirm spinal stability.
- *Flexion, combined flexion/distraction type fractures* are caused by rapid deceleration and flexion of the upper spine with respect to a restrained lower spine, for example, passengers restrained with a lap belt in MVCs. Due to the high-energy mechanism of trauma, additional injuries of the chest and abdomen are common.[21]

A *Chance fracture* is caused by combined flexion and distraction forces disrupting the supporting posterior structures of the spinal column, typically the interspinous ligaments or horizontal fracture through the spinous process (**Fig. 9**). A wedge fracture of the vertebral body can be seen; however, if there is no subluxation, the anterior longitudinal ligament usually remains intact. If there is no spinous process fracture, MR imaging is required to identify ligament injury to differentiate from simple compression fracture.[22]

Mimic: Chance fracture without associated horizontal fracture of the spinous process can be mistaken for a wedge compression fracture or a simple burst fracture if there is posterior displacement of the dorsal cortex of the vertebral body.

- *Translational and shear-type fractures* involve disruption of all 3 spinal columns with vertebral body subluxation. These are unstable injuries and are associated with spinal cord and intra-abdominal injury.[21] A shear-type fracture is characterized by disruption of the anterior longitudinal ligament and vertebral body subluxation (**Fig. 10**).
- *Facet joint dislocation* (eg, perched or jumped facets) can be on radiographs or CT. The mechanism is usually flexion/distraction with anterior translation of the upper spine. *Unilateral facet dislocation* results from combined flexion and rotation forces, and is associated with a lesser degree of vertebral body and spinal cord injury than bilateral facet dislocation

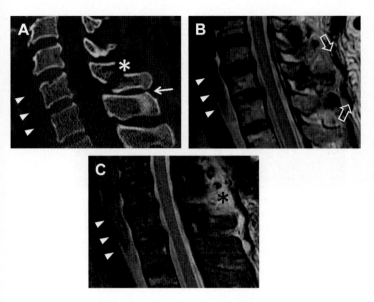

Fig. 8. Spinous process fracture, C7, with avulsed supraspinous ligament: 63-year-old woman presents with neck pain following injury to posterior neck. Sagittal CT (*A*) demonstrates displaced spinous process fracture (*asterisk*) and loss C7-T1 interspinous space (*arrow*). Prevertebral soft tissue thickening (*arrowheads*) is also present, suggesting hematoma. Sagittal T2WI (*B*) demonstrates a spinous process fracture and prevertebral hematoma (*arrowheads*); the supraspinous ligament is avulsed from the C6-T1 spinous processes (*arrows*). Sagittal T2WI-FS (*C*) demonstrates the prevertebral hematoma (*arrowheads*) and disruption of the supraspinous ligament (*asterisk*).

(**Fig. 11**).[23] *Bilateral facet dislocation* is caused by flexion injury with distraction of the posterior elements, compression of the vertebral body anteriorly with or without fracture, and variable anterior subluxation of the upper spine.

DISC INJURY AND HERNIATION

Injury of the disc, particularly in the lumbar spine, is a frequent cause of acute or worsening radiculopathy with or without neurologic deficit. The management of isolated low back pain is typically conservative and does not require imaging. Emergent MR imaging is reserved for severe cases in which surgical intervention may be indicated, such as new-onset or rapidly progressive

neurologic deficits, urinary retention, or saddle anesthesia. In the absence of focal neurologic deficits, emergent MR imaging is indicated in patients with suspected complication of cord or vertebral neoplasm, epidural abscess, or epidural hematoma.[24]

The term *disc herniation* is nonspecific and refers to extension of disc material beyond the normal confines of the annulus fibrosis, as defined by the peripheral margins of the adjoining vertebral endplates. *Protrusion* refers to herniated disc in which the greatest dimension of the herniated disc is smaller than the dimension of the hernia base. *Extrusion* refers to a herniated disc in which the greatest dimension of the herniated disc is greater than the dimension of the hernia base (**Fig. 12**). Disc extrusions in which the herniated

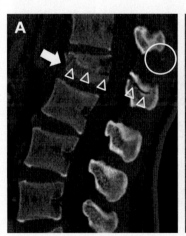
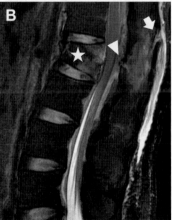

Fig. 9. Chance fracture, L1: 23-year-old man presents with lower extremity weakness and paresthesia following MVC. Sagittal CT (*A*) demonstrates loss of vertebral body height at L1 (*white arrow*) with fracture of the anterior and posterior cortex extending to spinous process of L1 (*arrowheads*). There is also a fragment at the site of interspinous and supraspinous ligament injury, consistent small avulsion fragment (*circle*). Sagittal T2WI-FS (*B*) demonstrates L1 vertebral body marrow edema (*star*) and increased signal in the spinous process marrow and interspinous ligaments. There is disruption of the ligamentum flavum (*arrowhead*) and interspinous ligament at the inferior margin of the T12 spinous process (*arrow*).

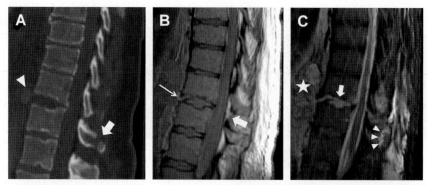

Fig. 10. Three-column shear-type fracture and ligament injury: 44-year-old woman presents following MVC. Sagittal CT image (*A*) demonstrates widening of the intervertebral space and hematoma anteriorly (*arrowhead*) and fracture involving the T12 spinous process (*arrow*). Sagittal PDWI (*B*) identifies anterior longitudinal ligament (*thin arrow*) and interspinous ligament (*thick arrow*) rupture. Sagittal STIR (*C*) clearly identifies fluid signal at site of disc injury (*arrow*), prevertebral hematoma (*star*), posterior soft tissue edema, and fluid signal at the spinous process fracture (*arrowheads*).

fragment is no longer contiguous with the donor disc are also referred to as *sequestered* or free disc fragments. *Disc migration* refers to disc material extending superiorly or inferiorly with respect to the donor disc as defined by the superior and inferior endplates, and is used to describe both contiguous and free disc fragments.[25]

Injury of the annulus fibrosis, the robust ligamentous structure retaining the intervertebral disc between the adjoining vertebral endplates, can result in acute back pain. Although injury to the annulus fibrosis may be inferred by the presence

of frank disc herniation/extrusion, isolated injury to the annulus fibrosis can occur without displacement of disc fragments and without focal neurologic symptoms. An *annular fissure or tear* is a small focus of T2 hyperintense signal at the margin of the disc, subjacent to the uniformly low signal annulus fibrosis (**Fig. 13**).

Failed back surgery syndrome (FBSS) refers to symptomatic recurrent protrusion/extrusion of disc material at a level of previous decompression. Although intravenous (IV) contrast is not required for the routine diagnosis of symptomatic disc

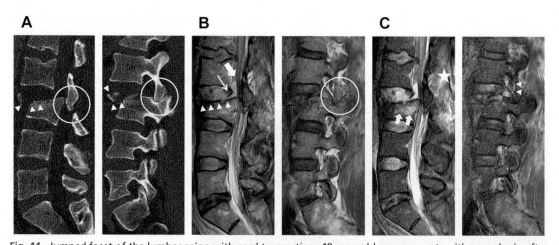

Fig. 11. Jumped facet of the lumbar spine with cord transection: 49-year-old man presents with paraplegia after MVC. Sagittal CT image (*A*) demonstrates compression fracture of the L2 with jumped L2 facet on the left (*circle, left*) and rotation of the right L2 facet into the spinal canal (*circle, right*). Compression L3 fracture is also present (*arrowheads*). The canal appears completely occluded. Sagittal T2WI (*B*) demonstrates widening of the disc space with increased fluid signal (*arrowheads*), disruption of the posterior longitudinal ligament (*thin arrow*), and abrupt discontinuity of the conus terminalis and cauda equina above the level of the fracture (*thick arrow*). Perched left facet is evident (*circle*). T2WI-FS (*C*) demonstrates increased marrow signal at site of L3 compression fracture (*arrows*) and linear fluid signal within the left L2 articular facet (*arrowheads*) corresponding to hairline fracture also faintly evident with extensive increased signal posteriorly (*star*) is consistent with ligamentous injury.

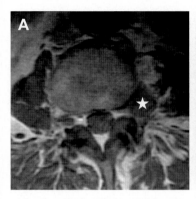

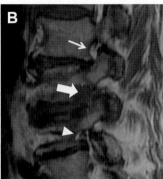

Fig. 12. Lateral disc herniation/extrusion, lumbar spine: 65-year-old woman presents with left lower extremity radiculopathy. Axial PDWI (*A*) demonstrates large left L3-L4 posterolateral disc extrusion (*star*). Parasagittal T1WI (*B*) demonstrates loss of the normal T1 hyperintense ring of fat surrounding the exiting nerve root (*thick arrow*) consistent with severe neuroforaminal stenosis at L3-L4. The left L2-L3 neural foramen is patent (*thin arrow*). There is moderate neuroforaminal stenosis at L4-L5 (*arrowhead*).

disease, precontrast and postcontrast T1WI is necessary to differentiate nonenhancing herniated disc material from the otherwise uniform enhancement of postprocedural granulation tissue at the site of previous disc resection (**Fig. 14**).

Mimics: Posterior endplate osteophyte, epidural fluid collection such as hemorrhage or abscess, and synovial cyst can all mimic acute disc herniation.

SPINAL CORD TRAUMA

Traumatic spinal cord injury is associated with injury to the vertebral column that may include vertebral fracture, dislocation, disc herniation, ligamentous injury, and evidence of penetrating injury or epidural hemorrhage. The cervical spinal cord is most commonly injured, representing approximately 50% of cases of reported cord injury.[26] CT and radiographs are insensitive for detecting spinal cord injury. Patterns of cord injury identified on MR imaging correspond to the prognosis for recovery.[24,26]

Acute contusion of the spinal cord is characterized by presence of increased signal on T2WI and STIR sequences and swelling of the cord, although initially can be normal (see **Fig. 1**). Superimposed *hemorrhage* (see **Fig. 5**) is detected as central hypointensity in T2*WI GRE or SWI, and suggest a worse prognosis than contusion alone.[27,28] *Transection* (see **Fig. 11**) of the spinal cord is characterized by discontinuity of the spinal cord with edema and hemorrhage. *Myelomalacia* of the spinal cord mimics cord contusion and hemorrhage; however, cord atrophy is usually present (**Fig. 15**). *Cauda equina syndrome* (**Fig. 16**) is a complication of severe nerve compression presenting as bilateral leg weakness, sciatica, and bowel and/or bladder dysfunction.

Isolated cervical spinal cord or ligamentous injury is characterized by disproportionate pain on physical examination or persisting neurologic deficit despite normal radiographic or CT evaluation of the spine and includes the syndrome of spinal cord injury without radiographic abnormality, or SCIWORA.[29] Prognosis is better than in injuries with fracture. MR imaging is a very sensitive examination to identifying ligamentous, disc, or spinal cord injuries (**Fig. 17**).[29]

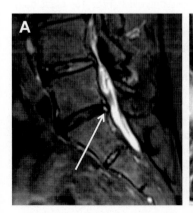

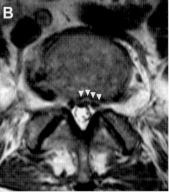

Fig. 13. Annular tear at L5-S1: 57-year-old woman presents with back pain after a fall. Sagittal T2WI-FS (*A*) demonstrates fluid signal deep to the annulus fibrosis at L5-S1 (*arrow*) consistent with age indeterminate annular fissure. Axial T2 (*B*) depicts increased T2 signal at this level (*arrowheads*).

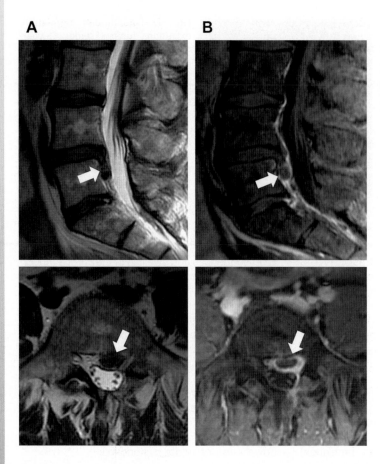

A **B**

Fig. 14. Recurrent posterior disc herniation/extrusion (FBSS): 40-year-old man with history of L4-L5 hemilaminectomy and partial discectomy presents with new right foot drop and lower back pain. T2WI (*A*; *top* = sagittal, *bottom* = axial) demonstrates large extrusion (*arrows*) eccentric to the left and inferiorly along the dorsal cortex of L5. T1WI-FS + Gd (*B*; *top* = sagittal, *bottom* = axial) demonstrates nonenhancing low-signal disc fragment (*arrows*) with peripheral enhancement typical of disc herniation. Postoperative scar and granulation tissue without disc fragment demonstrates uniform enhancement, distinguishing from FBSS.

SPINAL INFECTION

Emergent MR imaging of the spine is indicated in patients with new or worsening radiculopathy or neurologic deficits and signs or symptoms of infection, especially in patients with risk factors for infection, including recent instrumentation of the spine (eg, surgery, joint or epidural injections, device or catheter placement, lumbar puncture), immunocompromised status, or potential local or systemic source of infection (eg, infection elsewhere in the body, prosthetic valves, IV drug use).[30] Routes of infection include hematogenous spread, direct inoculation, or contiguous spread of disease.[31] Infection may involve the vertebrae, discs, joint spaces, epidural space, meninges, and spinal cord. Common organisms are *Staphylococcus aureus* and *Mycobacterium tuberculosis*.

Pyogenic osteomyelitis/discitis is the most common pattern of spinal infection. Vertebral segmental arteries supply the endplates on both sides of an intervertebral disc, which allows hematogenous seeding to contiguous vertebral bodies with possible extension to the disc.[31] Findings on MR imaging include decreased T1WI and increased T2WI marrow signal superior to and inferior to an intervertebral disc, similar signal changes in the affected disc with or without loss of disc height, and marrow and intervertebral disc enhancement. Abnormally increased T2WI signal, enhancement, or frank fluid collection in the paraspinal soft tissues or epidural space can be present. In advanced stages, the vertebral endplates and intervening disc can be destroyed with loss of height and kyphosis at the affected level.[31]

Tuberculosis osteomyelitis (**Fig. 18**) classically presents with chronic back pain or radiculopathy, fever, and weight loss. Compression fractures and epidural abscesses result in sudden neurologic deterioration including paraplegia and cauda equina syndrome. *Tuberculosis spondylitis* (Pott disease) arises from initial inoculation of the space adjacent to the anterior longitudinal ligament at the level of the disc or endplate, with extension to the anterior subchondral marrow of the adjacent vertebral bodies, and can appear similar to pyogenic osteomyelitis. In children, the intervertebral disc is often the initial site of infection due to direct inoculation of the immature vascular disc. The

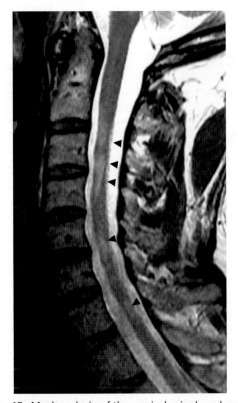

Fig. 15. Myelomalacia of the cervical spinal cord, multiple sclerosis: 33-year-old man with history of multiple sclerosis presents with recent fall, and increased lower extremity paresthesia. Sagittal T2WI demonstrates multiple regions of ill-defined hyperintensity within the cervical cord (*black arrowheads*) and cord atrophy. The presence of cord atrophy favors chronic gliosis over active demyelination or cord contusion.

lower thoracic and lumbar levels are most commonly affected. Paraspinal soft tissue involvement, such as the presence of an epidural and psoas abscesses, are often associated with pyogenic osteomyelitis.[32]

Epidural abscess (see **Fig. 18**) may be isolated or associated with other infections of the spine. Large abscesses can compress the spinal cord leading to reactive edema or, in rare instances, contiguous spread of infection or infarction.[33] Epidural abscesses typically demonstrate T1WI iso- or hypointensity, T2WI/STIR hyperintensity, and eccentric epidural thickening with peripheral enhancement in T1WI-FS+Gd imaging. Mild epidural thickening and enhancement may persist following treatment due to scar/granulation tissue. This finding is indistinguishable from epidural hematoma (see **Fig. 7**), thus a review of the patient's clinical presentation is required.[33]

Acute Complications of Spine Tumors

Spinal metastases

The frequency of *intramedullary metastases* is rising because of the improvements in cancer therapy and the increased survival of patients with cancer after initial diagnosis. Lung and breast cancer are the most common primary tumors that metastasize to the spine.[34] Dissemination to the spinal cord is typically hematogenous, although local spread of tumor from adjacent paraspinal soft tissues or bone and dissemination of disease through the CSF also can occur. Cervical and thoracic spinal cord lesions are more common

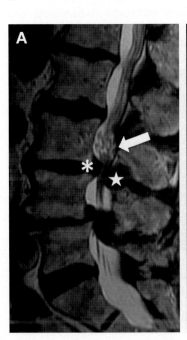
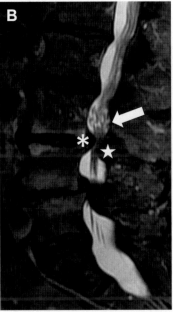

Fig. 16. Lumbar spinal stenosis with cauda equina compression: 89-year-old man presents with new onset of urinary retention and worsening sciatica. Sagittal T2WI (*A*) and T2WI-FS (*B*) demonstrate severe stenosis of the lumbar spinal canal at the level of a large L3-L4 posterior disc bulge-osteophyte complex (*asterisks*) with pronounced buckling of the ligamentum flavum posteriorly (*stars*). The cauda equina is clumped above the level of canal stenosis (*arrows*). Pseudonarrowing of the L4-L5 level is due to rotational scoliosis; the midline canal at L4-L5 is patent in adjacent sagittal images (not shown).

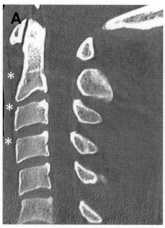
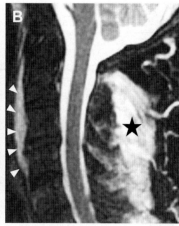

Fig. 17. An isolated ligamentous injury: 45-year-old man with neck pain fell from a ladder. Initial CT (*A*) demonstrates mild prevertebral soft tissue thickening suggestive of occult ligament injury (*asterisks*). T2WI-FS (*B*) indicates extensive injury involving the posterior interspinous and supraspinous ligaments (*star*) and prevertebral hematoma (*arrowheads*).

than lesions of the conus medullaris and cauda equina. The appearance on MR images is nonspecific and variable; intramedullary metastases are often T2 hyperintense, enhancing, and expansile in appearance. *Extramedullary/intradural metastases* also are highly variable in appearance. Lesions may be single, multiple, sessile, or nodular, with origins from the spinal cord, nerve roots, cauda equina, or dura (**Fig. 19**).[3]

Evaluation for *vertebral body metastases* as a cause of new or worsening back pain is a common indication for emergent MR imaging. Bone is a common site for metastatic disease, following the liver and lungs. Thoracic and lumbar vertebral bodies are most commonly affected due to the relative volume of vascularized marrow, and multiple levels of disease are often identified at the time of diagnosis (**Fig. 20**). Metastatic bone lesions are usually T1-hypointense due to replacement of marrow fat with tumor, associated edema, or

increased calcification secondary to sclerosis. T2WI signal is usually increased, although sclerotic lesions may appear hypointense. DWI will demonstrate restricted diffusion secondary to increased cellularity. Vertebral body metastases enhance on T1WI-FS + Gd sequence, differentiating metastatic lesions from simple marrow edema.[35]

Mimic: Osseous hemangiomata also can be T1 hypointense; however, the characteristic corrugated appearance on CT, loss of signal in T2WI-FS sequences, and lack of avid enhancement on T1WI-FS + Gd sequence are distinguishing features.

Mimic: Vertebral endplate discogenic marrow changes (ie, Modic-type changes) have a variable appearance and can mimic infiltrating marrow tumor.[36]

Mimic: Vertebral compression fractures may mimic infiltrating marrow tumor; however, the initial CT appearance and configuration of signal

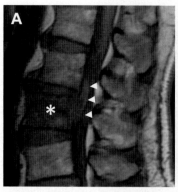
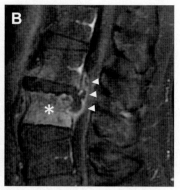

Fig. 18. Tuberculosis osteomyelitis with epidural abscess: 48-year-old man with back pain and history of tuberculosis. Sagittal T1WI (*A*) and T1WI-FS + Gd (*B*) demonstrate uniformly decreased marrow signal at L3 with marrow enhancement (*asterisks*). Disruption of the cortex posteriorly and associated epidural abscess is present, also common in tuberculosis (*arrowheads*). Tuberculosis osteomyelitis often differs in pattern from pyogenic osteomyelitis with less symmetric involvement of opposing endplates and the intervening disc, although advanced cases may demonstrate endplate and disc destruction indistinguishable from pyogenic osteomyelitis.

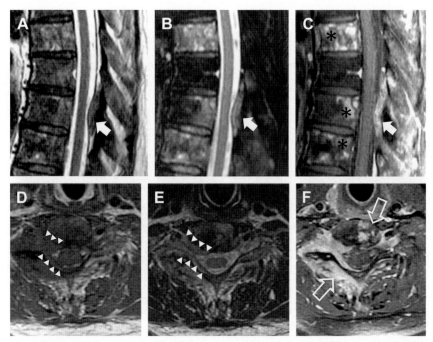

Fig. 19. Epidural metastasis, colon and lung cancer: 65-year-old man with history of colon cancer presents lower extremity paresthesias and back pain. Sagittal T1WI (*A*) and T2WI-FS (*B*) demonstrate T1-hypointense and T2-hyperintense thickening of the dorsal epidural soft tissues (*arrows*) and moderate narrowing of the spinal canal. Diffuse heterogeneity of the vertebral bodies is consistent with osseous metastases. T1WI-FS + Gd (*C*) depicts avid enhancement of both the epidural mass (*arrow*) and marrow (*asterisks*) consistent with tumor. Axial T1WI (*D*) and T2WI (*E*) from MR images of a 62-year-old woman with metastatic lung cancer and similar symptoms depict epidural thickening posteriorly with extension into and narrowing of the right neural foramen into the paraspinal soft tissues (*arrowheads*); T1WI-FS + Gd images (*F*) better demonstrate the extent of disease. These findings are consistent with metastasis (*arrows*).

changes in the context of a patient with history of trauma or risk factors for pathologic fractures (eg, osteoporosis) allow for proper differentiation.

PRIMARY SPINE NEOPLASMS

Primary spine neoplasms can present with radiculopathy and neurologic deficits. Lesions can be categorized as intramedullary, extramedullary/intradural, or extradural. A thorough discussion of primary bone neoplasms of the spine is beyond the scope of this review.

Although many primary neoplasms of the cord and spinal canal are of low-grade histology, small lesions can result in significant pain or neurologic deficit due to the confined anatomy of the spinal canal.[37]

Primary Intramedullary Neoplasms

Primary cord lesions are more common than intramedullary metastases. Imaging features are nonspecific, and histologic analysis is required

for diagnosis; however, MR imaging features may suggest the specific histology.[37] *Ependymomas* are most common and more frequently involve the lumbar and sacral levels than other primary tumors. Suggestive features include central location; involvement of at least 3 contiguous spinal segments, tumoral cysts, and/or syrinx; presence of hemosiderin without associated cord edema; and erosive changes of the spinal canal. *Astrocytomas* are less commonly associated with cystic changes, syrinx, and intralesional hemorrhage and may be indistinguishable from ependymoma; an eccentric location is suggestive of this diagnosis (**Fig. 21**). *Gangliogliomas* are more heterogeneous in appearance with a variable pattern of enhancement; calcifications, eccentric tumoral cysts, and involvement of fewer than 3 levels of the spinal cord suggest ganglioglioma over other tumors. *Hemangioblastomas* are nonglial tumors with highly variable appearance. Lesions range from small uniformly enhancing tumors to larger lesions involving multiple contiguous levels of the spinal cord with associated syrinx and evidence

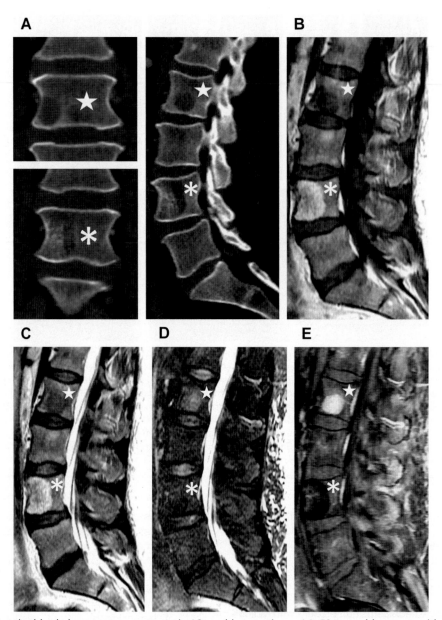

Fig. 20. Vertebral body breast cancer metastasis, L2, and hemangioma, L4: 59-year-old woman with history of breast cancer presents with acute back pain. On CT (*A*), lytic lesion at L2 (*star;* coronal = *top left* and sagittal = *right*) and corrugated-appearing lesion at L4 (*asterisk;* coronal = *bottom left* and sagittal = *right*) are noted, consistent with bone metastasis and osseous hemangioma, respectively. T1WI (*B*) and T2WI (*C*) also depict these lesions; the lytic lesion at L2 is T1 hypointense and slightly T2 hypointense with respect to adjacent marrow (*stars*), and the hemangioma is characteristically T1 and T2 hyperintense (*asterisks*). In T2WI-FS sequences (*D*), the lytic lesion at L2 is T2 hyperintense due to high fluid content (*star*), and the hemangioma (*asterisk*) becomes near isointense due to suppression of intralesional fat content. T1WI-FS + Gd (*E*) confirms the highly vascular lytic metastasis at L2 with avid enhancement (*star*), and the slow vascularity of the fat-containing L4 hemangioma (*asterisk*) is hypointense, relative to the surrounding marrow.

of large abnormal feeding arteries/draining veins. In patients with von Hippel-Lindau disease (one-third of cases), multiple lesions may be present at any level of the spinal cord.

Primary Extramedullary/Intradural Neoplasms

Schwannomas are the most common intradural extramedullary mass of the spinal canal.

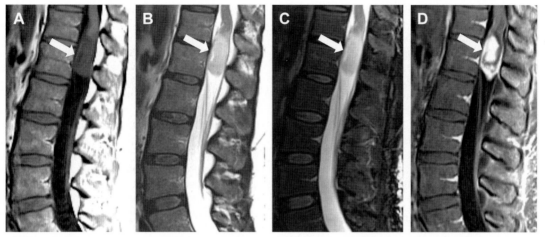

Fig. 21. Intramedullary mass, astrocytoma of the spinal cord: 47-year-old woman presents with lower back pain radiating to the lower extremities and urinary retention. Sagittal T1WI (*A*), T2WI (*B*), T2WI-FS (*C*), and T1WI-FS + Gd (*D*) demonstrate an expansile lesion of the conus medullaris (*arrows*) fills the entire spinal canal with splays of the cauda equina. The mass is intermediate on T1WI and hyperintense on T2WI and demonstrates near-homogeneous enhancement. This was a biopsy-proven high-grade (World Health Organization IV) astrocytoma.

Schwannomas can be intradural, transforaminal ("dumbbell" configuration), or extradural in configuration (**Fig. 22**). Lesions are usually T1 hypointense or isointense and heterogenously T2 hyperintense relative to the spinal cord, with or without intralesional cysts or hemorrhage, and demonstrate peripheral or uniform enhancement.[38] *Meningiomas* of the spinal canal are most commonly cervical or thoracic in location and are usually eccentric extramedullary masses

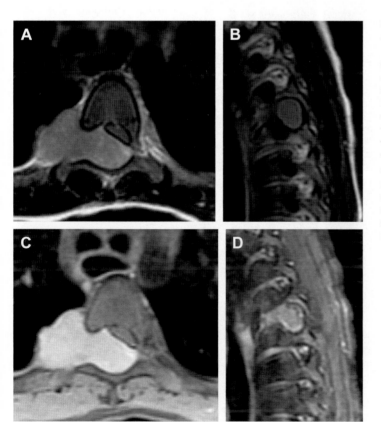

Fig. 22. Schwannoma, intraspinal and extraspinal, extradural, T3-T4: 12-year-old girl presents with progressive lower extremity weakness and hyperreflexia. Axial (*A*) and sagittal (*B*) T2WI demonstrate a large "dumbbell-shaped" intermediate signal intensity mass nearly filling the spinal canal, extending through the widened right neural foramen into the paraspinal soft tissues. There is compression and anterolateral displacement of the spinal cord. Axial PDWI + Gd (*C*) and sagittal T1WI-FS + Gd (*D*) demonstrate avid enhancement. Schwannoma was confirmed by biopsy.

with a broad-based dural attachment to the ventral or lateral canal; the MR imaging appearance is typically T1 and T2 hypointense, with uniform enhancement. *Paragangliomas* are uncommon neoplasms that occur mostly in the lower lumbar and sacral spinal canal; lesions are typically T1WI hypointense or isointense and T2WI hyperintense to the cord, enhancing, and may have associated feeding arteries/draining veins, intralesional cysts, and hemosiderin staining.

Mimic: Schwannomas are hyperintense on T2WI, which can mimic a perineural cyst, but schwannomas demonstrate avid enhancement.

NON-NEOPLASTIC SPINAL CORD LESIONS

MR imaging is also the preferred imaging modality for assessment of suspected infectious, inflammatory, autoimmune, and other non-neoplastic spinal cord lesions. Symptoms are sometimes nonspecific and vary according to degree of supratentorial and/or spinal cord involvement, but emergent presentations are not uncommon. The etiology varies and includes primary idiopathic conditions (such as idiopathic transverse myelitis), conditions related to central nervous system infection (eg, human immunodeficiency virus, herpes simplex virus [HSV], syphilis) (**Fig. 23**), parainfectious/autoimmune processes (eg, acute demyelinating encephalomyelitis),[39] systemic inflammatory conditions (eg, systemic lupus erythematosus, Sjögren syndrome, sarcoidosis), and primary demyelinating diseases (eg, multiple sclerosis) (**Fig. 24**).

Spinal cord infarction typically results from acute occlusion of the anterior spinal artery.[40] Although the cause is commonly idiopathic, vascular injury may also result from trauma, vasculitis, or neoplasm, systemic hypotension, iatrogenic injury or occlusion during catheter angiography, or acute complications of occlusive atherosclerotic disease of the aorta.[40] MR imaging features include expansion of the cord acutely, T2 hyperintense signal with restricted diffusion. Myelomalacia may demonstrate T2 hyperintensity with

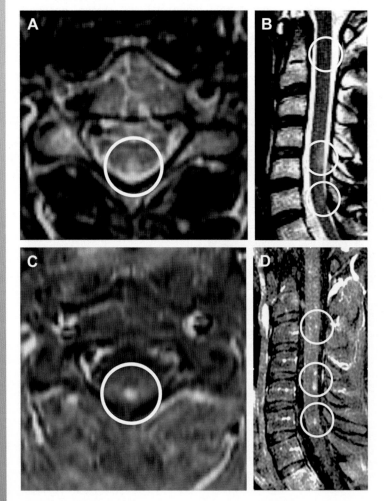

Fig. 23. Postinfectious transverse myelitis: 25-year-old man presents with progressive upper and lower extremity paresthesia, weakness, and penile vesicles on physical examination consistent with HSV. Axial, sagittal T2WIs (*A, B*) demonstrate ill-defined hyperintense cord lesions (*circles*). Axial and sagittal T1WI-FS + Gd images (*C, D*) demonstrate enhancement (*circles*). Findings are consistent with transverse myelitis.

A
B

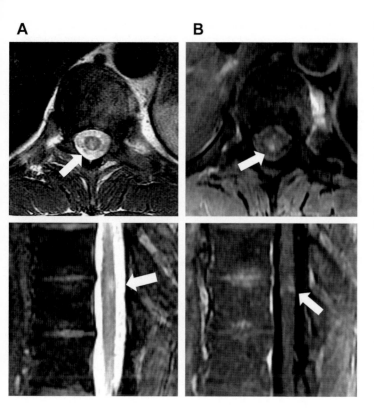

Fig. 24. Multiple sclerosis, enhancing plaque, thoracic spinal cord: 51-year-old man presents with new onset of paresthesia in the lower extremities. Axial T2WI (*A, top*) and sagittal T2WI-FS (*A, bottom*) demonstrate hyperintense cord lesion (*arrows*) at T9-T10; appearance is consistent with age-indeterminate plaque and may represent active demyelination or chronic gliosis. T1WI-FS + Gd axial (*B, top*) and sagittal (*B, bottom*) images demonstrate enhancement (*arrows*) consistent with active demyelination.

or without cord atrophy; however, restricted diffusion is absent.[41]

SUMMARY

MR imaging plays a critical role in the evaluation of disease of the spine and spinal cord in the emergent setting, including trauma, malignancy, infection, lesions of the spinal cord, and discogenic disease. Although MR imaging is sensitive and specific in the detection and diagnosis of these conditions, familiarity with common features is important for prompt and accurate diagnosis. The appropriate use of MR imaging in the emergent setting enables a higher standard of care and permits detection of spine conditions that require immediate medical or surgical intervention.

ACKNOWLEDGMENTS

Special thanks to Christopher Potter, MD, from Brigham and Women's Hospital, 75 Francis Street, Boston, MA, for contribution of cases.

REFERENCES

1. Arce D, Sass P, Abul-Khoudoud H. Recognizing spinal cord emergencies. Am Fam Physician 2001; 64(4):631–8.

2. Roudsari B, Jarvik JG. Lumbar spine MRI for low back pain: indications and yield. AJR Am J Roentgenol 2010;195(3):550–9.

3. Shah LM, Salzman KL. Imaging of spinal metastatic disease. Int J Surg Oncol 2011;2011:769753.

4. Claytor B, MacLennan PA, McGwin G Jr, et al. Cervical spine injury and restraint system use in motor vehicle collisions. Spine (Phila Pa 1976) 2004; 29(4):386–9 [discussion: Z382].

5. Sekhon LH, Fehlings MG. Epidemiology, demographics, and pathophysiology of acute spinal cord injury. Spine (Phila Pa 1976) 2001;26(24 Suppl):S2–12.

6. Wrathall JR, Pettegrew RK, Harvey F. Spinal cord contusion in the rat: production of graded, reproducible, injury groups. Exp Neurol 1985;88(1):108–22.

7. Greenbaum J, Walters N, Levy PD. An evidenced-based approach to radiographic assessment of cervical spine injuries in the emergency department. J Emerg Med 2009;36(1):64–71.

8. Denis F. The three column spine and its significance in the classification of acute thoracolumbar spinal injuries. Spine (Phila Pa 1976) 1983;8(8):817–31.

9. Munera F, Rivas LA, Nunez DB Jr, et al. Imaging evaluation of adult spinal injuries: emphasis on multidetector CT in cervical spine trauma. Radiology 2012;263(3):645–60.

10. Rojas CA, Bertozzi JC, Martinez CR, et al. Reassessment of the craniocervical junction: normal

values on CT. AJNR Am J Neuroradiol 2007;28(9): 1819–23.

11. Hall GC, Kinsman MJ, Nazar RG, et al. Atlanto-occipital dislocation. World J Orthop 2015;6(2): 236–43.

12. Dickman CA, Mamourian A, Sonntag VK, et al. Magnetic resonance imaging of the transverse atlantal ligament for the evaluation of atlantoaxial instability. J Neurosurg 1991;75(2):221–7.

13. Anderson LD, D'Alonzo RT. Fractures of the odontoid process of the axis. J Bone Joint Surg Am 1974;56(8):1663–74.

14. Grauer JN, Shafi B, Hilibrand AS, et al. Proposal of a modified, treatment-oriented classification of odontoid fractures. Spine J 2005;5(2):123–9.

15. Li XF, Dai LY, Lu H, et al. A systematic review of the management of hangman's fractures. Eur Spine J 2006;15(3):257–69.

16. Kwon BK, Vaccaro AR, Grauer JN, et al. Subaxial cervical spine trauma. J Am Acad Orthop Surg 2006;14(2):78–89.

17. Vaccaro AR, Lehman RA Jr, Hurlbert RJ, et al. A new classification of thoracolumbar injuries: the importance of injury morphology, the integrity of the posterior ligamentous complex, and neurologic status. Spine (Phila Pa 1976) 2005;30(20):2325–33.

18. Khurana B, Sheehan SE, Sodickson A, et al. Traumatic thoracolumbar spine injuries: what the spine surgeon wants to know. Radiographics 2013;33(7): 2031–46.

19. Denis F. Spinal instability as defined by the three-column spine concept in acute spinal trauma. Clin Orthop Relat Res 1984;(189):65–76.

20. Lee HM, Kim HS, Kim DJ, et al. Reliability of magnetic resonance imaging in detecting posterior ligament complex injury in thoracolumbar spinal fractures. Spine (Phila Pa 1976) 2000;25(16): 2079–84.

21. Bernstein MP, Mirvis SE, Shanmuganathan K. Chance-type fractures of the thoracolumbar spine: imaging analysis in 53 patients. AJR Am J Roentgenol 2006;187(4):859–68.

22. Radcliff K, Su BW, Kepler CK, et al. Correlation of posterior ligamentous complex injury and neurological injury to loss of vertebral body height, kyphosis, and canal compromise. Spine (Phila Pa 1976) 2012; 37(13):1142–50.

23. Hadley MN, Fitzpatrick BC, Sonntag VK, et al. Facet fracture-dislocation injuries of the cervical spine. Neurosurgery 1992;30(5):661–6.

24. Davis PC, Wippold FJ 2nd, Brunberg JA, et al. ACR Appropriateness Criteria on low back pain. J Am Coll Radiol 2009;6(6):401–7.

25. Fardon DF, Williams AL, Dohring EJ, et al. Lumbar disc nomenclature: version 2.0: Recommendations of the combined task forces of the North American Spine Society, the American Society of Spine Radiology and the American Society of Neuroradiology. Spine J 2014;14(11):2525–45.

26. Devivo MJ. Epidemiology of traumatic spinal cord injury: trends and future implications. Spinal Cord 2012;50(5):365–72.

27. Selden NR, Quint DJ, Patel N, et al. Emergency magnetic resonance imaging of cervical spinal cord injuries: clinical correlation and prognosis. Neurosurgery 1999;44(4):785–92 [discussion: 792–3].

28. Bozzo A, Marcoux J, Radhakrishna M, et al. The role of magnetic resonance imaging in the management of acute spinal cord injury. J Neurotrauma 2011; 28(8):1401–11.

29. Kothari P, Freeman B, Grevitt M, et al. Injury to the spinal cord without radiological abnormality (SCI-WORA) in adults. J Bone Joint Surg Br 2000;82(7): 1034–7.

30. Darouiche RO. Spinal epidural abscess. N Engl J Med 2006;355(19):2012–20.

31. Tali ET, Oner AY, Koc AM. Pyogenic spinal infections. Neuroimaging Clin N Am 2015;25(2):193–208.

32. Jung NY, Jee WH, Ha KY, et al. Discrimination of tuberculous spondylitis from pyogenic spondylitis on MRI. AJR Am J Roentgenol 2004;182(6): 1405–10.

33. Eastwood JD, Vollmer RT, Provenzale JM. Diffusion-weighted imaging in a patient with vertebral and epidural abscesses. AJNR Am J Neuroradiol 2002; 23(3):496–8.

34. Harrington KD. Metastatic disease of the spine. J Bone Joint Surg Am 1986;68(7):1110–5.

35. Guillevin R, Vallee JN, Lafitte F, et al. Spine metastasis imaging: review of the literature. J Neuroradiol 2007;34(5):311–21.

36. Modic MT, Ross JS. Lumbar degenerative disk disease. Radiology 2007;245(1):43–61.

37. Koeller KK, Rosenblum RS, Morrison AL. Neoplasms of the spinal cord and filum terminale: radiologic-pathologic correlation. Radiographics 2000;20(6): 1721–49.

38. Abul-Kasim K, Thurnher MM, McKeever P, et al. Intradural spinal tumors: current classification and MRI features. Neuroradiology 2008;50(4):301–14.

39. Noorbakhsh F, Johnson RT, Emery D, et al. Acute disseminated encephalomyelitis: clinical and pathogenesis features. Neurol Clin 2008;26(3):759–80, ix.

40. Novy J, Carruzzo A, Maeder P, et al. Spinal cord ischemia: clinical and imaging patterns, pathogenesis, and outcomes in 27 patients. Arch Neurol 2006;63(8):1113–20.

41. Vargas MI, Gariani J, Sztajzel R, et al. Spinal cord ischemia: practical imaging tips, pearls, and pitfalls. AJNR Am J Neuroradiol 2015;36(5):825–30.

Magnetic Resonance Imaging of Acute Head and Neck Infections

Neil Thayil, MD[a], Margaret N. Chapman, MD[a,b], Naoko Saito, MD, PhD[c],
Akifumi Fujita, MD, PhD[d], Osamu Sakai, MD, PhD[a,*]

KEYWORDS

• Infections • MR imaging • Head and neck • Complications

KEY POINTS

- The severity of head and neck infections can often be ascertained from the clinical history and physical examination.
- In some sinus and periorbital infections, MR imaging is crucial for identifying spread of infection into the orbital and intracranial compartments and helps to guide management.
- MR imaging is unsurpassed in its ability to identify and evaluate complications of middle ear and temporal bone infections.
- MR imaging detects osteomyelitis and is useful to differentiate osteomyelitis from acute bone infarction in the setting of sickle cell disease.
- MR imaging is an invaluable tool to pinpoint the exact origin and extent of retropharyngeal and prevertebral infections and to identify possible associated complications.

INTRODUCTION

Acute head and neck infections can evolve as slowly progressive smoldering processes, or advance as rapidly debilitating entities with clinical consequences that can often be life threatening. The clinical presentation of the infectious process in question varies depending on the specific head and neck compartment that is primarily affected. The severity and aggressive nature of the disease process can usually be sufficiently elucidated though the clinical examination and history.

Imaging is often relied upon to assist in the evaluation of the anatomic extent of the acute infection and to identify any pertinent complications that could contribute to patient morbidity and mortality if left unidentified and untreated. Although computed tomography (CT) is the first-line modality in the acute setting of many uncomplicated infectious processes, MR imaging is the modality of choice in examining the exact scope of certain complicated infections owing to its superior delineation of soft tissue contrast, particularly when intracranial complications are suspected. MR imaging is unquestionably the modality of choice for high-resolution evaluation of multiple entities including facial neuritis, optic neuritis, labyrinthitis, petrous apicitis, and acute osteomyelitis. MR imaging is also a valuable tool to evaluate the bone marrow and differentiate between entities such as osteomyelitis and bone infarct. MR imaging also detects vascular complications caused by acute infections, such as sinus venous thrombosis. The ability to identify these dreaded complications and drastically influence clinical management confirms the utility of MR imaging in the evaluation of acute head and neck infections.

The authors have nothing to disclose.

[a] Department of Radiology, Boston Medical Center, Boston University School of Medicine, FGH Building, 3rd Floor, 820 Harrison Avenue, Boston, MA 02118, USA; [b] Radiology Service, VA Boston Healthcare System, 1400 VFW Parkway, West Roxbury, MA 02132, USA; [c] Department of Radiology, Saitama International Medical Center, Saitama Medical University, 1397-1 Yamane, Hidaka, Saitama 350-1298, Japan; [d] Department of Radiology, Jichi Medical University School of Medicine, 3311-1 Yakushiji, Shimotsuke, Tochigi 329-0498, Japan
* Corresponding author.
E-mail address: osamu.sakai@bmc.org

Magn Reson Imaging Clin N Am 24 (2016) 345–367
http://dx.doi.org/10.1016/j.mric.2015.11.003
1064-9689/16/$ – see front matter © 2016 Elsevier Inc. All rights reserved.

This article discusses the use of MR imaging in various acute infectious diseases of the head and neck, with particular emphasis on situations where MR imaging provides additional information that can significantly impact treatment decisions and outcomes. MR imaging findings of various disease processes are discussed, based on the head and neck compartments from which they originate. Specifically, infectious entities of the orbit, paranasal sinuses, pharynx, oral cavity (including periodontal disease), salivary glands, temporal bone, and lymph nodes are described in detail.

ORBITS
Periorbital and Orbital Infections

The orbital septum is the anatomic landmark that distinguishes the periorbital (preseptal) tissues from the orbit proper (postseptal tissues). The orbital septum is a thin membranous sheet extending from the orbital periosteum. Superiorly, it inserts and blends with the aponeurosis of the levator palpebrae superioris, and inferiorly it blends with the tarsal plates. This structure is not readily demonstrated on imaging, but it serves as a barrier to posterior spread of infections from the periorbital tissues into the orbit proper.[1–3]

Periorbital cellulitis typically occurs secondary to a nearby sinonasal, facial, or dental infection that spreads to involve the periorbital tissues. Local trauma may also serve as an etiology. Typical presenting symptoms include pain, eyelid swelling and erythema, conjunctivitis, and fever. On MR imaging, periorbital cellulitis usually manifests as edema, soft tissue swelling, and diffuse periorbital soft tissue enhancement. A loculated abscess within the periorbital or surrounding facial soft tissues may also be present.[3–5]

In contrast, orbital cellulitis usually results as a complication of adjacent paranasal sinusitis (Fig. 1) and occasionally from a dental infection.[6] Embedded posttraumatic foreign bodies can also contribute to this process. Typical presenting symptoms are similar to periorbital cellulitis, with the addition of proptosis as a predominant feature.[3,4] Orbital cellulitis is associated with an increased risk of devastating neurologic sequelae, including ophthalmic vein thrombosis, venous sinus thrombosis, mycotic aneurysm, meningitis, and intracranial abscess.[2,3] Thus, identifying an infection in the orbit is of paramount importance to help guide management and prevent poor outcomes.

The MR imaging findings of orbital cellulitis include fat stranding and rim-enhancing abscess formation, which can be intraconal or extraconal (often subperiosteal) and edema and abnormal enhancement of the extraocular muscles.[3,5]

Noninfectious conditions, including idiopathic orbital inflammatory syndrome ("pseudotumor"; Fig. 2), and immunoglobulin G4 (IgG4)-related disease can mimic this infection. Grave's ophthalmopathy is also a differential consideration, but can be differentiated by noting the classic sparing of the tendinous insertions.[3]

Treatment of orbital cellulitis typically involves hospital admission with administration of intravenous antibiotics and possible drainage of loculated orbital collections, if present. In contrast, uncomplicated periorbital cellulitis can be treated on an outpatient basis with oral antibiotics.[3]

Of note, dacryocystitis is an infection that results from obstruction of the medial nasolacrimal duct that can be complicated by periorbital and, rarely, orbital cellulitis. Infection from *Streptococcus pneumoniae* accounts for almost 25% of the cases, although other microorganisms from the *Streptococcus* and *Staphylococcus* families can also be responsible.[7,8] Typical clinical presentation involves focal swelling along the medial canthus, conjunctivitis, and purulent drainage. MR imaging may demonstrate a dilated fluid-filled lacrimal sac along the medial canthus with peripheral rim enhancement on postcontrast images. When clinical assessment is limited owing to concurrent periorbital and orbital cellulitis, the value of MR imaging is its ability to accurately depict these complications. Treatment may be either medical or surgical, depending on patient symptomatology and the presence of associated complications.[3,8]

PARANASAL SINUSES
Bacterial Infection

A variety of organisms have been implicated as causes of acute and chronic sinusitis, including *S pneumoniae* and other *Streptococcus* strains, *Staphylococcus aureus*, *Moraxella catarrhalis*, *Pseudomonas* species, particularly in immunosuppressed and diabetics, and anaerobic bacteria.[9] Differentiating between acute and chronic sinusitis can only be made by considering the timeframe during which it has been present. Inflammation of the paranasal sinus mucosa present for fewer than 4 weeks is defined as acute sinusitis, whereas chronic sinusitis refers to disease that is present for longer than 12 weeks.[9] Both entities clinically present with nasal congestion, purulent discharge, headache, maxillary and dental pain, and reduced sense of taste or smell.

Imaging is not typically necessary to diagnose sinusitis, particularly in the acute phase. Although CT is the first-line modality, MR imaging can be performed when intracranial or intraorbital complications are suspected clinically. MR imaging is sensitive in identifying inflammation of the paranasal

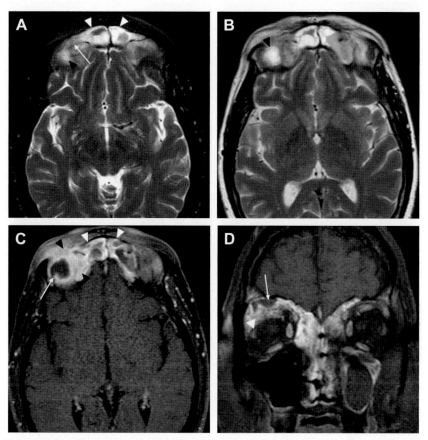

Fig. 1. Frontal sinusitis complicated by orbital cellulitis. Axial fat-suppressed T2-weighted image (*A*) demonstrates complete opacification of the frontal sinuses (*white arrowheads*). There is a focal region of dehiscence involving the lateral wall of the right frontal sinus with absence of the usual T2 dark cortical signal (*white arrow*). The sinus debris extends through this defect into the right superior orbit (*black arrowhead*). Axial T2-weighted image (*B*) at an adjacent level shows a rounded T2 hyperintense collection in the region of the right superior orbit (*black arrowhead*). Axial post-contrast fat-suppressed T1-weighted image (*C*) shows peripheral enhancement of the fluid collection, compatible with a subperiosteal abscess. There is inflammation in the adjacent soft tissues, seen as the adjacent asymmetric enhancement (*black arrowheads*) and extensive mucosal enhancement within the frontal sinuses (*white arrowheads*). Coronal post-contrast fat-suppressed T1-weighted image (*D*) through the orbits shows the extensive inflammatory change within the superior right orbit resulting in mass effect with downward displacement of the inflamed, thickened, and enhancing right superior rectus muscle (*white arrowhead*). The subperiosteal abscess is seen as the non-enhancing round collection adjacent to the orbital roof (*white arrow*).

sinus mucosa. Although the diagnosis of sinusitis should not be based solely on imaging findings, greater than 4 mm of sinus mucosal thickening suggests a greater likelihood of sinusitis.[10] Findings that increase the diagnostic confidence of acute sinusitis include the presence of air–fluid levels or complete fluid opacification of one or more of the paranasal sinuses. If there is an underlying obstructing tumor, fluid-sensitive sequences can be useful in demonstrating the relatively hypointense mass adjacent to hyperintense inflamed sinus mucosa and fluid.[9,11] In the chronic stage of sinusitis, much of the sinus fluid becomes inspissated with an increase in protein concentration. As a result, fluid signal on T1-weighted images, which is initially hypointense,

becomes hyperintense, and signal on T2-weighted images becomes progressively darker.[11]

Sinus infection may result in orbital and intracranial complications owing to their proximity to the sinonasal cavities (see **Fig. 1**). Approximately 3% of patients with sinusitis (especially ethmoid sinusitis) can develop orbital complications, particularly in children or young adults.[12] Orbital complications, including periorbital/orbital cellulitis or subperiosteal abscess formation, are well depicted on MR imaging (described in greater detail in the Orbits section). Orbital complications are much more common than intracranial complications.[9]

Neurologic complications, including meningitis, cavernous sinus thrombosis, and subperiosteal

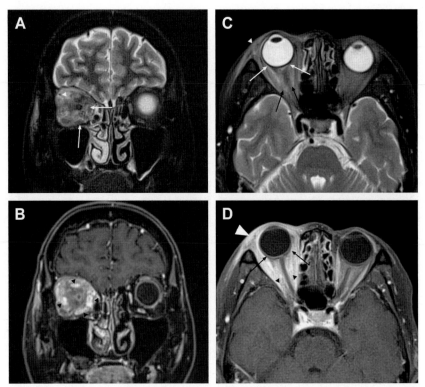

Fig. 2. Orbital pseudotumor with posterior scleritis. Coronal fat-suppressed T2-weighted image (*A*) demonstrates extensive heterogeneous signal abnormality and infiltration involving the right orbit, resulting in right proptosis (*white arrowhead*). The infiltrative lesion surrounds the extraocular muscles (*white arrows*), which are asymmetrically thickened relative to the left. Coronal post-contrast fat-suppressed T1-weighted image (*B*) demonstrates extensive enhancement of the orbital soft tissues, abnormal enlargement and enhancement of the extraocular muscles (*black arrowheads*), and enhancement of the optic nerve sheath. Axial fat-suppressed T2-weighted image (*C*) demonstrates thickening of the posterior sclera (*white arrows*). Abnormal signal in the right retrobulbar region (*black arrows*) and periorbital soft tissues (*white arrowhead*) results in right proptosis. Corresponding enhancement of the thickened posterior sclera (*black arrows*), as well as of the orbital and periorbital soft tissues (*arrowheads*), is seen on the axial fat-suppressed post-contrast T1-weighted image (*D*).

and intracranial abscesses, can also be readily identified with MR images.[3,12] Pott's puffy tumor is a complication of sinusitis characterized by subperiosteal abscess and osteomyelitis of the frontal bone, resulting from spread of infection beyond the confines of the sinus into the surrounding bone via infectious thrombophlebitis of penetrating valveless emissary veins. On clinical examination, this entity presents as a fluctuant mass overlying the eyebrow. MR imaging is not only useful in demonstrating the extent of osteomyelitis, subperiosteal abscess, and surrounding soft tissue inflammation, but more valuable in identifying intracranial complications such as intraaxial or extraaxial abscess (**Fig. 3**), or venous sinus thrombosis.[12–14]

Fungal Infection

Fungal sinusitis can be classified into two groups: noninvasive and invasive. The noninvasive category is further classified into allergic fungal sinusitis and

mycetoma (fungus ball). Both subtypes of the noninvasive category are characterized by disease involvement that is limited to the lumen of the affected sinus without penetration past the mucosa, and is seen typically in immunocompetent patients.[15,16]

Allergic fungal sinusitis is the most common form of fungal sinusitis, and typically occurs in younger patients with a history of atopy, asthma, nasal polyposis, and aspirin intolerance. *Aspergillus* species are commonly responsible for allergic fungal sinusitis. Patients present with complaints of chronic nasal congestion and headaches.[14,15] Characteristic MR imaging findings (**Fig. 4**) include near complete sinus opacification of multiple sinuses with T2-hypointense material owing to its low water and high protein content and the high concentration of paramagnetic substances.[15]

Mycetoma is characterized by the presence of a fungus ball limited to the cavity of an affected sinus and is also most commonly secondary to

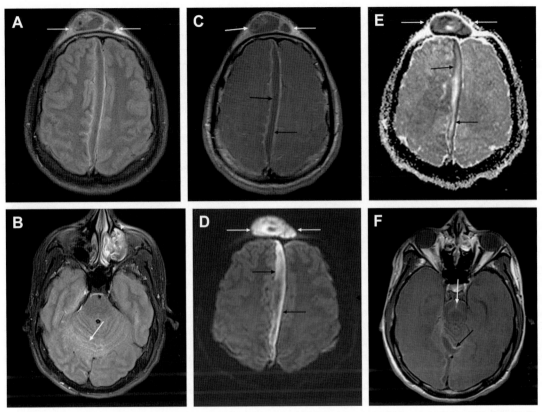

Fig. 3. Pott's puffy tumor. Axial fat-suppressed FLAIR image (*A*) demonstrates a heterogeneous collection in the extracranial frontal soft tissue (*white arrows*) in a 17 year old boy with left-sided sinusitis (*white arrowhead in B*). The collection demonstrates peripheral enhancement (*white arrows*) on post-contrast fat-suppressed T1-weighted images (*C*) and diffusion restriction (*white arrows, D* and *E*), consistent with an abscess. Associated intracranial complications are seen, including a peripherally enhancing subdural empyema (*black arrows, C–F*), and meningitis, characterized by abnormal leptomeningeal signal and enhancement overlying the cerebellar folia and within the interpeduncular cistern (*white arrows, B* and *F*).

Aspergillus species. Clinical symptoms are usually minimal.[15,16] Characteristic MR imaging findings include an intraluminal mass that is usually T1 and T2 hypointense owing to lack of water content, with scattered areas of susceptibility artifact secondary to calcification and paramagnetic substances such as manganese, iron, and magnesium. Usually, a single sinus is involved, most

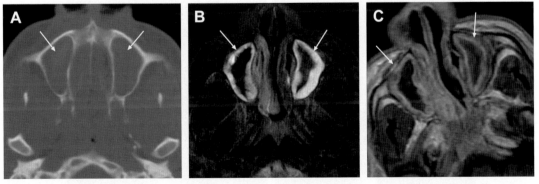

Fig. 4. Allergic fungal sinusitis. Axial CT image (*A*) shows complete opacification of the both maxillary sinuses (*white arrows*) with high density debris and mucosal thickening. Axial fat-suppressed T2-weighted (*B*) and post-contrast T1-weighted (*C*) images demonstrate corresponding submucosal edema, mucosal thickening and enhancement in the bilateral maxillary sinuses (*white arrows*). Note the low signal filling the central maxillary sinuses bilaterally. The low signal on T1 and T2-weighted images is secondary to a combination of proteinaceous mucus and concentration of heavy metals such as iron, manganese, and magnesium.

commonly the maxillary sinus (**Fig. 5**), followed by the sphenoid sinus.[15]

Invasive fungal sinusitis is characterized by spread of disease beyond the mucosa, with invasion of penetrating vessels that allows the infection to infiltrate into the surrounding osseous structures, orbital, and intracranial compartments (**Fig. 6**).[15,16] Acute invasive fungal sinusitis is a rapidly progressive and deteriorating infection with a 50% to 80% fatality rate, most often afflicting immunocompromised and poorly controlled diabetic patients.[17] Zygomycetes such as *Rhizopus* and *Mucor* are the organisms classically involved in this form of sinusitis.[15,16] In addition to the usual symptoms of sinusitis, invasive fungal sinusitis often presents with neurologic symptoms including cranial nerve impairment, seizures, mental status changes, coma, proptosis, and visual field defects secondary to intracranial and orbital invasion.[17] Chronic invasive fungal sinusitis differs from its acute counterpart in that it progresses slowly over the course of months to years. Characteristic MR imaging findings of invasive fungal sinusitis include unilateral erosive/destructive changes of the osseous walls of the affected sinuses with extension into the orbit and brain, resulting in orbital cellulitis, cranial nerve impairment, and cavernous sinus thrombosis. Internal carotid artery invasion may cause occlusion or pseudoaneurysm formation, with an associated increased risk of cerebral infarct and hemorrhage.[17]

SALIVARY GLANDS
Sialadenitis

Sialadenitis refers to infection or inflammation of the salivary glands (**Fig. 7**). Viral sialadenitis, often secondary to mumps infection from paramyxovirus, is more common and typically presents as bilateral parotitis (**Fig. 8**).[18] Acute bacterial causes, most commonly *Staphylococcus* or *Streptococcus* species, usually present unilaterally and occur in elderly, debilitated, or postoperative dehydrated patients.[14,18,19] Sialolithiasis is a major risk factor for development of bacterial sialadenitis (**Fig. 9**), and most commonly affects the submandibular glands, possibly as result of increased viscosity of submandibular secretions. Thus, the submandibular glands are most commonly affected by bacterial sialadenitis.[12,18] Oral cavity or floor of mouth malignancy may also cause outflow duct obstruction and associated inflammation of the affected salivary gland (**Fig. 10**). Typical presentation involves swelling and pain or focal tenderness. In the case of bacterial sialadenitis associated with an obstructing sialolith, pain can often be exacerbated by activities that stimulate saliva production ("salivary colic").[18,19]

Sialadenitis is well-depicted on MR imaging, characteristically demonstrating any combination of the following features: (1) edema and abnormal enhancement within the affected salivary gland(s) sometimes associated with a rim-enhancing abscess (**Fig. 11**), (2) inflammation of the periglandular fat and soft tissues, and (3) associated sialolithiasis which demonstrates signal void within the obstructed ducts, most commonly Wharton's duct.[18,19]

TEMPORAL BONE
Acute Otitis Media/Otomastoiditis

Acute otitis media refers to middle ear infection or inflammation and fluid opacification, typically occurring in patients younger than 5 years of age. Presenting symptoms include otalgia and otorrhea, and affected children often exhibit

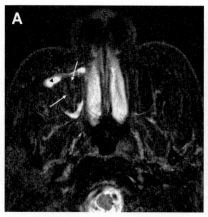
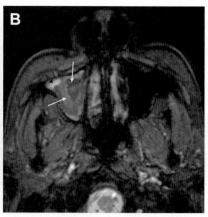

Fig. 5. Mycetoma. Axial fat-suppressed T2-weighted (*A*) and gradient echo (*B*) images show mucosal thickening within the right maxillary sinus (*black arrowhead*). Note the lobulated T2 hypointense lesion within the central right maxillary sinus with heterogeneous signal on gradient echo image (*white arrows*), representing a fungus ball (mycetoma), which could be easily mistaken for air on T2-weighted images.

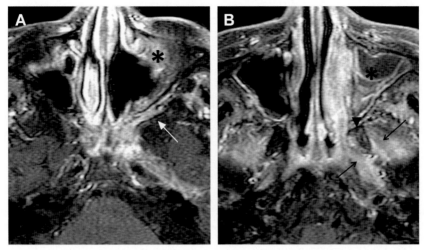

Fig. 6. Invasive fungal sinusitis. Axial post-contrast fat-suppressed T1-weighted images (*A* and *B*) through the maxillary sinuses demonstrate partial opacification and mucosal thickening within the left maxillary sinus with mild associated enhancement (*asterisks*). Asymmetric enhancement within the left retroantral fat (*white arrow*, *A*) is consistent with infiltration. There is spread of the infection into the adjacent soft tissues, with asymmetric enhancement within the left medial and lateral pterygoid muscles (*black arrows*, *B*) and left pterygoid plate (*black arrowhead*, *B*). Compare with the normal pterygoid plate on the right. Pathology revealed invasive mucormycosis. (*Courtesy of* Yoshimi Anzai, MD, MPH, University of Washington Medical Center, Seattle, WA.)

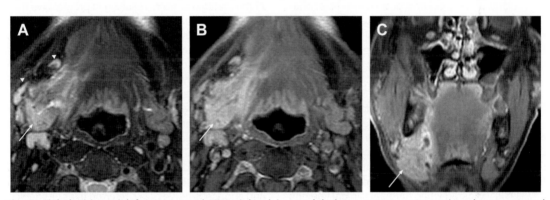

Fig. 7. Sialadenitis. Axial fat-suppressed T2-weighted image (*A*) demonstrates asymmetric enlargement and increased signal of the right submandibular gland (*white arrow*) relative to the normal appearing left submandibular gland. There are surrounding enlarged level IB lymph nodes (*white arrowheads*), likely reactive. Homogeneous avid enhancement is seen on the axial and coronal post-contrast fat-suppressed T1-weighted images (*white arrows*, *B* and *C*). Although minimal dilatation of the intraglandular duct is seen, there is no evidence of extraglandular ductal dilation, or focal region of signal void to suggest a sialolith as etiology for this process.

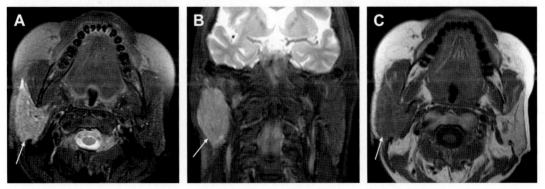

Fig. 8. Parotitis. Axial and coronal fat-suppressed T2-weighted images (*A* and *B*) demonstrate asymmetric enlargement and increased signal involving the entire right parotid gland (*white arrow*). There is associated diffuse hypointense signal seen on the axial T1-weighted image (*white arrow*, *C*), in comparison to the fatty left parotid gland. Imaging features are consistent with diffuse inflammation of the right parotid gland.

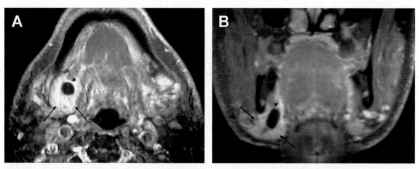

Fig. 9. Sialadenitis of the right submandibular gland with an obstructing sialolith. Axial (*A*) and coronal (*B*) post-contrast fat-suppressed T1-weighted images demonstrate asymmetric enhancement and enlargement of the right submandibular gland relative to the left (*black arrows*), consistent with sialoadenitis. Note the ovoid signal void in the region of the submandibular duct, consistent with an obstructing stone (*black arrowhead*).

tugging at their ears, increased irritability, and sleep disturbance.[12,20,21]

Acute otitis media typically occurs in the setting of concurrent upper respiratory tract infection, particularly in the pediatric population. Nasopharyngeal mucosal edema associated with upper respiratory infection often results in Eustachian tube obstruction, leading to accumulation of fluid in the middle ear and subsequent superimposed infection.[12,20,21] The infection is most often bacterial, with typical culprits including *S pneumoniae, Haemophilus influenzae, and M catarrhalis*.[21]

The diagnosis of acute otitis media should be made clinically with a bulging and erythematous tympanic membrane seen on otoscopic examination. Imaging is not typically indicated for evaluation of uncomplicated otitis media; however, MR imaging is indicated when atypical clinical findings and a strong clinical suspicion for intracranial complications exist.

Temporal bone complications of otitis media occur with increased frequency in the setting of prolonged or recurrent infection. Otomastoiditis (**Fig. 12**) occurs secondary to persistent obstruction of the mastoid antrum, resulting in progressive fluid accumulation and superimposed infection of the mastoid air cells. Petrous apicitis (**Fig. 13**) refers to infection/inflammation of the petrous apex secondary to otomastoiditis. Cranial neuropathy is often present clinically. MR imaging demonstrates inflammatory changes in the petrous apex, which may or may not be pneumatized. MR imaging is superior to CT in demonstrating marrow abnormality and extension of infection to the cavernous sinus and paracavernous region (see **Fig. 13**). Middle ear infection extending to the petrous apex, Meckel's cave, and Dorello's canal may result in facial pain and abducens nerve palsy, referred to as Gradenigo syndrome.[12,20,21] Coalescent mastoiditis (**Fig. 14**) is another complication of otomastoiditis, resulting

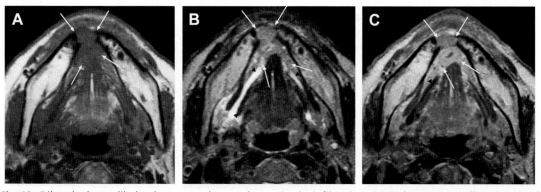

Fig. 10. Dilated submandibular ducts secondary to obstruction by infiltrating gingival squamous cell carcinoma of the floor of the mouth. Axial pre-contrast T1-weighted image (*A*) shows hypointense gingival mass (*white arrows*) eroding through the mandibular symphysis into the floor of the mouth. Axial T2-weighted image (*B*) and axial post-contrast T1-weighted image (*C*) show dilation of the bilateral submandibular ducts right more pronounced than left (*black arrowheads*), secondary to obstruction by the aforementioned floor of mouth tumor (*white arrows*) which demonstrates mild enhancement.

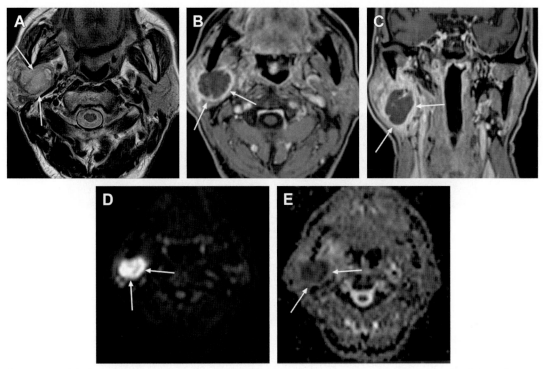

Fig. 11. Parotid abscess. (*A*) Axial T2-weighted image demonstrates a heterogeneous, mostly T2 hyperintense, lesion located within the right parotid gland (*white arrows*). Associated peripheral enhancement is well depicted on the axial (*B*) and coronal (*C*) post-contrast fat-suppressed T1-weighted images (*white arrows*, *B* and *C*), and there is restricted diffusion on diffusion-weighted (*D*) and ADC (*E*) images (*white arrows*, *D*, *E*).

from erosion of the mastoid septa with abscess formation. If left untreated, this complication may eventually result in cortical erosion and destruction of the temporal bone as well as spread of infection to the soft tissues of the neck deep to the sternocleidomastoid muscle, known as Bezold's abscess.[12,20,21] Otomastoiditis may result in dural sinus thrombosis, commonly involving the sigmoid sinus, with or without adjacent abscess formation.[12,20,21] Absence of flow voids on spin echo images or lack of flow-related enhancement on gradient echo sequences is indicative of dural sinus thrombosis. MR venogram and diffusion-weighted images are also useful to detect dural sinus

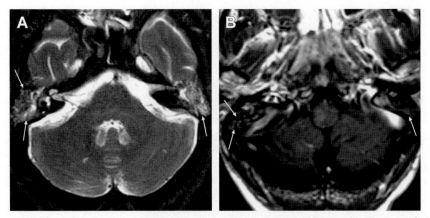

Fig. 12. Otomastoiditis. (*A*) Axial T2-weighted image through the temporal bones demonstrates fluid opacification of the bilateral mastoid air cells (*white arrows*), right slightly greater than left. (*B*) Axial post-contrast T1-weighted image demonstrates corresponding mild enhancement of the mastoid air cells (*white arrows*), also right greater than left.

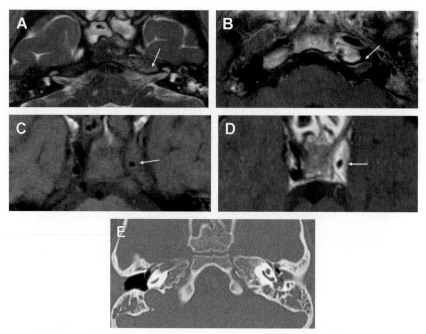

Fig. 13. Petrous apicitis secondary to otomastoiditis. Axial fat-suppressed T2-weighted image (*A*) through the bilateral internal auditory canals demonstrates bilateral mastoid opacification. There is increased T2 signal within the left petrous apex (*white arrow*). Axial post-contrast T1-weighted image (*B*) shows enhancement within the bilateral mastoid air cells, left greater than right. There is associated enhancement along the dura of the left internal auditory canal, resulting as a complication of the adjacent infection. In addition, axial pre- (*C*) and post-contrast (*D*) fat-suppressed T1-weighted images at the level of the cavernous sinuses show abnormal signal and enhancement involving the left cavernous sinus, with encasement of the left cavernous ICA (*white arrow*). (*E*) Axial CT image in bone windows through the mastoid air cells shows bilateral opacification without apparent abnormality in the petrous apices.

thrombosis (**Fig. 15**). Careful evaluation of the intracranial structures, including the dural venous sinus as well as brain parenchyma, is crucial.

Chronic otomastoiditis is commonly associated with formation of cholesteatoma (**Fig. 16**), demonstrated as a lesion with restricted diffusion on diffusion-weighted image. However, an abscess can also demonstrate restricted diffusion; therefore, the clinical presentation and history are extremely important in making the diagnosis.

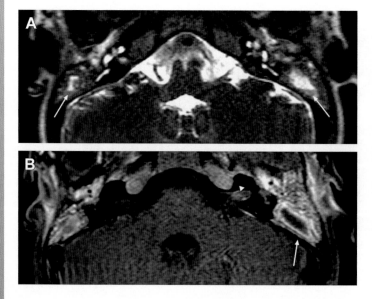

Fig. 14. Coalescent mastoiditis. Axial T2-weighted image (*A*) through the temporal bones shows bilateral mastoid opacification (*white arrows*), left greater than right, with absence of the mastoid septae on the left. (*B*) Axial post-contrast fat-suppressed T1-weighted image shows peripheral enhancement of the left mastoid fluid collection (*white arrow, B*), consistent with an abscess and coalescent mastoiditis. Enhancement of the right mastoid air cells is also present, without peripheral enhancing fluid collection to suggest an abscess. Also noted is enhancement within the left internal auditory canal (*white arrowhead*), indicating extension of the infection and inflammation.

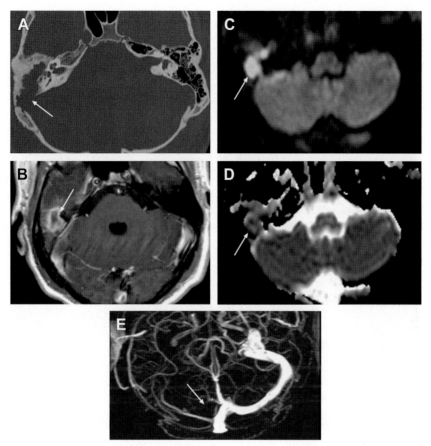

Fig. 15. Dural sinus thrombosis secondary to otomastoiditis. (Axial unenhanced CT image (*A*) through the temporal bones shows right mastoid opacification (*white arrow*). There is destruction of the mastoid septa, and dehiscence of the posterior aspect of the right temporal bone, in the region of the right sigmoid/transverse sinus junction. Axial post-contrast T1-weighted image (*B*) at a corresponding level shows a peripherally enhancing fluid collection (*white arrow*) with associated diffusion restriction (*white arrows, C* and *D*), consistent with an abscess. (*E*) Phase-contrast MRV MIP image demonstrates lack of flow related enhancement of the right transverse and sigmoid sinuses (*white arrow*), indicating sinus thrombosis.

Labyrinthitis

Labyrinthitis refers to infection/inflammation of the membranous labyrinth, usually resulting from viral infections such as herpes simplex, cytomegalovirus, varicella zoster, and influenza. In a minority of cases, bacterial labyrinthitis may occur secondary to trauma, surgery, or otitis media. Patients typically present with vertigo and sensorineural hearing loss.[21] The key imaging finding is membranous labyrinth enhancement (**Fig. 17**); therefore, postcontrast high-resolution imaging is necessary to make the diagnosis. Although imaging findings are present, in some cases the exact cause of labyrinthitis remains unknown.[22,23] Ramsay Hunt syndrome (herpes zoster oticus) is a form of labyrinthitis that affects the facial nerve along with the membranous labyrinth. MR imaging demonstrates avid enhancement of the internal auditory canal, membranous labyrinth, and facial nerve (**Fig. 18**).

Acute labyrinthine hemorrhage is a distinct acute pathology of the membranous labyrinth, characterized by blood filling the normally fluid-filled labyrinth, which may result from leukemia, sickle cell disease, infection, trauma, anticoagulation therapy, and prior head/neck radiation.[24–27] The classic presentation includes the sudden onset of sensorineural hearing loss and vertigo. MR imaging demonstrates high signal from methemoglobin on T1-weighted images (**Fig. 19**). Therefore, it is important to evaluate precontrast images as well as postcontrast images.

Labyrinthitis ossificans (**Fig. 20**) is a chronic form of labyrinthitis with ossification or calcification of the labyrinth from any cause, most commonly from bacterial meningitis, followed by direct infection from otitis media, surgery, trauma, and rarely sickle cell disease. MR imaging demonstrates loss of normal fluid signal in the membranous labyrinth on high resolution T2-weighted

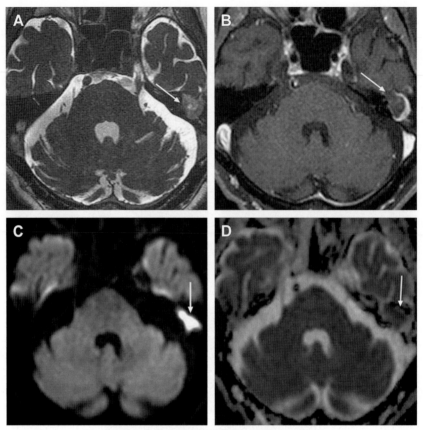

Fig. 16. Cholesteatoma. Axial T2-weighted image through the temporal bones (*A*) demonstrates heterogeneous slightly hyperintense signal in the region of the left middle ear (*white arrow*), with associated heterogeneous enhancement on corresponding postcontrast fat-suppressed T1-weighted image (*B*). Axial diffusion-weighted (*C*) and corresponding apparent diffusion coefficient (*D*) images through a similar level show restricted diffusion, consistent with a cholesteatoma.

images such as constructive interference in the steady state (CISS), fast imaging employing steady-state acquisition (FIESTA), and driven equilibrium radio frequency reset pulse (DRIVE), and is more sensitive than CT.[21,27–31]

Facial Neuritis (Bell's Palsy)

Bell's palsy is an infectious/inflammatory process that results in the loss of function of the facial nerve peripherally, typically presenting with paralysis of the innervated facial muscles. Historically, Bell's palsy has been considered as idiopathic in nature; however, recent evidence points to possible reactivation of the herpes simplex virus in the geniculate ganglion as a potential cause. Additionally, herpes zoster reactivation (Ramsay Hunt syndrome) and other infectious etiologies such as cytomegalovirus, *Borrelia burgdorferi*, and Epstein–Barr virus have also been implicated as causes of facial nerve dysfunction.[32]

Although imaging is not necessarily indicated to diagnose Bell's palsy in the classic clinical scenario, MR imaging may be helpful in atypical clinical presentations or in the setting of persistent palsy despite treatment (**Fig. 21**). Abnormal enhancement of the facial nerve, typically affecting the canalicular, labyrinthine, and tympanic segments, can be seen on MR imaging.[33] Differential considerations including perineural tumor spread or facial nerve schwannoma may appear similar on imaging.[21,34]

PHARYNGEAL AND LARYNGEAL INFECTIONS
Acute Tonsillitis/Peritonsillar Abscess

Acute tonsillar infections predominate in patients in their teenage and early adult years, with approximately 45,000 cases of acute tonsillitis occurring annually in the United States. Approximately one-third of all head and neck soft tissue abscesses are of peritonsillar origin.[12,18,35] *S aureus*, *S pneumoniae*, beta-hemolytic streptococcus species, and *H influenzae* are the most common bacterial agents responsible for tonsillitis and peritonsillar infections. Typical presenting symptoms

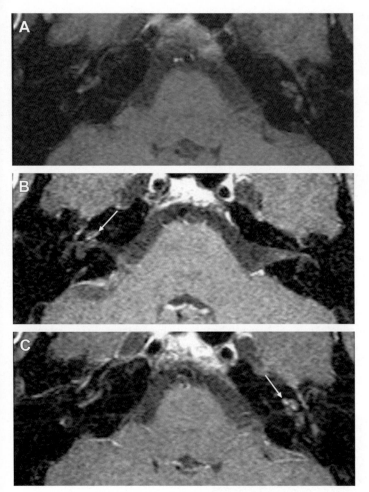

Fig. 17. Labyrinthitis. Axial precontrast (*A*) and axial postcontrast (*B*, *C*) T1-weighted images through the temporal bones demonstrate subtle abnormal enhancement of the cochlea bilaterally (*white arrows*), indicative of labyrinthitis.

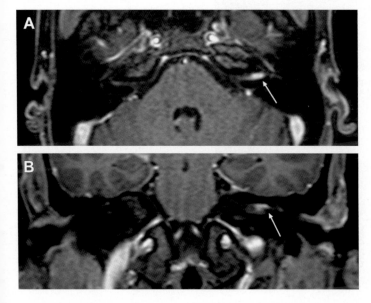

Fig. 18. Ramsay Hunt syndrome. A 17-year-old female with left facial nerve palsy, ear pain, and facial blister. Axial (*A*) and coronal (*B*) postcontrast fat-suppressed T1-weighted images demonstrate abnormal enhancement of the intracanalicular segment of the left facial nerve (*white arrows*).

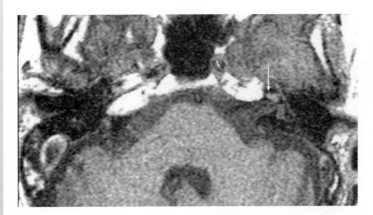

Fig. 19. Labyrinthine hemorrhage. Axial precontrast T1-weighted image through the temporal bones demonstrates increased signal within the left cochlea (*arrow*) and, to a lesser degree, the semicircular canals and vestibule, consistent with labyrinthine hemorrhage.

include dysphagia, fever, and cervical lymphadenopathy.[18,36] The infected tonsils may rarely undergo cavitary necrosis resulting in intratonsillar abscess formation. More commonly, suppuration between the tonsillar capsule and the tonsillar pillar can occur, giving rise to a peritonsillar abscess. Identification of this complication is essential, because its presence will alter clinical management and necessitate drainage in addition to routine antibiotic therapy.[12,18]

Imaging is not typically indicated in cases of uncomplicated acute tonsillitis. However, if performed, MR imaging demonstrates enlargement and diffuse enhancement of the affected tonsil (Fig. 22). Imaging features are nonspecific, and similar or identical to other processes, such as benign lymphoid hyperplasia, viral infections such as mononucleosis, and neoplasms such as lymphoma or squamous cell carcinoma.[12,18] In the setting of a peritonsillar abscess, MR imaging

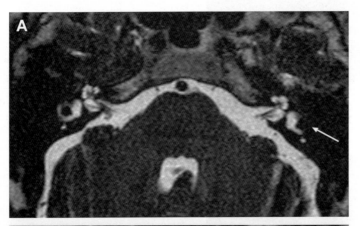

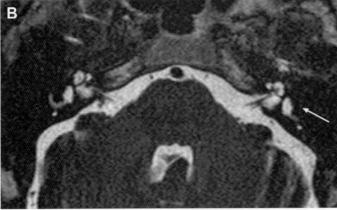

Fig. 20. Labyrinthitis ossificans. Consecutive axial T2-weighted images (*A* and *B*) through the temporal bones demonstrate asymmetric signal loss of the left lateral semicircular canal in comparison to the right side, consistent with labyrinthitis ossificans.

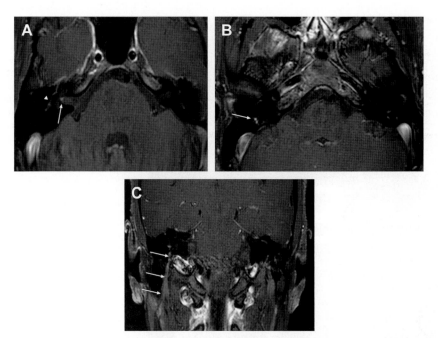

Fig. 21. Bell's palsy. Axial postcontrast fat-suppressed T1-weighted image through the temporal bones (*A*) shows an asymmetric focus of enhancement at the fundus of the right internal auditory canal (*white arrow*) and within the region of the genu and tympanic segments of the right facial nerve (*white arrowhead*). At a more inferior level of the right temporal bone (*B*), enhancement is seen along the expected course of the mastoid segment of the right facial nerve (*white arrow*). The asymmetric enhancement is well-depicted on a coronal fat-suppressed postcontrast image (*C*), which shows the long segment region of enhancement, extending through the stylomastoid foramen (*white arrows*).

shows a rim-enhancing loculated fluid collection within the peritonsillar fossa. The diagnosis can be further solidified by the presence of restricted diffusion on diffusion-weighted imaging (**Fig. 23**).[12,13,18]

Retropharyngeal Abscess

The retropharyngeal space is a potential space. Although lateral retropharyngeal nodes (nodes of Rouvière) are seen in both children and adults in the nasopharynx, medial retropharyngeal nodes are not commonly seen after 6 years of age, and are often only present at the oropharyngeal level. Retropharyngeal nodes in children serve as a major nidus for infection and can become secondarily infected as a result of lymph drainage from a primary focus of infection, typically from the oral cavity, oropharynx, middle ear, or sinuses. The affected lymph nodes can then undergo suppuration (**Fig. 24**) and surrounding perinodal inflammation sometimes results in cellulitis. Rupture of the lymph nodes may eventually ensue if treatment is not instituted expeditiously, giving rise to a retropharyngeal abscess (**Fig. 25**). In adults, the primary etiology of infection in the retropharyngeal space is a penetrating injury.[12,18,37]

The most common offending organisms include *S aureus, H influenzae,* and *beta-hemolytic Streptococcus.* Patients usually present with symptoms of fever, throat and neck pain, dysphagia, limited neck range of motion, and difficulty breathing. Retropharyngeal cellulitis and small abscesses are usually treated with antibiotics, whereas drainage is typically indicated in the setting of larger collections.[12,18,37]

In the absence of disease, the retropharyngeal space is not easily identifiable on imaging.[12,18] Scrutiny of the retropharyngeal region, better accomplished with MR imaging, is crucial to identify both the primary infective process and dreaded complications such as mediastinitis because early treatment is necessary to reduce patient morbidity and mortality. Typical MR imaging features include (1) bow-tie–shaped distention of the retropharyngeal space causing displacement of the posterior pharyngeal wall anteriorly, (2) retropharyngeal T2 hyperintensity and T1 hypointensity indicating edema/cellulitis, (3) loculated rim-enhancing fluid collection on postcontrast imaging indicative of abscess, and (4) restricted diffusion in the area of the collection.[12,18,37]

Spinal epidural abscess occurring secondary to a directly spreading retropharyngeal infection is

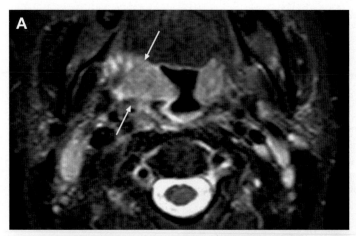

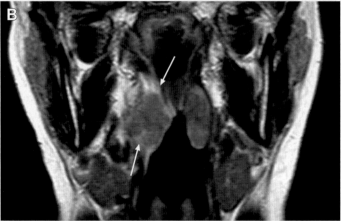

Fig. 22. Uncomplicated right tonsillitis. Axial fat-suppressed T2-weighted (*A*) and coronal T2-weighted (*B*) images demonstrate asymmetric enlargement and inflammation of the right palatine tonsil (*white arrows*) indicative of uncomplicated tonsillitis. There is mild to moderate associated narrowing of the oropharynx. No evidence of a focal fluid collection or draining sinus tract.

relatively rare in comparison with its occurrence secondary to infection in the prevertebral space and discitis–osteomyelitis (**Fig. 26**). Nonetheless, MR imaging is valuable in identifying the source of infection as arising in the retropharyngeal space versus the prevertebral space, because the former requires otolaryngology intervention and the latter requires neurosurgical intervention, particularly in the setting of cord compression.[38]

CERVICAL LYMPHADENITIS
Suppurative Lymphadenopathy

Lymph node infection may result in a pyogenic immune response, leading to progressive enlargement of nodes filled with purulent material. This form of infection is most often seen in children between one to four years old.[39,40] Group A *Streptococcus* and *S aureus* account for the majority of offending organisms. Patients typically present with swollen and tender cervical lymph nodes, fever, and possible difficulty swallowing or breathing depending on the location of affected nodes.

On MR imaging, suppurative lymphadenitis (**Fig. 27**) is demonstrated as enlarged lymph nodes with intranodal fluid/abscess, peripheral enhancement, and inflammatory changes in the perinodal tissues. Associated retropharyngeal abscesses may also be identified with MR imaging (see retropharyngeal abscess section above). Identifying this complication is crucial as its presence may necessitate drainage in addition to antibiotic treatment, depending on its size.[6,39–41]

Tuberculous Lymphadenitis

An estimated 12% to 15% of extrapulmonary tuberculosis cases occur within the head and neck. The most common manifestation is lymphadenitis, more often affecting adults in the third and fourth decades of life.[39–42] Unlike suppurative lymphadenitis, tuberculous lymph node enlargement is typically painless and more often bilateral and symmetric. Posterior triangle (level V) and internal jugular chain lymph nodes are more commonly affected, and patients usually present with few constitutional symptoms.[6,39–42]

Lymph nodes affected by tuberculosis demonstrate variable appearance (**Fig. 28**), with signal and enhancement pattern varying depending on

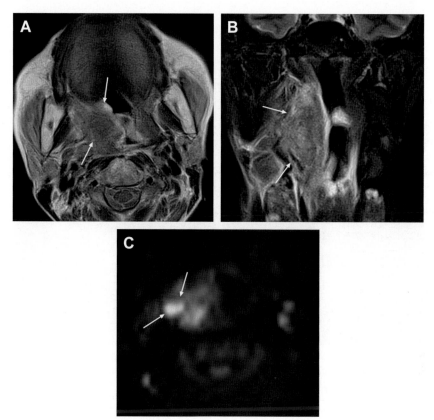

Fig. 23. Peritonsillar abscess. Axial (*A*) and coronal (*B*) T2-weighted MR images demonstrate irregular enlargement and edema signal of the right palatine tonsil (*white arrows*). Axial diffusion-weighted image (*C*) shows restricted diffusion of the lesion (*white arrows*), representing peritonsillar abscess.

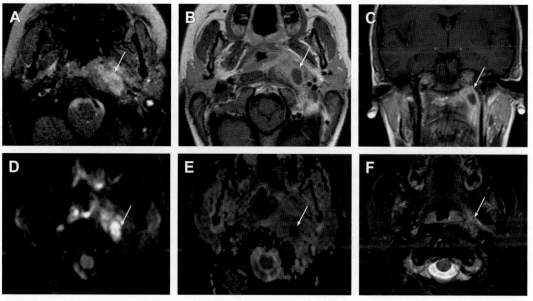

Fig. 24. Retropharyngeal intranodal abscess. Axial T2-weighted image (*A*) shows edema within the left retropharyngeal space extending into the left parapharyngeal space and left prevertebral space involving the longus coli muscle (*white arrow*). Axial (*B*) and coronal (*C*) postcontrast T1-weighted images demonstrate a peripherally enhancing collection within the left lateral retropharyngeal lymph node (*white arrow*). There is restricted diffusion (*white arrow*) on axial diffusion-weighted (*D*) and apparent diffusion coefficient (*E*) images, consistent with an intranodal abscess. There is resolution of this collection with mild residual inflammation in surrounding regions after completion of a course of antibiotics, demonstrated on the axial fat-suppressed T2-weighted image (*F*) acquired 2 weeks later.

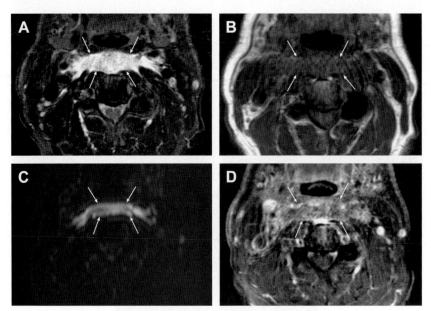

Fig. 25. Retropharyngeal abscess. Axial fat-suppressed T2-weighted image (*A*) demonstrates bright fluid collection within the retropharyngeal space (*white arrows*). Axial precontrast T1-weighted image (*B*) shows collection as isointense to hypointense (*white arrows*). Axial diffusion-weighted image (*C*) demonstrates corresponding diffusion hyperintensity (*white arrows*), and there is demonstration of subtle peripheral enhancement of the retropharyngeal collection (*white arrows*) on the axial postcontrast fat-suppressed T1-weighted image (*D*).

the phase of clinical presentation. Three phases of tuberculous lymphadenitis are recognized on imaging, namely, acute, subacute, and chronic. The various phases are associated with the following imaging findings: (1) acute phase is inflammation without central necrosis, homogenous signal on T1- and T2-weighted imaging with homogenous enhancement, (2) subacute phase is inflammation with central necrosis of affected lymph nodes with rim enhancement, and (3) chronic phase is posttreatment fibrocalcific change, T1 and T2 hypointensity without enhancement.[6,39–42] Chronic phase

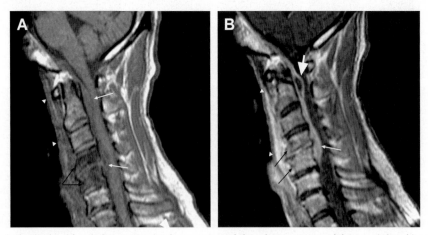

Fig. 26. Cervical spinal epidural abscess. Sagittal precontrast (*A*) and postcontrast (*B*) T1-weighted images demonstrate a large fluid collection within the ventral epidural space extending from the level of C1 to approximately C5-C6 level (*thin white arrows, A*). Maximal thickness of the collection is at the C1-C2 level, where there is demonstration of peripheral enhancement and mild cord compression (*thick white arrow, B*). More homogeneously enhancing phlegmonous component is seen at C4-5 level (*thin white arrow, B*). Additionally, there is note of an enhancing prevertebral collection along levels of C1 to C5-6 (*arrowheads, A and B*). Furthermore, there is increased abnormal enhancement of the C4 and C5 vertebral bodies as well as the C4-C5 disc, indicative of discitis–osteomyelitis (*black arrows, A and B*).

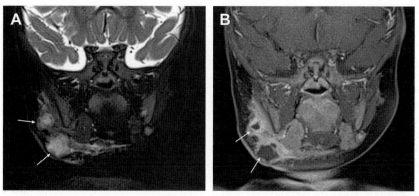

Fig. 27. Suppurative lymphadenopathy. Coronal fat-suppressed T2-weighted image (*A*) demonstrates enlargement and inflammation of right-sided cervical lymph nodes (*white arrows*). Coronal postcontrast fat-suppressed T1-weighted image (*B*) shows corresponding central necrosis and suppuration of lymph nodes (*white arrows*) with enhancement and inflammation within the surrounding soft tissues adjacent to the right mandible and right submandibular gland. No draining sinus tract is seen.

fibrocalcific changes are seen less frequently with cervical lymph nodes in comparison with mediastinal lymph nodes. Additionally, necrotic lymphadenopathy can also result from nodal metastasis from squamous cell carcinoma or papillary thyroid carcinoma. Correlation with clinical history and a search for a primary head and neck cancer should be performed to exclude malignancy.

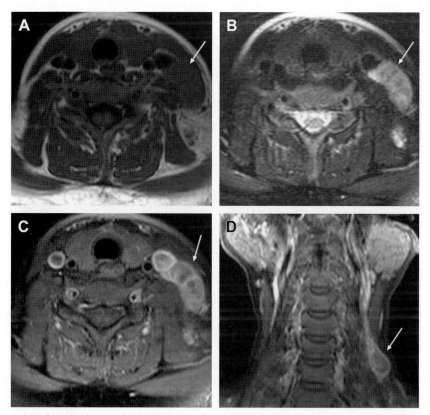

Fig. 28. Tuberculous lymphadenopathy. Isointense soft tissue thickening (*white arrow*) posterolateral to the left internal jugular vein is shown on the axial T1-weighted image (*A*), which is further delineated on the axial fat-suppressed T2-weighted image (*B*) to represent a conglomerate of cervical lymph nodes (*white arrow*) with mild surrounding inflammatory change. Axial (*C*) and coronal (*D*) postcontrast fat-suppressed T1-weighted images further demonstrate peripheral enhancement and central necrosis (*white arrow*) of the lymph node conglomerate.

Viral and Other Lymphadenitis

Viral, inflammatory, idiopathic, and neoplastic etiologies are differential considerations for cervical lymph node enlargement that can also exhibit some of the imaging findings described. For example, neoplastic etiologies such as lymphoma or metastases, and viral etiologies such as mononucleosis or human immunodeficiency virus (HIV) can cause diffuse cervical lymph node enlargement, but with a much lesser degree of surrounding inflammatory changes than a suppurative process. Cervical lymph node enlargement can also be seen with inflammatory conditions such as sarcoidosis, and usually presents with other classic pulmonary and mediastinal findings. Idiopathic entities such as Kimura disease, Kawasaki disease, or Kikuchi–Fujimoto disease may demonstrate lymphadenopathy with perinodal inflammation and also serve as etiologies in the appropriate clinical setting.[39–41]

ODONTOGENIC INFECTIONS

Odontogenic infections may occur via two major pathways. A dental cavity may facilitate the entry of organisms to a particular tooth root, predisposing to apical periodontitis and abscess formation. Infection may also occur via bacterial overgrowth and chronically poor hygiene, predisposing to gingivitis and periodontitis. Chronic inflammation over time increases risk for osteomyelitis, intraosseous abscesses, and perimandibular cellulitis and abscesses.[6,12]

Responsible organisms include anaerobes such as gram positive (*Streptococcus milleri* group, *Peptostreptococcus*) and gram negative (*Bacteroides*) bacteria. Symptoms include tooth/jaw pain, facial pain and swelling, fever, dysphagia, and trismus. Antibiotic treatment is typically sufficient for uncomplicated infections and associated acute osteomyelitis. However, chronic osteomyelitis may require antibiotics along with curettage, debridement, and/or sequestrectomy. Drainage and antibiotics may also be necessary to treat periodontal abscess. Long-term definitive treatment typically entails tooth extraction or root canal.[6,12]

Periapical lucencies and periodontal abscesses are often adequately evaluated with CT. However, MR imaging is more sensitive for evaluation of complications such as osteomyelitis and extraosseous abscess (**Fig. 29**). Of note, bone infarct with intramedullary/subperiosteal hemorrhage in the

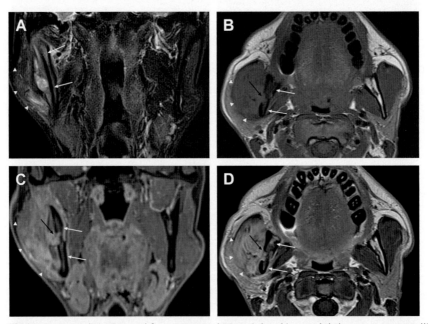

Fig. 29. Mandibular osteomyelitis. Coronal fat-suppressed T2-weighted image (*A*) demonstrates swelling and heterogeneously hyperintense edema signal within the right masseter muscle (*white arrowheads*) and associated hyperintense signal within the right mandibular ramus (*white arrows*). Precontrast T1-weighted image (*B*) demonstrates these areas of signal abnormality within the right masseter muscle (*white arrowheads*) and right mandibular ramus (*white arrows*) as hypointense. Coronal postcontrast fat-suppressed (*C*) and axial postcontrast (*D*) T1-weighted images demonstrate avid enhancement of the swollen right masseter muscle (*white arrowheads*), indicative of myositis. There is also mild enhancement of the right mandible, consistent with osteomyelitis (*white arrows, C and D*). An avidly enhancing sinus tract (*black arrow, B, C and D*) is also seen extending through the lateral cortex of the right mandibular ramus into the adjacent muscle.

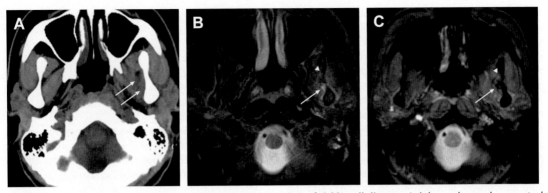

Fig. 30. Bone infarct with subperiosteal hemorrhage in setting of sickle cell disease. Axial unenhanced computed tomography image (*A*) demonstrates ill-defined soft tissue/water density (*white arrows*) adjacent to the left lateral pterygoid muscle, suggesting edema. On the corresponding axial fat-suppressed T2-weighted (*B*) and gradient echo (*C*) images, cortical irregularity and mildly increased osseous signal (*white arrowheads*) is seen, consistent with a bone infarct. The fat-suppressed T2-weighted image shows a small hyperintense collection with susceptibility artifact on the gradient echo image, consistent with subperiosteal hemorrhage (*white arrows*, *B* and *C*).

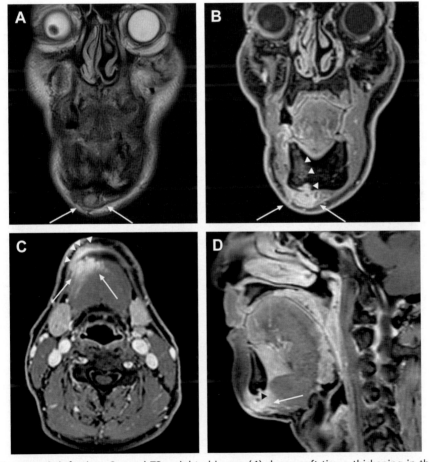

Fig. 31. Actinomycosis infection. Coronal T2-weighted image (*A*) shows soft tissue thickening in the right submental region (*white arrows*), with corresponding avid enhancement seen on postcontrast fat-suppressed T1-weighted images (*B–D*). Postcontrast fat-suppressed T1-weighted images (*B–D*) localize the enhancement to the region of the right anterior belly of the digastric muscle and the right mylohyoid muscle (*white arrows*, *B–D*). There is also cortical disruption and enhancement within the adjacent mandibular symphysis extending to the body of the right mandible (*white arrowheads*, *B–D*), secondary to osteomyelitis.

setting of sickle cell disease (**Fig. 30**) may present with clinical and CT imaging findings similar to osteomyelitis and subperiosteal abscess, and MR imaging may be useful to differential these two conditions.[6,25,43–47] Ludwig's angina can be a complication of periodontal disease, characterized as a necrotizing soft tissue infection of the floor of mouth, with MR imaging demonstrating edema and swelling, and presence of a rim-enhancing abscess.[12,43,48] Actinomycosis (**Fig. 31**) is an uncommon infection caused by *Actinomyces israelii*, typically manifesting as a chronic disease with multiple abscesses, firm soft tissue masses, and the presence of sulfur granules in exudates or tissues. Clinical findings are often similar to neoplasms. Intralesional gas, osteolytic changes with extensive surrounding inflammatory changes extending to the skin surface, fistula formation, and an absence of lymphadenopathy are frequently seen and are helpful in narrowing the differential diagnosis.[41,49,50]

SUMMARY

For a significant proportion of head and neck infections, evaluation of the severity and nature of the infectious processes is done with detailed history taking and physical examination. Due to its superior delineation of soft tissue contrast, MR imaging plays a crucial role in the accurate assessment of the anatomic extent of disease processes and for the detection of possible complications. The ability to identify morbid complications and drastically alter clinical management strongly confirms the importance of MR imaging in the evaluation of acute head and neck infections.

REFERENCES

1. Meyer DR, Linberg JV, Wobig JL, et al. Anatomy of the orbital septum and associated eyelid connective tissues. Ophthal Plast Reconstr Surg 1991;7:104–13.
2. Cunnane ME, Sepahdari AR, Gardiner M, et al. Pathology of the eye and orbit. In: Som PM, Curtin HD, editors. Head and neck imaging. 5th edition. St Louis (MO): Mosby Inc; 2011. p. 591–756.
3. LeBedis CA, Sakai O. Nontraumatic orbital conditions: diagnosis with CT and MR imaging in the emergent setting. Radiographics 2008;28:1741–53.
4. Eustis HS, Mafee MF, Walton C, et al. MR imaging and CT of orbital infections and complications in acute rhinosinusitis. Radiol Clin North Am 1998; 36(6):1165–83.
5. Sepahdari AR, Aakalu VK, Kapur R, et al. MRI of Orbital cellulitis and orbital abscess: the role of diffusion-weighted imaging. AJR Am J Roentgenol 2009;193:W244–50.
6. Chapman MN, Nadgir RN, Akman AS, et al. Periapical lucency around the tooth: radiologic evaluation and differential diagnosis. Radiographics 2013; 33(1):E15–32.
7. Kebede A, Adamu Y, Bejiga A. Bacteriological study of dacryocystitis among patients attending in Menelik II Hospital, Addis Ababa, Ethiopia. Ethiop Med J 2010;48(1):29–33.
8. Kassel EE, Schatz CJ. Anatomy, imaging, and pathology of the lacrimal apparatus. In: Som PM, Curtin HD, editors. Head and neck imaging. 5th edition. St Louis (MO): Mosby Inc; 2011. p. 757–854.
9. Eggesbø HB. Radiological imaging of inflammatory lesions in the nasal cavity and paranasal sinuses. Eur Radiol 2006;16:872–88.
10. Rak KM, Newell JD, Yakes WF, et al. Paranasal sinuses on MR images of the brain: significance of mucosal thickening. Am J Roentgenol 1991;156: 381–4.
11. Som PM, Brandwein MS, Wang BY. Inflammatory diseases of the sinonasal cavities. In: Som PM, Curtin HD, editors. Head and neck imaging. 5th edition. St Louis (MO): Mosby Inc; 2011. p. 167–252.
12. Aribandi M, McCoy VA, Bazan C III. Imaging features of invasive and noninvasive fungal sinusitis: a review. Radiographics 2007;27:1283–96.
13. Mishra AM, Gupta RK, Saksena S, et al. Biological correlates of diffusivity in brain abscess. Magn Reson Med 2005;54:878–85.
14. Epstein VA, Kern RC. Invasive fungal sinusitis and complications of rhinosinusitis. Otolaryngol Clin North Am 2008;41(3):497–524.
15. DeShazo RD, Chapin K, Swain RE. Fungal sinusitis. N Engl J Med 1997;337(4):254–9.
16. Gillespie MB, O'Malley BW Jr, Francis HW. An approach to fulminant invasive fungal rhinosinusitis in the immunocompromised host. Arch Otolaryngol Head Neck Surg 1998;124(5):520–6.
17. Ludwig BJ, Foster BR, Saito N, et al. Diagnostic imaging in nontraumatic pediatric head and neck emergencies. Radiographics 2010;30:781–99.
18. Capps EF, Kinsella JJ, Gupta M, et al. Emergency imaging assessment of acute, nontraumatic conditions of the head and neck. Radiographics 2010; 30:1335–52.
19. Som PM, Brandwein-Gensler MS. Anatomy and pathology of the salivary glands. In: Som PM, Curtin HD, editors. Head and neck imaging. 5th edition. St Louis (MO): Mosby Elsevier; 2011. p. 2449–610.
20. Vazquez E, Castellote A, Piqueras J, et al. Imaging of complications of acute mastoiditis in children. Radiographics 2003;23(2):359–72.
21. Swartz JD, Hagiwara M. Inflammatory disease of the temporal bone. In: Som PM, Curtin HD, editors. Head and neck imaging. 5th edition. St Louis (MO): Mosby Inc; 2011. p. 1183–230.

22. Dubrulle F, Kohler R, Vincent C, et al. Differential diagnosis and prognosis of T1-weighted post-gadolinium intralabyrinthine hyper-intensities. Eur Radiol 2010;20(11):2628–36.

23. Seltzer S, Mark AS. Contrast enhancement of the labyrinth on MR scans in patients with sudden hearing loss and vertigo: evidence of labyrinthine disease. AJNR Am J Neuroradiol 1991;12(1):13–6.

24. Kothari M, Knopp E, Jonas S, et al. Presumed vestibular hemorrhage secondary to warfarin. Neuroradiology 1995;37(4):324–5.

25. Schuknecht HF, Igarashi M, Chasin WD. Inner ear hemorrhage in leukemia. A case report. Laryngoscope 1965;75:662–8.

26. Poh AC, Tan TY. Sudden deafness due to intralabyrinthine haemorrhage: a possible rare late complication of head and neck irradiation. Ann Acad Med Singapore 2007;36(1):78–82.

27. Saito N, Watanabe M, Liao J, et al. Clinical and radiologic findings of inner ear involvement in sickle cell disease. AJNR Am J Neuroradiol 2011; 32:2160–4.

28. Saito N, Nadgir RN, Flower EN, et al. Clinical and radiologic manifestations of sickle cell disease in the head and neck. Radiographics 2010;30: 1021–35.

29. Collins WO, Younis RT, Garcia MT. Extramedullary hematopoiesis of the paranasal sinuses in sickle cell disease. Otolaryngol Head Neck Surg 2005; 132(6):954–6.

30. Stamataki S, Behar P, Brodsky L. Extramedullary hematopoiesis in the maxillary sinus. Int J Pediatr Otorhinolaryngol 2009;4(1):32–5.

31. Demirbas AK, Aktener BO, Unsal C. Pulpal necrosis with sickle cell anaemia. Int Endod J 2004;37(9): 602–6.

32. Kanerva M, Nissinen J, Moilanen K, et al. Microbiologic findings in acute facial palsy in children. Otol Neurotol 2013;34(7):e82–7.

33. Engstrom M, Abdsaleh S, Ahlstrom H, et al. Serial GD-enhanced MRI and assessment of facial nerve involvement in Bell's palsy. Otolaryngol Head Neck Surg 1997;117:559–66.

34. Caldemeyer KS, Mathews VP, Righi PD, et al. Imaging features and clinical significance of perineural spread or extension of head and neck tumors. Radiographics 1998;18(1):97–110.

35. Herzon FS. Harris P. Mosher award thesis. Peritonsillar abscess: incidence, current management practices, and a proposal for treatment guidelines. Laryngoscope 1995;105(8 Pt 3 Suppl 74):1–17.

36. Tewfik TL, Garni MA. Tonsillopharyngitis: clinical highlights. J Otolaryngol 2005;34(Suppl 1):S45–9.

37. Chong VF, Fan YF. Radiology of the retropharyngeal space. Clin Radiol 2000;55(10):740.

38. Lang IM, Hughes DG, Jenkins JP, et al. MR imaging appearances of cervical epidural abscess. Clin Radiol 1995;50:466–71.

39. Som PM, Brandwine-Gensler MS. Lymph nodes of the neck. In: Som PM, Curtin HD, editors. Head and neck imaging. 5th edition. St Louis (MO): Mosby; 2011. p. 2287–384.

40. Ludwig BJ, Wang J, Nadgir RN, et al. Imaging of cervical lymphadenopathy in children and young adults. AJR Am J Roentgenol 2012;199:1105–13.

41. Sakai O, Curtin HD, Romo LV, et al. Lymph node pathology: benign proliferative, lymphoma, and metastatic disease. Radiol Clin North Am 2000;38(5): 979–98.

42. Moon WK, Han MH, Chang KH, et al. CT and MR imaging of head and neck tuberculosis. Radiographics 1997;17:391–402.

43. Kaneda T, Weber AL, Scrivani SJ, et al. Cysts, tumors and nontumorous lesions of the jaw. In: Som PM, Curtin HD, editors. Head and neck imaging. 5th edition. St Louis (MO): Mosby Elsevier; 2011. p. 1469–546.

44. Watanabe M, Saito N, Nadgir RN, et al. Craniofacial bone infarcts in sickle cell disease: clinical and radiological manifestations. J Comput Assist Tomogr 2013;37(1):91–7.

45. Jain R, Sawhney S, Rizvi SG. Acute bone crises in sickle cell disease: the T1 fat-saturated sequence in differentiation of acute bone infarcts from acute osteomyelitis. Clin Radiol 2008;63:59–70.

46. Al-Mujaini A, Ganesh A, William R, et al. Orbital wall infarction versus infection in sickle cell disease. Can J Ophthalmol 2009;44:101.

47. Nwawka OK, Nadgir R, Fujita A, et al. Granulomatous disease in the head and neck: developing a differential diagnosis. Radiographics 2014;34(5): 1240–56.

48. Vieira F, Allen SM, Stocks RM, et al. Deep neck infection. Otolaryngol Clin North Am 2008;41(3): 459–83.

49. Park JK, Lee HK, Ha HK, et al. Cervicofacial actinomycosis: CT and MR imaging findings in seven patients. AJNR Am J Neuroradiol 2003;24:331–5.

50. Sasaki Y, Kaneda T, Uyeda JW, et al. Actinomycosis in the mandible: CT and MR findings. AJNR Am J Neuroradiol 2014;35(2):390–4.

Magnetic Resonance Imaging of Nontraumatic Musculoskeletal Emergencies

CrossMark

Andrew Kompel, MD*, Akira Murakami, MD,
Ali Guermazi, MD, PhD

KEYWORDS

- Osteomyelitis • Osteonecrosis • Stress fracture • Pathologic fracture • Rhabdomyolysis
- Septic arthritis • Compartment syndrome • Necrotizing fasciitis

KEY POINTS

- MR imaging is highly sensitive and sometimes specific in the diagnosis of many nontraumatic musculoskeletal emergencies.
- Imaging should not delay the treatment of acute compartment syndrome and necrotizing fasciitis.
- T1-weighted and fat-suppressed fluid-sensitive sequences (T2-weighted or STIR) are the critical MR imaging protocol components.

BONES

Osteomyelitis

Osteomyelitis is an infection of bone that can involve cortical bone and bone marrow.[1,2] Typical causes include direct extension from overlying soft tissue including ulcers and posttraumatic infections, and hematologic spread.[3] Delay in diagnosis can lead to significant morbidity, making early detection and diagnosis critically important.

Diabetic ulcers and posttraumatic infections are frequent clinical presentations that may lead the clinician to suspect osteomyelitis from direct extension. A physical examination demonstrates cellulitis and soft tissue defects, although imaging is often performed to evaluate for associated abscess and osseous involvement.[4] These additional imaging findings may affect treatment management.

Hematologic spread of bacteria to bone usually presents with fever and lethargy. Depending on which bone is involved, localized soft tissue swelling, decreased range of motion, and focal pain are additional symptoms. These localizing findings provide an indication of field of view coverage for imaging.

Normal anatomy and imaging technique

MR imaging is useful for suspected cases of osteomyelitis because of its high sensitivity for detection of disease, for evaluating early changes in bone marrow composition, and for determining the extent of the disease[5] (**Fig. 1**). MR imaging has been shown to be capable of detecting changes in bone marrow within 3 days of infection.[6] Protocols include T1-weighted and fluid-sensitive sequences, including T2-weighted fat-suppressed or short-tau inversion recovery (STIR). Precontrast and postcontrast T1-weighted sequences are often performed, although osteomyelitis can be diagnosed without such sequences.[7,8]

Beyond its usefulness for diagnosis, MR imaging can affect how the patient is to be treated.

Drs A. Kompel and A. Murakami have nothing to disclose. Dr A. Guermazi is the President of Boston Imaging Core Lab, LLC, and is a consultant to Merck Serono, Genzyme, TissueGene, and OrthoTrophix.
Section of Musculoskeletal Imaging, Department of Radiology, Boston Medical Center, Boston University School of Medicine, 820 Harrison Ave, FGH Building 3rd Floor, Boston, MA 02118, USA
* Corresponding author.
E-mail address: Andrew.Kompel@bmc.org

Magn Reson Imaging Clin N Am 24 (2016) 369–389
http://dx.doi.org/10.1016/j.mric.2015.11.005
1064-9689/16/$ – see front matter
© 2016 Elsevier Inc. All rights reserved.

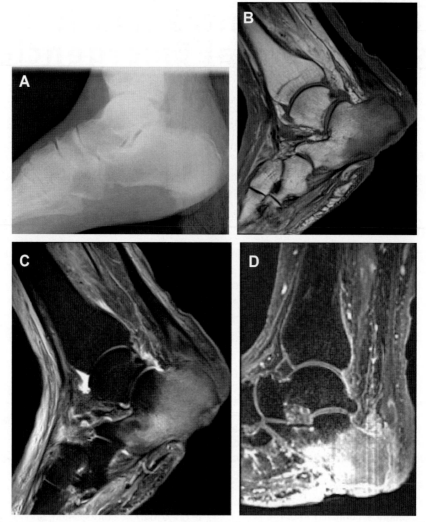

Fig. 1. (A) Lateral radiograph shows increased sclerosis in the plantar aspect of the calcaneus. The overlying bandage limits evaluation of the mineralization and soft tissues of the heel. MR imaging clearly shows the soft tissue defect over the heel extending to bone. The adjacent bone demonstrates geographic T1-weighted hypointensity in the marrow and loss of the low signal cortical bone, which is diagnostic of osteomyelitis (B). T2-weighted fat-suppressed (C) and postcontrast images (D) demonstrate edema and enhancement of the calcaneus, which extend beyond the regions of T1-weighted signal abnormality, indicating reactive changes.

Compared with other modalities, the higher sensitivity of MR imaging leads to earlier treatment and potentially improved patient outcomes. If antibiotics fail and surgery is warranted, the amount of devitalized tissue and adjacent critical structures can be identified, modifying the approach accordingly to minimize complications and morbidity.[9] Imaging planes should include a short axis (axial) and at least one long axis (sagittal or coronal).

One particular anatomic consideration should be raised when dealing with hematologic spread in pediatric cases. The metaphyses of long bones are highly vascularized; with an open physis, vessels do not cross the growth plate. The result is slower flow in the metaphysis and more chances

for bacterial seeding in this region of bone in the pediatric population[6] (Fig. 2).

Imaging Protocols
Primary Protocol
- T1-weighted non-fat-suppressed
- Fluid-sensitive sequence (T2-weighted fat-suppressed or STIR)
Additional Sequences
- Precontrast and postcontrast T1-weighted fat-suppressed

Imaging findings and pathology
The characteristic signal of normal fatty bone marrow is critical for the evaluation of

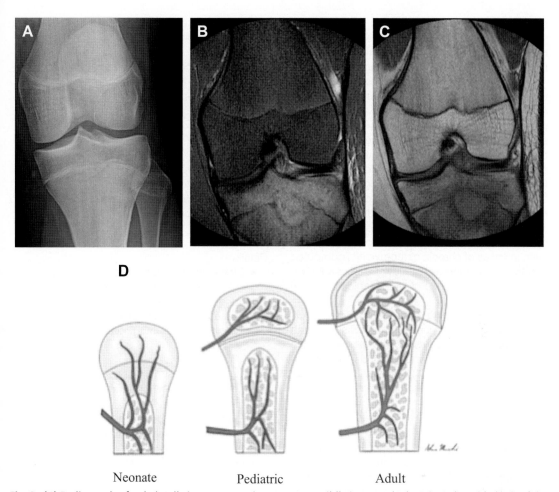

Neonate   Pediatric   Adult

Fig. 2. (*A*) Radiograph of a skeletally immature patient suggests mildly increased sclerosis at the mid physis of the tibia, although it is a subtle finding. MR imaging shows marked bone marrow edema (*B*) in the proximal tibia with corresponding T1-weighted hypointensity (*C*) centered at the mid physeal line. These findings along with symptoms of pain and fever were diagnostic of osteomyelitis. In pediatric patients, there is slower blood flow at the metaphysis, increasing the potential for bacterial seeding. (*D*) Osteomyelitis caused by hematogenous spread is the most common cause in the pediatric population. Initially, vascular connections to the cartilaginous epiphysis in neonates and infants can lead to spread of infection to involve the joint. When the physis opens, there is slower blood flow in the metaphyseal vessels, which can lead to bacteria seeding this portion of the bone. Physeal closure diminishes the risk of infection in this portion of the bone because of the improved blood supply.

osteomyelitis. On T1-weighted sequences, fatty marrow is hyperintense. On fat-suppressed sequences, the signal becomes hypointense. When bone becomes infected, the medullary cavity is filled with bacterial cells, exudative debris, and edema leading to alterations in the normal appearance of the marrow. A T1-weighted sequence demonstrates a geographic, confluent, low signal-intensity, and fluid-sensitive sequences show high signal intensity.[10]

Reactive bone marrow edema from surrounding soft tissue infection or postinfectious granulation tissue within the marrow space may complicate the diagnosis. In these cases, the bone marrow signal demonstrates T2-weighted hyperintensity that is related to osteitis but there is no active bone infection. T1-weighted sequences demonstrate hazy, reticular, and subcortical hypointensity with osteitis.[10]

After the appropriate treatment of osteomyelitis, abnormal marrow signal changes persist for months. A low signal remains on T1-weighted sequences, which can lead to difficulty in evaluating for persistent infection. Comparison with prior examinations or serial MR imaging examinations evaluating the extent of involved bone may provide the only imaging clue to decipher postinfectious granulation tissue from persistent, active infection. However, in these situations, the clinical response to therapy may supersede the imaging findings.[11]

The imaging findings in chronic osteomyelitis vary from those observed in acute osteomyelitis.[12] Acute osteomyelitis is an aggressive process with osteolysis and marked edema. Chronic osteomyelitis demonstrates cortical thickening, sequestrum (a small piece of dead bone with low signal on T1- and T2-weighted sequences), involucrum (periosteal new bone surrounding the sequestrum), and cloaca (sclerotic margin at the periosteal interface surrounding a draining sinus) (**Fig. 3**). MR imaging is the more desirable modality for the evaluation of acute osteomyelitis. However, in cases of chronic osteomyelitis, computed tomography is more sensitive for detecting a sequestrum, the presence of which indicates active infection.[12,13]

Postcontrast imaging offers no additional information for the diagnosis of osteomyelitis, although it can help diagnose an associated abscess in the adjacent soft tissues or intraosseous (Brodie abscess).[14] This finding is critically important because interventional or surgical drainage may be required.

Diagnostic Criteria
- Primary: geographic, medullary, confluent area of T1-weighted hypointensity
- Secondary: bone marrow edema, periosteal reaction, ulcer, cellulitis, sinus tract, abscess, cortical interruption
- Chronic osteomyelitis: sequestrum, involucrum, and cloaca

Differential Diagnosis
- Charcot joint
- Osteitis
- Stress reaction
- Metastatic lesion
- Primary bone neoplasm
- Langerhans cell histiocytosis of bone

Pearls
- Highly sensitive
- Early diagnosis
- Evaluate for abscess and other associated complications

Pitfalls
- Distinguishing postinfectious granulation tissue versus persistent, active infection
- Imaging orthopedic hardware
- Acute neuropathic osteolysis and osteomyelitis have similar imaging appearance[15]

What the Referring Physician Needs to Know
- MR imaging is highly useful for the diagnosis of osteomyelitis
- Diagnosis can be made without intravenous contrast, although contrast helps evaluate for adjacent abscess
- Localizing the area of suspected osteomyelitis can lead to increased diagnostic accuracy (high resolution)
- Orthopedic hardware and neuropathic joints decrease the sensitivity and specificity of diagnosis

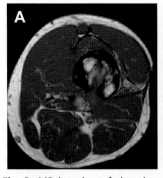 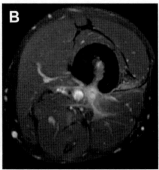 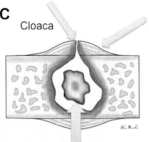

Fig. 3. MR imaging of chronic osteomyelitis shows cortical thickening, which is more conspicuous on the T1-weighted sequence (*A*), and sclerosis at the margins of a draining sinus tract. (*B*) The sinus tract is better seen on the T2-weighted fat-suppressed image. A sequestrum may be difficult to detect on MR imaging because of its small size and low signal intensity. Computed tomography may offer additional diagnostic information on the presence of a sequestrum because of the increased conspicuity of the sclerotic fragment. (*C*) Chronic osteomyelitis demonstrates cortical thickening, sequestrum (dead bone within the cavity), involucrum (periosteal new bone surrounding the sequestrum), and cloaca (sclerotic margin at the periosteal interface surrounding a draining sinus).

- Persistent, active infection can appear similar to posttreatment changes and comparison or serial examinations may be needed

Summary

MR imaging allows for the early detection of osteomyelitis with high sensitivity in the appropriate clinical setting. In addition to diagnosis, MR imaging is useful for guiding patient management and to assess complications that could modify the treatment regime. Postcontrast imaging provides additional information, primarily about the surrounding soft tissues. Difficulties in diagnosis arise in assessing for persistent, active infection, in patients with orthopedic hardware, and in neuropathic joints.

Osteonecrosis of the Femoral Head

The incidence of osteonecrosis of the femoral head (ONFH) is increasing, with causes including exogenous steroid use and trauma. Initially, patients may be asymptomatic, but joint destruction may result if the condition is not recognized early.[16] Once hip pain is present, joint replacement is usually required within 3 years.[17] This may occur in patients younger than 50, but it is not limited by age. Traumatic causes of ONFH are unilateral. When other causes (eg, exogenous steroids, alcohol, smoking, hemoglobinopathies) are suspected, imaging should include both hips to evaluate for clinically occult ONFH.

Normal anatomy and imaging technique

The major blood supply to the epiphysis of the femoral head is the posterior-superior retinacular arteries (**Fig. 4**E). The vessels are within the joint capsule as they cross the femoral neck and branch into the lateral epiphyseal vessels, which supply the femoral head. Trauma to the femoral head/neck area results in disruption or kinking of the distal posterior superior reticular arteries, whereas other etiologies cause occlusion of the vessels.[18,19]

MR imaging is a markedly sensitive and specific modality.[20] Protocols should include a large field of view covering both hips given the high incidence of bilateral disease (**Fig. 4**A, B). T1-weighted and fluid-sensitive sequences (T2-weighted fat-suppressed or STIR) are commonly used for diagnosis. Postcontrast sequences are not routinely acquired, although they may provide additional detail when the diagnosis is not definitive.[21]

Imaging Protocols
  Large field of view (both hips)
  - T1-weighted non-fat-suppressed coronal
  - Fluid-sensitive fat-suppressed coronal

- Fluid-sensitive fat-suppressed axial
- T1-weighted non-fat-suppressed axial (optional)

Small field of view (affected hip)
  - T1-weighted non-fat-suppressed (two planes)
  - Fluid-sensitive fat-suppressed (two planes)

Imaging findings and pathology

A specific staging system (Ficat[22]) for ONFH includes radiography, MR imaging, and bone scan findings. An MR imaging classification of avascular necrosis has also been developed based on the central avascular segment signal. Earliest changes in the femoral head are usually subchondral at the superior femoral head and starting at the anterior portion.

Ficat Classification (MR imaging findings)
  Stage 0: normal
  Stage 1: bone marrow edema
  Stage 2: geographic defect
  Stage 3: crescent sign with possible cortical collapse
  Stage 4: secondary degenerative changes

MR Imaging Avascular Necrosis Classification[23]
  Class A: signal analogous to fat; hyperintense T1-weighted; intermediate to high T2-weighted signal
  Class B: signal analogous to blood; hyperintense T1-weighted and T2-weighted signal
  Class C: signal analogous to fluid; hypointense T1-weighted; high T2-weighted signal
  Class D: signal analogous to fibrous tissue; hypointense T1-weighted and T2-weighted

T1-weighted findings vary depending on the underlying pathology. If there is subchondral edema then T1-weighted signal is low. With blood products, T1-weighted signal is high. In both cases, there is a peripheral hypointense band outlining the area of osteonecrosis extending to the subchondral plate.[18] This band represents the junction between reparative and necrotic zones.

On T2-weighted sequences, a double-line sign is diagnostic of ONFH. There is a peripheral hypointense band similar to T1-weighted sequences with an additional high signal inner peripheral band. The inner hyperintense band represents granulation tissue and is present in up to 80% of cases.[20] Focal areas of T2-weighted low signal represent necrotic or fibrous tissue (**Fig. 4**C, D). Occasionally a focal lesion may not be present in the femoral head, which makes the diagnosis more difficult. Edema may be the only finding if imaged before an identifiable reactive/necrotic zone interface develops. Contrast imaging may

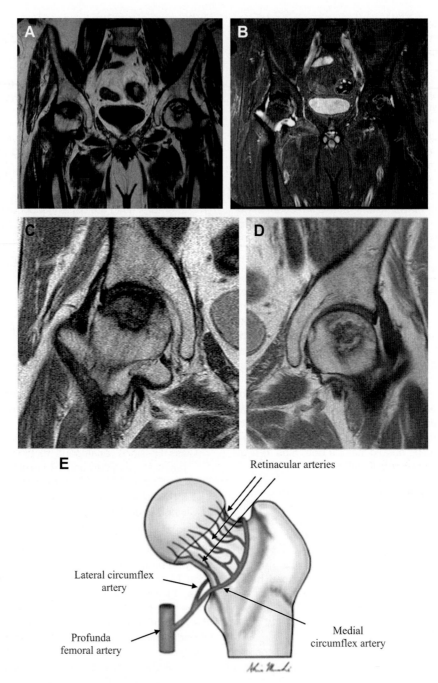

Fig. 4. Large field of view images of the bilateral hips demonstrate osteonecrosis of the femoral heads with crescent sign. The left hip has signal corresponding to fat and the right hip has mixed signal representing blood and fibrous tissue in the areas of osteonecrosis. (*A*) There is a peripheral hypointense band outlining the osteonecrosis that extends to the subchondral plate. (*B*) The right hip also has an effusion. (*C*) The right hip has a partial collapse of the femoral head involving the superior lateral aspect. (*D*) The left femoral head maintains the normal convex contour. (*E*) The major blood supply to the femoral head epiphysis is the posterior-superior retinacular arteries within the joint capsule as they cross the femoral neck. At the neck they branch into the lateral epiphyseal vessels, which supply the femoral head.

provide additional detail for distinguishing osteonecrosis from transient edema (nonviable from viable tissue).[21]

Diagnostic Criteria
- Variable central T1-weighted signal at the superior femoral head with a low signal peripheral rim
- Variable central T2-weighted signal at the superior femoral head with low signal peripheral rim; double line sign, if present, is pathognomonic

Differential Diagnosis
- Transient osteoporosis of the hip
- Transient bone marrow syndrome
- Bone contusion
- Subchondral fracture

Pearls
- Most sensitive modality
- Larger MR imaging lesions have a greater tendency for femoral head collapse[24]
- Low signal peripheral rim and double line sign provide high diagnostic accuracy

Pitfalls
- MR imaging classification has low predictive value in femoral head collapse
- Failure to identify associated subchondral fracture
- T1-only protocols have higher false-negative rate[25]

What the Referring Physician Needs to Know
- In addition to history and physical examination, MR imaging is a critical component for evaluation, especially in younger patients
- Stage, extent of necrosis, and degree of joint involvement have prognostic value[26]
- Comprehensive quantitative staging system allows for optimal evaluation and treatment, unlike older nonquantitative systems

Summary

ONFH may initially be asymptomatic but can progress to joint destruction if not appropriately identified and treated. MR imaging is the most sensitive and specific modality and screening of both hips should be performed to diagnose clinically occult disease. Imaging with T1- and T2-weighted sequences is optimal for evaluation. Peripheral low signal intensity band and double line sign represent the junction of necrotic and fibrous tissue and are critically important diagnostic criteria. The extent of necrosis and joint involvement has

prognostic value compared with older staging methods.

Stress Fracture

Stress fractures encompass two different types of injuries: fatigue fractures and insufficiency fractures. Fatigue fractures arise from abnormal stress on normal bone, seen commonly in young, active individuals.[27] These injuries occur frequently in athletes engaging in repetitive activity, often when the activity is first begun.[28] Running and gymnastics are popular activities that result in fatigue fractures.[29] The lower extremities, more specifically the medial neck of the femur and pelvic ring, are commonly affected and may demonstrate bilateral abnormalities. Upper extremity injuries are less common and typically unilateral.

Insufficiency fracture is normal stress on abnormal bone and is common in elderly women. Pathologic conditions that weaken bone are the leading risk factor, with osteoporosis and long-term bisphosphonate use being common etiologies.[30] This injury occurs almost exclusively in weight-bearing locations including the spine, sacrum, and femurs.

Stress fractures present with pain regardless of cause. With fatigue fractures, performing a repetitive activity exacerbates the pain, which improves with rest. Insufficiency fractures are most commonly atraumatic or result from low-impact mechanisms.

Normal anatomy and imaging technique

MR imaging is the most sensitive and specific modality for stress fractures.[31] Similar to imaging of traumatic injuries, T1- and T2-weighted fat-suppressed sequences are essential to the diagnosis.[32,33] When imaging the extremities, axial and coronal planes are frequently used. For example, fatigue fractures of the femoral neck are commonly medial and insufficiency fractures lateral, and are most conspicuous in the coronal plane. However, the sagittal plane may provide the most diagnostic information for sternal and vertebral insufficiency fractures.

Imaging Protocols
- T1-weighted: coronal and axial planes (sagittal for sternum and spine)
- Fluid-sensitive sequence (T2-weighted fat-suppressed or STIR): coronal and axial planes (sagittal for sternum and spine)
- Precontrast and postcontrast sequences: performed if pathologic fracture is suspected (discussed separately)

Imaging findings and pathology

MR imaging's increased sensitivity over radiography and superior specificity compared with bone scan make it the optimal imaging decision. Diagnosis is based on linear T1-weighted hypointensity with associated T2-weighted hyperintensity that commonly extends into the surrounding soft tissues[32] (**Figs. 5** and **6**). Insufficiency fractures follow a pattern where the lateral periosteum and cortex are initially affected and may present as incomplete fractures.[27]

Bisphosphonate-related insufficiency fractures are typically located at the proximal third of the femur. These fractures have an atypical fracture pattern and are a diagnosis of exclusion.[34] This fracture pattern occurs more frequently in older women treated continuously with bisphosphonates.[30] The causative mechanism is unknown. One theory proposes that long-term bisphosphonate therapy limits bone remodeling from microtrauma, leading to fragility.[35]

Diagnostic Criteria
- T1-weighted linear low marrow signal intensity usually arising from the cortex and perpendicular to the surface of bone
- Diffuse T2-weighted hyperintensity with low signal fracture line

Differential Diagnosis
- Traumatic fracture
- Stress reaction
- Pathologic fracture
- Osteoid osteoma

Pearls
- MR imaging is highly sensitive and specific

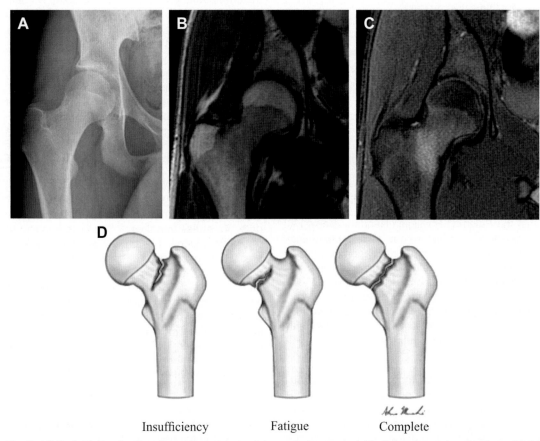

Insufficiency   Fatigue   Complete

Fig. 5. (*A*) On initial evaluation, the radiograph was interpreted as normal. (*B, C*) Subsequent evaluation with MR imaging demonstrates its superior sensitivity by showing an area of edema in the femoral neck. In addition, there is a small linear hypointensity at the medial femoral neck diagnostic of a stress fracture. Early diagnosis can help to prevent progression to a complete fracture through the femoral neck that would necessitate surgical intervention. (*D*) Fatigue fractures of the femoral neck are commonly medially and insufficiency fractures laterally. They are most conspicuous in the coronal plane. Early diagnosis and treatment is critical to prevent progression to a complete fracture.

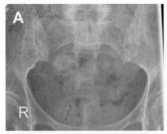 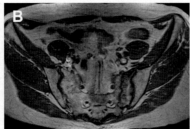 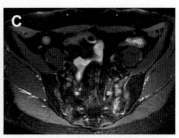

Fig. 6. Sacral insufficiency fractures are not uncommon among the elderly. Diagnosis on radiography (*A*) and computed tomography may be challenging. On a T1-weighted sequence (*B*), there is a vertical hypointensity through the left sacral ala representing the fracture line with corresponding T2-weighted hyperintensity (*C*). In retrospect, there is a subtle vertical sclerotic line on the radiograph (*A*) in the left sacrum that correlates with the MR imaging findings.

- Identify other causes (soft tissue, bone, or joint) for pain
- Linear low signal component is classic criteria for stress fracture (bone contusion is microfracture without discrete low signal line)

Pitfalls
- Failure to identify underlying lesion with insufficiency fracture (pathologic fracture)
- Delay in obtaining diagnosis (with MR imaging) may lead to a worse outcome, such as complete fracture and lengthened recovery time

What the Referring Physician Needs to Know
- Radiographs are frequently normal for suspected stress fractures
- MR imaging provides superior sensitivity and the ability to diagnose other causes for pain
- MR imaging is performed without contrast unless pathologic fracture is a clinical concern

Summary
Stress fractures encompass fatigue and insufficiency fractures. Fatigue fracture is abnormal stress on normal bone. Insufficiency fracture is normal stress on abnormal bone. Radiographs are frequently normal and MR imaging provides better diagnostic capabilities. T1-weighted and fluid-sensitive sequences provide high diagnostic accuracy and ability to diagnose other etiologies for pain.

Pathologic Fracture

Pathologic fractures are a type of insufficiency fracture. An underlying lesion within the bone weakens the structure so that normal stress leads to fracture. Frequently, these fractures are associated with malignant lesions, with metastasis the most common.[36] Benign lesions, including bone

cysts and fibrous lesions, have also been seen with pathologic fractures.

When a patient presents with a fracture, it is important to exclude an underlying lesion. Patient history, atypical fracture pattern, and radiographic findings can lead to suspicion of an underlying lesion. Recent advancements in MR imaging protocols have made this evaluation more sensitive and specific.[37]

Normal anatomy and imaging technique
Typical appearance of fatty bone marrow (high signal) on T1-weighted sequences is useful for detecting the presence of an underlying lesion. A lesion replaces the normal bone marrow, leading to well-defined T1-weighted marrow signal hypointensity. T1-weighted in-phase and opposed-phase (chemical shift) sequences can assist in the diagnosis[37,38] especially when the fracture site has a heterogeneous T1-weighted signal secondary to hemorrhage (**Fig. 7**). Fluid-sensitive and contrast sequences are less specific given potential similarities between stress and pathologic fractures.[38,39] Diffusion-weighted imaging (DWI) is another sequence that may help the radiologist determine the presence of an underlying lesion.[37]

Imaging Protocols
- T1-weighted: axial and long-axis planes
- T2-weighted fat-suppressed or STIR: axial and long-axis planes
- Chemical shift (in-phase and opposed-phase): axial plane
- Diffusion imaging with ADC mapping: axial plane
- Precontrast and postcontrast T1-weighted fat-suppressed axial, sagittal, and coronal
- Precontrast and postcontrast subtraction images

Imaging findings and pathology
Evaluation with T1-weighted, T2-weighted, and postcontrast sequences can be confusing when

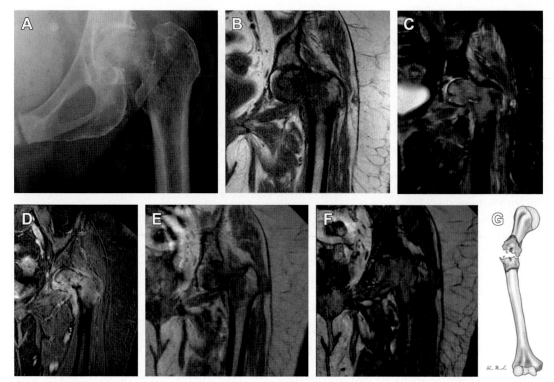

Fig. 7. (A) Radiograph shows osseous demineralization most prominent in the proximal femur with a suspicious permeative pattern. Shortening of the femoral neck with a valgus angulation could be a fracture. MR imaging demonstrates a fracture through the femoral neck with surrounding edema (B, C) and enhancement (D). Heterogeneous signal at the fracture site corresponds to hemorrhage. However, the T1-weighted signal hypointensity (B) extends into the femoral head and intertrochanteric regions, which raises the possibility of an underlying lesion. Chemical shift imaging (T1-weighted in-phase [E] and opposed-phase [F]) confirms the presence of an underlying lesion. The lack of signal drop on the opposed-phase sequence excludes the possibility that the T1-weighted signal hypointensity represented edema or hemorrhage within the marrow adjacent to the fracture site. (G) Pathologic fractures are a type of insufficiency fracture. An underlying lesion within the bone weakens the structure so that normal stress leads to fracture. A lesion replaces the normal bone marrow, leading to well-defined T1-weighted marrow signal hypointensity. T1-weighted in-phase and opposed-phase sequences can assist in the diagnosis especially when the fracture site has a heterogeneous T1-weighted signal secondary to hemorrhage.

trying to determine whether a fracture is pathologic. MR imaging signal intensities of an uncomplicated fracture and pathologic fracture can be much alike. T1-weighted sequences are optimal for evaluating the extent of a marrow-replacing tumor because of the contrast between tumor and fatty marrow.[40] However, in the acute phase of a fracture, edema and hemorrhage replace the normal marrow signal resulting in T1-weighted hypointensity and T2-weighted hyperintensity. After contrast administration, there is enhancement at the fracture site. Secondary imaging findings, including endosteal scalloping and adjacent soft tissue abnormalities, have been shown to help with the diagnosis in these cases.[39]

Chemical shift is a fast imaging technique that can distinguish marrow-replacing tumor from

hematopoietic marrow or hemorrhage within the medullary cavity.[38] In normal fatty marrow, in-phase demonstrates additive signal from water and fat in the same voxel, but opposed-phase shows dropped signal. When a marrow-replacing tumor is present, the opposed-phase sequence does not show a decreased signal when compared with the in-phase image.

DWI is a method of functional imaging commonly used when evaluating the central nervous system.[41] DWI measures the movement of water in the intracellular and extracellular spaces.[42] Within a tumor there is restricted diffusion because of the high cellularity that limits water motion.[43] Correlation with an ADC map is essential to provide a quantitative assessment of the cellularity of a region rather than relying only on the qualitative assessment of DWI.[37]

Diagnostic Criteria
- Well-defined T1-weighted focal hypointensity at the fracture site (chemical shift and DWI imaging may provide additional diagnostic information)
- Endosteal scalloping
- Associated soft tissue component

Differential Diagnosis
- Traumatic fracture
- Stress fracture

Pearls
- MR imaging increases sensitivity and specificity for diagnosis
- Chemical shift and DWI imaging provide additional tools to increase diagnostic accuracy

Pitfalls
- Hemorrhage at the fracture site can lead to confusion in interpretation

What the Referring Physician Needs to Know
- Pathologic fracture is a type of insufficiency fracture
- Patient history, atypical fracture pattern, or radiographic findings may lead to suspicion of a pathologic fracture
- MR imaging can be used in indeterminate cases

Summary
Pathologic fracture is a subtype of insufficiency fracture. T1-weighted and chemical shift sequences are important for evaluating changes in the normal marrow signal. If there is clinical or radiographic suspicion of an underlying lesion, MR imaging frequently can assist in the diagnosis and, perhaps, alter the treatment.

JOINTS
Septic Arthritis

Septic arthritis is an intra-articular infection. Modes of inoculation include direct extension and hematologic spread (**Fig. 8**D). Early diagnosis is critical to avoid damage to the cartilage and irreversible destruction of the joint.[44] Risk factors include bacteremia (intravenous drug use), joint injections, prosthetic joints, and an immunocompromised state. Patients present with joint pain and clinical signs of infection including fever, elevated inflammatory markers, and white blood cell count. Diagnosis is made with joint aspiration[45] and culture. However, MR imaging can provide evidence to support the clinical diagnosis.

Normal anatomy and imaging technique
Similar to imaging in osteomyelitis, T1-weighted and fluid-sensitive sequences are the mainstay for evaluating musculoskeletal infections (**Fig. 8**A, B). Postcontrast T1-weighted fat-suppressed images are obtained if there are no contraindications (**Fig. 8**C). In addition to bone, evaluation of the synovium and surrounding soft tissues helps to suggest septic arthritis from other causes of joint effusion.[46]

Imaging Protocols
Primary Protocol
- T1-weighted non-fat-saturated
- Fluid-sensitive sequence (T2-weighted fat-suppressed or STIR)
Additional Sequences
- Precontrast and postcontrast T1-weighted fat-suppressed

Imaging findings and pathology
On noncontrast MR imaging, joint effusion and perisynovial edema are commonly seen with septic joints.[46] Unlike other etiologies for joint effusion, with infection the surrounding soft tissues demonstrate marked inflammation/edematous change including fasciitis and myositis (**Fig. 9**). However, the fluid signal in a joint effusion from noninfectious causes has the same signal intensity as a joint effusion from an infected joint. Also, the smaller joints of the hands and feet may not demonstrate an effusion with a septic joint.[46] Postcontrast imaging helps to evaluate the degree of synovial inflammation and the presence of perisynovial abscess. These associated findings increase the degree of confidence in suggesting septic arthritis.[46]

When septic arthritis is suspected, evaluation of the surrounding osseous structures frequently demonstrates edema. Differential considerations include reactive edema from the synovial inflammation and osteomyelitis[46] (**Fig. 10**). Diagnosing osteomyelitis adjacent to a joint is like diagnosing osteomyelitis at other locations and is discussed separately.

Diagnostic Criteria
MR imaging findings associated with septic arthritis[46]
- Synovial enhancement
- Perisynovial edema
- Joint effusion
- Fluid decompressing from joint
- Fluid enhancement
- Synovial thickening

Differential Diagnosis
- Inflammatory arthritis

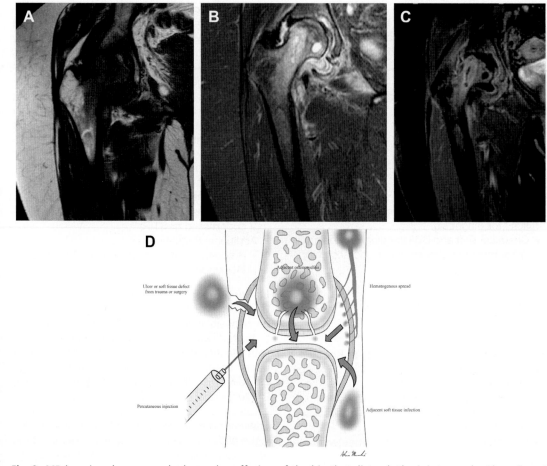

Fig. 8. MR imaging shows a marked complex effusion of the hip that distends the joint capsule. There is peri-synovial edema (*A, B*), synovial enhancement, and thickening (*C*). Edema extends to involve the gluteal and adductor muscle compartments (*B*). There is associated osteomyelitis in the femoral head and neck (*A*) with an intraosseous abscess in the femoral neck (*C*) (a geode is incidentally noted in the inferior aspect of the femoral head). (*D*) Septic arthritis is an intra-articular infection. Modes of inoculation include direct extension (adjacent soft tissue infection, ulcer, or osteomyelitis), percutaneous injection, surgical procedure, and hematologic spread.

- Degenerative arthritis
- Posttraumatic effusion/inflammation

Pearls
- Joint effusion and synovial enhancement are frequently present
- Smaller joints of the extremities may not have a joint effusion
- Imaging protocol should include T1-weighted sequences to evaluate for concomitant osteomyelitis

Pitfalls
- Although MR imaging findings may correlate with septic arthritis, there is a lack of specificity

- Most joint effusions are noninfectious

What the Referring Physician Needs to Know
- Joint aspiration and culture should be performed in suspected cases
- MR imaging findings can support the diagnosis and evaluate for concomitant osteomyelitis

Summary
In clinically suspected cases of septic arthritis, joint aspiration and culture should be performed. MR imaging findings, including joint effusion and synovial enhancement, have a high correlation, although not specific for an infected joint. Early diagnosis and treatment is critical to prevent cartilage damage and joint destruction.

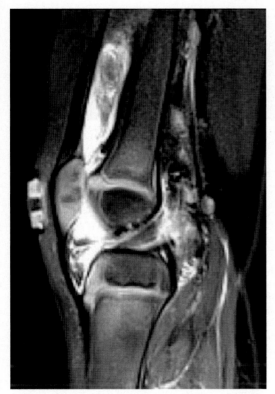

Fig. 9. Although joint effusion is a highly sensitive indicator of septic arthritis, the large complex effusion in this pediatric patient was secondary to juvenile idiopathic arthritis. Note that despite the complexity and size of the effusion, there is a lack of the soft tissue inflammation surrounding the joint that would be typical of an infected joint.

MUSCLE
Rhabdomyolysis

Rhabdomyolysis is the breakdown of skeletal muscle from traumatic and nontraumatic causes. With muscle cell injury or death, the intracellular components are released into the bloodstream leading to serious adverse events (**Fig. 11**D). The syndrome usually manifests with muscle pain, weakness, and dark urine. Early diagnosis and treatment can prevent long-term complications and be life saving.[47]

Nontraumatic causes include drugs (cocaine, common in the western world), ischemia, infection, and immobilization. The release of myoglobin can result in acute kidney injury, cardiac arrhythmias, and tetanus. On clinical testing, creatinine kinase,[48] potassium, and urine myoglobin levels are elevated.

Normal anatomy and imaging technique

Skeletal muscle has a characteristic appearance on MR imaging. On T1-weighted sequences, signal from skeletal muscle is much lower than fat and slightly higher than water. On fat-suppressed fluid-sensitive sequences, the signal is much lower than water and higher than fat. Muscle size and shape can be evaluated on other modalities, but MR imaging provides the advantage of also showing changes in muscle signal.

The muscle cell injury leads to alterations in the normal signal characteristics making MR imaging useful given its sensitivity to soft tissue abnormalities. T1-weighted, fluid-sensitive sequences, and gadolinium-enhanced sequences are typically performed. However, given the potential for kidney injury and a rare complication of nephrogenic systemic sclerosis, the glomerular filtration rate needs to be checked before the administration of contrast. Given the potential for subtle abnormalities, the field of view may be increased to include the opposite extremity for comparison.

Imaging Protocols
- T1-weighted: axial and long axis
- Fat-suppressed fluid-sensitive sequence (T2-weighted fat-suppressed or STIR): axial and long axis

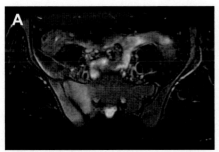
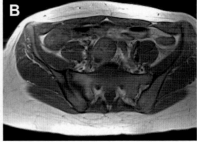

Fig. 10. (*A*) Effusion and bone marrow edema at the right sacroiliac joint were the result of an inflammatory arthropathy, not infection. (*B*) The corresponding T1-weighted hypointensity involving the sacrum and ilium adjacent to the right sacroiliac joint represent noninfectious sclerosis. Final diagnosis was made after joint aspiration, bone biopsy, and patient history.

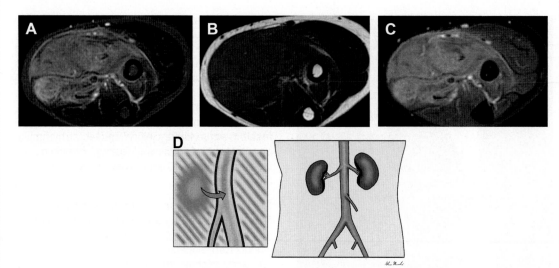

Fig. 11. Drug-induced rhabdomyolysis. There is relatively homogenous increased signal (*A*, *B*) and enhancement (*C*) involving the supinator, pronator teres, flexor carpi radialis, and flexor digitorum superficialis, compatible with type 1 rhabdomyolysis. Traumatic muscle injury or other inflammatory myopathies may have a similar imaging appearance; the clinical context is important when interpreting the study. (*D*) With muscle cell injury or death, the intracellular components are released into the bloodstream leading to serious adverse events. Given the potential for kidney injury and a rare complication of nephrogenic systemic sclerosis, the glomerular filtration rate needs to be checked before the administration of intravenous contrast for imaging.

- Precontrast and postcontrast T1-weighted fat-saturated

Imaging findings and pathology
Rhabdomyolysis represents damage to skeletal muscle resulting in release of potentially harmful intracellular contents into the bloodstream. MR imaging of skeletal muscle may be nonspecific without clinical context.[49] In cases where rhabdomyolysis is suspected, MR imaging can help differentiate between various myopathies; evaluate the extent of disease; and show the presence of muscle necrosis, which is referred to as the "stipple" sign.[50]

Two types of rhabdomyolysis have been described based on muscle signal intensity and presence of myonecrosis.[50] In type 1, there is homogenous signal abnormality on all sequences (**Fig. 11**A–C). Findings are difficult to differentiate from other causes of muscle edema, such as myositis and myopathy (ie, muscle tear, infection).[49] In type 2, more severe muscle damage leads to heterogeneous signal on T1 and fluid-sensitive sequences. Postcontrast images demonstrate peripheral enhancement in the regions of myonecrosis (**Fig. 12**). Areas with type 1 lesions have been shown to be reversible; type 2 lesions result in permanent damage.[51]

Diagnostic Criteria
    Type 1

- T1-weighted: homogenously isointense to hyperintense
- Fluid-sensitive: homogenously hyperintense
- Postcontrast T1-weighted: homogenously enhancing

Type 2
- T1-weighted: variable isointense to hyperintense
- Fluid-sensitive: heterogeneously hyperintense
- Postcontrast T1-weighted: peripherally enhancing

Differential Diagnosis
- Infectious/inflammatory/traumatic myositis
- Early myositis ossificans
- Neuropathic changes
- Infiltrating neoplasm

Pearls
- MR imaging is highly sensitive for detecting muscle abnormalities including distribution and extent of disease
- MR imaging can detect areas of myonecrosis

Pitfalls
- MR imaging findings are nonspecific
- Failure to diagnose can lead to long-term complications

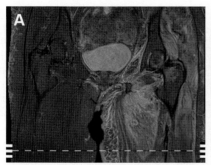
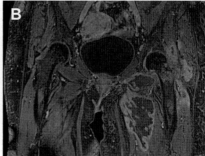

Fig. 12. Drug-induced (acetaminophen) rhabdomyolysis. (*A*) There is marked edema throughout the left adductor and gluteal muscle compartments. On the fat-suppressed fluid-sensitive sequence (*A*) there is a suggestion of heterogeneous areas in the adductor muscles. (*B*) Postcontrast image shows peripheral enhancement in these regions indicating areas of myonecrosis (type 2 rhabdomyolysis). Both lower extremities were included in the field of view for comparison and evaluation for subtle muscle signal changes.

What the Referring Physician Needs to Know
- Rhabdomyolysis is a clinical and laboratory diagnosis
- MR imaging is highly sensitive for detecting muscle abnormalities including extent of disease and presence of myonecrosis

Summary
Rhabdomyolysis is the breakdown of skeletal muscle from traumatic and nontraumatic causes. Two types of rhabdomyolysis have been described on MR imaging that correlate with the degree of severity and reversibility. Type 1 shows homogenous signal abnormalities on all sequences. Type 2 shows heterogeneous signal abnormalities with areas of rim enhancement. Early diagnosis and treatment is critical to preventing long-term complications.

Compartment Syndrome

Fascia is a connective tissue that invests muscles providing protection and acting as a supportive structure for myofibril attachments. Compartment syndrome occurs when the pressure within a muscle compartment exceeds the perfusion pressure.[52–55] The result is ischemia of the muscles and nerves, which can lead to necrosis if left untreated.

Acute and chronic compartment syndromes vary in their presentation and cause.[55] Acute compartment syndrome is most commonly caused by trauma including fractures and penetrating injury. Other etiologies resulting in muscle edema or muscle compartment expansion[56] (ie, hematoma, burns, rhabdomyolysis, muscle hypertrophy, autoimmune vasculitis, deep venous thrombosis/muscle ischemia) can lead to acute compartment syndrome.

Chronic exertional compartment syndrome (CECS) frequently occurs in younger patients

who participate in sports. Presenting symptoms include recurrent bouts of pain after exercise that improve with rest.[55,57] They may worsen over time leading to severe limitations in activity.[55] There may be residual tenderness or weakness and sensory abnormalities of an involved nerve may be present. Symptoms may mimic other causes of exercise-induced pain including shin splints. Along with clinical history, MR imaging can help in the diagnosis and in considering other causes of pain.

Normal anatomy and imaging technique
Diagnosing acute compartment syndrome is critically important to prevent long-term complications. The standard for diagnosis is measurement of intracompartmental pressure. Imaging does not have a role in the initial diagnosis, but can evaluate for other disorders once compartment syndrome is excluded.

CECS can be a difficult diagnosis, often unsuspected on initial presentation.[58,59] The syndrome usually presents in younger athletes, with lower extremity pain that is often bilateral.[60] Most sports usually require intensive exercise of the lower extremity muscles; the anterior compartment of the lower leg is most commonly affected in CECS.[61]

Out-of-scanner and in-scanner exercise protocols are used to induce the patient's symptoms for imaging.[52] T1-weighted and fat-suppressed fluid-sensitive sequences are used to evaluate changes in muscle signal; involved compartments; and concurrent pathology, such as shin splints.

Imaging Protocols
- T1-weighted: axial and coronal plane
- T2-weighted fat-suppressed or STIR: axial and coronal plane

Imaging findings and pathology

Compartment syndrome occurs when intracompartmental pressure exceeds the perfusion pressure (**Fig. 13**E). When fluid is introduced into a compartment or a muscle swells, the interstitial pressure rises, which can lead to capillary collapse and tissue ischemia. The result is increased vascular permeability leading to more interstitial fluid and higher pressure.[62] This cycle of events worsens muscle perfusion and can lead to necrosis.

MR imaging is highly sensitive for detecting changes in muscle edema and interstitial fluid[57,62,63] (**Fig. 13**A–D). Fat-suppressed fluid-sensitive sequences demonstrate hyperintensity in the affected muscles and possibly muscle enlargement. The degree of T2-weighted signal abnormality has been shown to correlate with elevated intracompartmental pressures.[60,62,63]

On T1-weighted sequences, with an increase in interstitial fluid, a loss in the expected fat-striated appearance of muscle may be observed along with an increased relaxation time.[64–66] MR imaging protocols have demonstrated high sensitivity and specificity[62] with CECS. Symptom-provoking exercise either immediately before imaging or during the scan is a potential alternative to invasive testing.[57,62,63]

Diagnostic Criteria
- Fat-suppressed fluid-sensitive sequence: muscular edema; possible muscular enlargement/swelling
- T1-weighted sequence: increased relaxation time
- Anterior and lateral compartment of the lower extremity most commonly affected
- Frequently bilateral

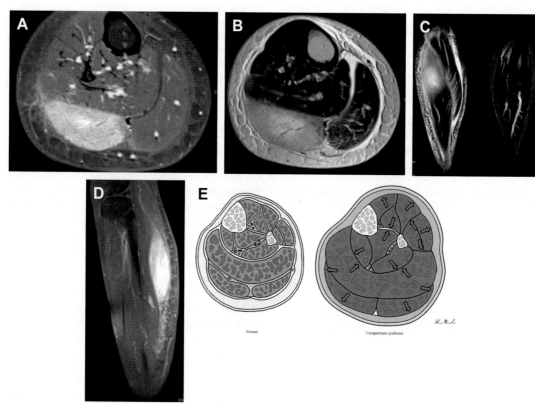

Fig. 13. Proton-density fat-suppressed (*A*) and T2-weighted axial sequences (*B*) show marked edema in the lateral gastrocnemius and muscle enlargement. (*B, C*) There is mild edema of the medial gastrocnemius muscle and fluid tracking along the deep fascial compartments predominantly involving the superficial posterior compartment. T1-weighted fat-suppressed contrast-enhanced sagittal image (*D*) shows avid homogenous enhancement corresponding to the marked edema in the lateral gastrocnemius muscle. (*E*) Compartment syndrome occurs when intracompartmental pressure exceeds the perfusion pressure. When fluid is introduced into a compartment or a muscle swells, the interstitial pressure rises, which can lead to capillary collapse and tissue ischemia. The result is increased vascular permeability leading to more interstitial fluid and higher pressure. This cycle of events worsens muscle perfusion and can lead to necrosis. (*Courtesy of [A–D]* Frank Roemer, MD, Klinikum Augsburg, Germany.)

Differential Diagnosis
- Repetitive stress injury (medial tibial stress syndrome)
- Popliteal artery entrapment syndrome
- Nerve entrapment
- Muscle herniation
- Baker cyst rupture

Pearls
- MR imaging is a potential alternative to invasive testing for CECS
- MR imaging has been shown to be highly sensitive and specific for CECS
- Allows for detection of alternative or concomitant pathologies

Pitfalls
- Nonexercise protocol may fail to diagnose CECS
- In suspected acute compartment syndrome, intracompartmental pressure measurement is the standard for diagnosis, not imaging

What the Referring Physician Needs to Know
- In patients with recurring lower extremity pain with activity, CECS should be a differential consideration
- MR imaging can be considered for evaluation; however, specify suspected CECS so an exercise protocol is performed

Summary

Acute and CECS vary in their presentation and cause. Acute compartment syndrome is most frequently caused by trauma and diagnosed by intracompartmental pressure measurements. CECS presents with pain during activity, usually in the lower extremities, that improves with cessation of the activity. An exercise protocol MR imaging is a potential alternative to invasive testing for CECS. In addition, other causes or concomitant pathologies can be diagnosed.

SOFT TISSUES
Necrotizing Fasciitis

Necrotizing fasciitis is an infection of the subcutaneous tissues and deep fascia that progresses rapidly.[67] Initially, the underlying muscle is not typically involved. Early in the disease process, necrotizing fasciitis may present similarly to cellulitis,[68] although, accurate diagnosis and surgical debridement lead to improved survival.[69] Single organism and polymicrobial infections can cause necrotizing fasciitis.[70] The organisms are frequently toxin-producing, resulting in systemic failure and rapid death.

Normal anatomy and imaging technique

Infections can involve various layers of the soft tissues including skin, subcutaneous fat, subcutaneous fascia, deep fascia, and muscle (**Fig. 14F**). The fascia, connecting skin and muscle, is a conduit for the spread of infection.[71] Cellulitis is an infection of multiple soft tissue layers but it usually spares the deep fascia, unlike necrotizing fasciitis.[72] Rapid diagnosis is critical for successful treatment. Computed tomography scan can be performed quickly to evaluate for gas, thickened fascia, muscle edema, and fluid tracking along deep fascial sheaths[73,74] (**Fig. 14A, B**). If further imaging evaluation is warranted, MR imaging is a sensitive tool for detecting involvement of the deep fascia[73] (**Fig. 14C–E**).

Fat-suppressed fluid-sensitive and contrast-enhanced T1-weighted sequences are frequently used in the evaluation. Axial and long axis plane imaging (depending on the site of involvement) should be performed. A detailed examination for abnormal muscle signal, necrosis, fascial thickness, fluid along the fascia, and abscess is critical.[73,75]

Imaging Protocol
- Fluid-sensitive sequence (T2-weighted fat-suppressed or STIR): axial and a long axis plane
- T1-weighted: axial and a long axis plane
- Precontrast and postcontrast fat-suppressed T1-weighted: axial and long axis

Imaging findings and pathology

Necrotizing fasciitis is a bacterial infection usually involving the deep fascia that can be rapidly fatal. Gas (signal void on MR imaging) within the necrotic fascia is characteristic of the disease but is not always present.[75,76] MR imaging is highly sensitive for detecting abnormalities of the fascia including thickening, enhancement, and tracking fluid.[77] Fluid-sensitive sequences are highly sensitive for detecting abnormalities of the fascia, although they may overestimate the extent of infected tissue. Alternatively, postcontrast images may underestimate the degree of involvement because of necrosis and hypoperfusion.[78] Also, other infectious, inflammatory, or traumatic etiologies can present with fascial abnormalities.[77] Clinical history, physical examination findings, and laboratory testing can assist in narrowing the differential diagnosis.

Diagnostic Criteria
- Fat-suppressed fluid-sensitive sequences: thick (>3 mm) hyperintense signal in the deep fascia

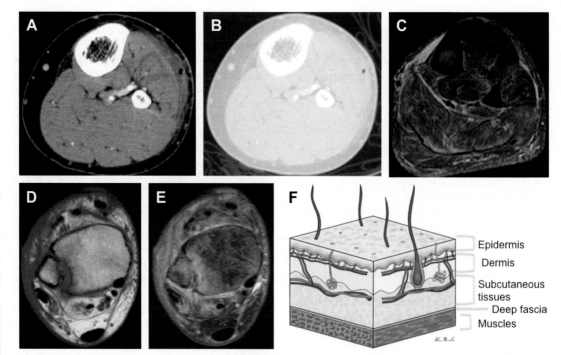

Fig. 14. Soft tissue gas on computed tomography (*A, B*—gas is in the soft tissues overlying the anterior/lateral compartments) is more conspicuous when compared with MR imaging (*C, D, E*—focus of gas [signal void] is posterior to the tibialis anterior tendon). Differential considerations for a signal void on MR imaging include gas but the void may also represent calcium, vessel flow void, or an artifact from surgical material/foreign body. (*C*) Fluid tracking along fascial planes, fascial thickening, and associated muscle changes are more clearly demonstrated on MR imaging. (*F*) Infections can involve various layers of the soft tissues including skin, subcutaneous fat, subcutaneous fascia, deep fascia, and muscle. Cellulitis is an infection of multiple soft tissue layers but it usually spares the deep fascia, unlike necrotizing fasciitis. Initially, the underlying muscle is not typically involved in necrotizing fasciitis.

- Fat-suppressed T1-weighted postcontrast sequences: mixed pattern of enhancement along a thickened fascia
- Involvement of multiple myofascial compartments
- Gas (signal void) within the necrotic fascia is characteristic, although not always present

Differential Diagnosis
- Cellulitis
- Infectious myositis/pyomyositis
- Posttraumatic changes (ie, muscle or tendon tear, soft tissue contusion, degloving injury)

Pearls
- MR imaging has a high sensitivity
- Necrotizing fasciitis usually involves the deep fascia

Pitfalls
- MR imaging has a low specificity

- Gas (signal voids) within the soft tissues is characteristic, although not always present

What the Referring Physician Needs to Know
- Necrotizing fasciitis can be rapidly fatal, so early diagnosis is critical
- Early in the disease process, gas along the necrotic fascia may not be present
- MR imaging findings can assist in the diagnosis especially in cases that are indeterminate based on clinical presentation

Summary
Necrotizing fasciitis is a bacterial infection usually involving the deep fascia that progresses rapidly. Surgical debridement can improve the outcome. Diagnosis may be difficult because of early presentation or confounding clinical findings. MR imaging, although extremely sensitive for detecting fascial disease, lacks specificity. Imaging should not delay treatment, but can facilitate the diagnosis in difficult cases.

REFERENCES

1. Tehranzadeh J, Wang F, Mesgarzadeh M. Magnetic resonance imaging of osteomyelitis. Crit Rev Diagn Imaging 1992;33(6):495–534.
2. Pineda C, Vargas A, Rodríguez AV. Imaging of osteomyelitis: current concepts. Infect Dis Clin North Am 2006;20(4):789–825.
3. Waldvogel FA, Medoff G, Swartz MN. Osteomyelitis: a review of clinical features, therapeutic considerations and unusual aspects. N Engl J Med 1970; 282(4):198–206.
4. Schweitzer ME, Daffner RH, Weissman BN, et al. ACR Appropriateness Criteria on suspected osteomyelitis in patients with diabetes mellitus. J Am Coll Radiol 2008;5(8):881–6.
5. Kapoor A, Page S, Lavalley M, et al. Magnetic resonance imaging for diagnosing foot osteomyelitis: a meta-analysis. Arch Intern Med 2007; 167(2):125–32.
6. Kocher MS, Lee B, Dolan M, et al. Pediatric orthopedic infections; early detection and treatment. Pediatr Ann 2006;35:112–22.
7. Morrison WB, Schweitzer ME, Bock GW, et al. Diagnosis of osteomyelitis: utility of fat-suppressed contrast-enhanced MR imaging. Radiology 1993; 189(1):251–7.
8. Craig JG, Amin MB, Wu K, et al. Osteomyelitis of the diabetic foot: MR imaging–pathologic correlation. Radiology 1997;203:849–55.
9. Flemming D, Murphey M, McCarthy K. Imaging of the foot and ankle: summary and update. Curr Opin Orthop 2005;16:54–9.
10. Collins MS, Schaar MM, Wenger DE, et al. T1-weighted MRI characteristics of pedal osteomyelitis. AJR Am J Roentgenol 2005;185(2):386–93.
11. Kowalski TJ, Layton KF, Berbari EF, et al. Follow-up MR imaging in patients with pyogenic spine infections: lack of correlation with clinical features. AJNR Am J Neuroradiol 2007;28(4):693–9.
12. Pineda C, Espinosa R, Pena A. Radiographic imaging in osteomyelitis: the role of plain radiography, computed tomography, ultrasonography, magnetic resonance imaging, and scintigraphy. Semin Plast Surg 2009;23(2):80–9.
13. Gold RH, Hawkins RA, Katz RD. Bacterial osteomyelitis: findings on plain radiography CT, MR and scintigraphy. AJR Am J Roentgenol 1991; 157:365–70.
14. Morrison WB, Schweitzer ME, Batte WG, et al. Osteomyelitis of the foot: relative importance of primary and secondary MR imaging signs. Radiology 1998;207(3):625–32.
15. Marcus CD, Ladam-Marcus VJ, Leone J, et al. MR imaging of osteomyelitis and neuropathic osteoarthropathy in the feet of diabetics. Radiographics 1996; 16(6):1337–48.
16. Chan K, Mok C. Glucocorticoid-induced avascular bone necrosis: diagnosis and management. Open Orthop J 2012;6:449–57.
17. Yochum T, Rowe L. Essentials of skeletal radiology. 2nd edition. Baltimore (MD): Williams & Wilkins; 1996. p. 260–3.
18. Karantanas AH, Drakonaki EE. The role of MR imaging in avascular necrosis of the femoral head. Semin Musculoskelet Radiol 2011;15(3):281–300.
19. Khanna AJ, Yoon TR, Mont MA, et al. Femoral head osteonecrosis: detection and grading by using a rapid MR imaging protocol. Radiology 2000;217(1): 188–92.
20. Glickstein MF, Burk DL, Schiebler ML, et al. Avascular necrosis versus other diseases of the hip: sensitivity of MR imaging. Radiology 1988;169(1): 213–5.
21. Lee JH, Dyke JP, Ballon D, et al. Assessment of bone perfusion with contrast-enhanced magnetic resonance imaging. Orthop Clin North Am 2009; 40(2):249–57.
22. Ficat RP, Arlet J. Necrosis of the femoral head. In: Hungerford DS, editor. Ischemia and necrosis of bone. Philadelphia: Lippincott Williams & Wilkins; 1980. p. 171.
23. Mitchell DG, Rao VM, Dalinka MK, et al. Femoral head avascular necrosis: correlation of MR imaging, radiographic staging, radionuclide imaging, and clinical findings. Radiology 1987;162(3):709–15.
24. Shimizu K, Moriya H, Akita T. Prediction of collapse with magnetic resonance imaging of avascular necrosis of the femoral head. J Bone Joint Surg Am 1994;76:215–33.
25. Gruson KI, Kwon YW. Atraumatic osteonecrosis of the humeral head. Bull NYU Hosp Jt Dis 2009; 67(1):6–14.
26. Lee GC, Steinberg ME. Are we evaluating osteonecrosis adequately? Int Orthop 2012;36(12):2433–9.
27. Pommering TL, Kluchurosky L. Overuse injuries in adolescents. Adolesc Med State Art Rev 2007; 18(1):95–120, ix.
28. Daffner RH. Stress fractures: current concepts. Skeletal Radiol 1978;2:221–9.
29. Burgener FA, Kormano M, Pudas T. Bone and joint disorders. New York: Thieme; 2006.
30. Porrino JA, Kohl CA, Taljanovic M, et al. Diagnosis of proximal femoral insufficiency fractures in patients receiving bisphosphonate therapy. AJR Am J Roentgenol 2010;194(4):1061–4.
31. Lee JK, Yao L. Stress fractures: MR imaging. Radiology 1988;169(1):217–20.
32. Umans HR, Kaye JJ. Longitudinal stress fractures of the tibia: diagnosis by magnetic resonance imaging. Skeletal Radiol 1996;25(4):319–24.
33. Torbet JT, Lackman RD. Pathological fractures. Chapter 2. In: Pignolo RJ, Keenan MA, Hebela NM, editors. Fractures in the elderly. A

guide to practical management. New York: Springer; 2011. p. 43–53, XII.

34. Haworth AE, Webb J. Skeletal complications of bisphosphonate use: what the radiologist should know. Br J Radiol 2012;85(1018):1333–42.

35. Yoon RS, Hwang JS, Beebe KS. Long-term bisphosphonate usage and subtrochanteric insufficiency fractures: a cause for concern? J Bone Joint Surg Br 2011;93(10):1289–95.

36. Hage WD, Aboulafia AJ, Aboulafia DM. Incidence, location and diagnostic evaluation of metastatic bone disease. Orthop Clin North Am 2000;31: 515–28.

37. Fayad LM, Jacobs MA, Wang X, et al. Musculoskeletal tumors: how to use anatomic, functional, and metabolic MR techniques. Radiology 2012;265(2): 340–56.

38. Zajick DC Jr, Morrison WB, Schweitzer ME, et al. Benign and malignant processes: normal values and differentiation with chemical shift MR imaging in vertebral marrow. Radiology 2005;237(2):590–6.

39. Fayad LM, Kawamoto S, Kamel IR, et al. Distinction of long bone stress fractures from pathological fractures on cross-sectional imaging: how successful are we? Am J Roentgenol 2005;185(4):915–24.

40. Richardson ML, Amparo EG, Gillespy T 3rd, et al. Theoretical considerations for optimizing intensity differences between primary musculoskeletal tumors and normal tissue with spin-echo magnetic resonance imaging. Invest Radiol 1985;20(5):492–7.

41. Chenevert TL, Meyer CR, Moffat BA, et al. Diffusion MRI: a new strategy for assessment of cancer therapeutic efficacy. Mol Imaging 2002;1(4):336–43.

42. Szafer A, Zhong J, Gore JC. Theoretical model for water diffusion in tissues. Magn Reson Med 1995; 33(5):697–712.

43. Dudeck O, Zeile M, Pink D, et al. Diffusion-weighted magnetic resonance imaging allows monitoring of anticancer treatment effects in patients with soft-tissue sarcomas. J Magn Reson Imaging 2008; 27(5):1109–13.

44. Learch TJ, Farooki S. Magnetic resonance imaging of septic arthritis. Clin Imaging 2000;24:236–42.

45. Gilbert MS, Aledort LM, Seremetis S, et al. Long term evaluation of septic arthritis in hemophilic patients. Clin Orthop Relat Res 1996;(328):54–9.

46. Karchevsky M, Schweitzer ME, Morrison WB, et al. MRI findings of septic arthritis and associated osteomyelitis in adults. AJR Am J Roentgenol 2004; 182(1):119–22.

47. Moratalla MB, Braun P, Fornas GM. Importance of MRI in the diagnosis and treatment of rhabdomyolysis. Eur J Radiol 2008;65(2):311–5.

48. Khan FY. Rhabdomyolysis: a review of the literature. Neth J Med 2009;67:272–83.

49. May DA, Disler DG, Jones EA, et al. Abnormal signal intensity in skeletal muscle at MR imaging: patterns, pearls, and pitfalls. Radiographics 2000; 20:S295–315.

50. Lu CH, Tsang YM, Yu CW, et al. Rhabdomyolysis: magnetic resonance imaging and computed tomography findings. J Comput Assist Tomogr 2007;31(3): 368–74.

51. Cheng YC, Lan HH, Shih CH, et al. Magnetic resonance imaging of rhabdomyolysis: muscle necrosis versus ischemia. J Radiol Sci 38:143–8.

52. Ringler MD, Litwiller DV, Felmlee JP, et al. MRI accurately detects chronic exertional compartment syndrome: a validation study. Skeletal Radiol 2013; 42(3):385–92.

53. Detmer DE, Sharpe K, Sufit RL, et al. Chronic compartment syndrome: diagnosis, management, and outcomes. Am J Sports Med 1985;13(3):162–9.

54. Leversedge FJ, Casey PJ, Seiler JG, et al. Endoscopically assisted fasciotomy: description of technique and in-vitro assessment of lower-leg compartment decompression. Am J Sports Med 2002;30(2):272–8.

55. Blackman PG. A review of chronic exertional compartment syndrome in the lower leg. Med Sci Sports Exerc 2000;32(3 Suppl):S4–10.

56. Mubarak SJ, Hargens AR. Acute compartment syndromes. Surg Clin North Am 1983;63(3):539–65.

57. Lecocq J, Isner-Horobeti ME, Dupeyron A, et al. Exertional compartment syndrome. Ann Readapt Med Phys 2004;47(6):334–45.

58. Tekwani K, Sikka R. High-risk chief complaints III: abdomen and extremities. Emerg Med Clin North Am 2009;27(4):747–65, x.

59. George CA, Hutchinson MR. Chronic exertional compartment syndrome. Clin Sports Med 2012; 31(2):307–19.

60. Tucker AK. Chronic exertional compartment syndrome of the leg. Curr Rev Musculoskelet Med 2010;3(1–4):32–7.

61. Schubert AG. Exertional compartment syndrome: review of the literature and proposed rehabilitation guidelines following surgical release. Int J Sports Phys Ther 2011;6(2):126–41.

62. Litwiller DV, Amrami KK, Dahm DL, et al. Chronic exertional compartment syndrome of the lower extremities: improved screening using a novel dual birdcage coil and in-scanner exercised protocol. Skeletal Radiol 2007;36(11):1067–75.

63. Amendola A, Rorabeck CH, Vellett D, et al. The use of magnetic resonance imaging in exertional compartment syndromes. Am J Sports Med 1990; 18(1):29–34.

64. Fleckenstein JL, Canby RC, Parkey RW, et al. Acute effects of exercise on MR imaging of skeletal muscle in normal volunteers. AJR Am J Roentgenol 1988; 151(2):231–7.

65. Adams GR, Duvoisin MR, Dudley GA. Magnetic resonance imaging and electromyography as

indexes of muscle function. J Appl Physiol 1992; 73(4):1578–83.

66. Paz Maya S, Dualde Beltrán D, Lemercier P, et al. Necrotizing fasciitis: an urgent diagnosis. Skeletal Radiol 2014;43(5):577–89.

67. Fugitt JB, Puckett ML, Quigley MM, et al. Necrotizing fasciitis. Radiographics 2004;24(5):1472–6.

68. Becker M, Zbaren P, Hermans R, et al. Necrotizing fasciitis of the head and neck: role of CT in diagnosis and management. Radiology 1997;202:471–6.

69. Voros D, Pissiotis C, Georgantas D, et al. Role of early and extensive surgery in the treatment of severe necrotizing soft tissue infections. Br J Surg 1993;80:1190–1.

70. Callahan E, Adal K, Tomecki K. Cutaneous (non HIV) infections. Dermatol Clin 2000;18:497–508.

71. Kothari NA, Pelchovitz DJ, Meyer JS. Imaging of musculoskeletal infections. Radiol Clin North Am 2001;39(4):653–71.

72. Malghem J, Lecouvet FE, Omoumi P, et al. Necrotizing fasciitis: contribution and limitations of diagnostic imaging. Joint Bone Spine 2013;80(2): 146–54.

73. Schmid MR, Kossman T, Duewell S. Differentiation of necrotizing fasciitis and cellulitis using MR imaging. AJR Am J Roentgenol 1998;170:615–20.

74. Wu CM, Davis F, Fishman EK. Musculoskeletal complications of the patient with acquired immunodeficiency syndrome (AIDS): CT evaluation. Semin Ultrasound CT MR 1998;19:200–8.

75. Struk D, Munk P, Lee M, et al. Imaging of soft tissue infections. Radiol Clin North Am 2001;39:277–301.

76. Rehman J, Kaynan A, Samadi D, et al. Air on radiography of perirenal necrotizing fasciitis indicates testis involvement. J Urol 1999;162:2101.

77. Ali SZ, Srinivasan S, Peh WC. MRI in necrotizing fasciitis of the extremities. Br J Radiol 2014;87(1033): 20130560.

78. Miller T, Randolph D, Staron R, et al. Fat-suppressed MRI of musculoskeletal infection: fast T2-weighted techniques versus gadolinium-enhanced T1-weighted images. Skeletal Radiol 1997;26:654–8.

Emergency Magnetic Resonance Imaging of Musculoskeletal Trauma

Manickam Kumaravel, MD[a],*, William M. Weathers, MD[b]

KEYWORDS

- MR imaging • Musculoskeletal trauma • Morel-Lavalléelesion • Internal derangement knee
- Fracture • Osteochondral defects • Ligament injury • Tendon injury

KEY POINTS

- Magnetic resonance (MR) imaging is a superior modality for assessment of musculoskeletal (MSK) soft tissue injury in both high-velocity and low-velocity trauma.
- Understanding of normal anatomy in the MSK system is critical to interpretation.
- Any increased T2-weighted signal should alert the radiologist to abnormality at that site.
- MR imaging is the most appropriate modality for evaluation of subtle bone injury.
- MR imaging with short, rapid sequences is paramount in the setting of trauma.

INTRODUCTION

Musculoskeletal (MSK) trauma is commonly encountered in emergency departments. The degree of MSK trauma ranges from trivial injuries to significant life-threatening injuries. Imaging plays an integral role in diagnosis and management of these injuries. The most commonly used modality in the diagnosis of MSK injuries continues to be plain radiographs. For more complex injuries, computed tomography (CT) is still the most commonly available and widely used cross-sectional imaging tool. Although CT has many advantages, the soft tissue detail offered by CT scanning is limited in the evaluation of MSK injuries. Magnetic resonance (MR) imaging produces excellent soft tissue contrast and fine anatomic detail. The availability of MR imaging in emergency centers has gradually increased over the years, and, in major trauma centers, the availability of MR imaging 24 hours a day, 7 days a week, is now standard. A corresponding increase in subspecialist availability in orthopedics and

trauma and increased reliance on complex MSK trauma evaluation has further contributed to the increased use of MR imaging in the emergency room (ER) setting. MR imaging provides definitive diagnosis of soft tissue and bony injury both in low-velocity and high-velocity trauma. It acts as an excellent tool in problem solving in repetitive trauma as well as in complex sports injuries.

This article introduces the applications of MR imaging in an emergency setting in the evaluation of MSK trauma. Given the wide range of presenting injuries in MSK trauma in the ER, this article provides an overview of some of the most common injuries, but is not comprehensive. The aim is to educate the reader about recognition of these injuries and mechanisms to avoid pitfalls.

MAGNETIC RESONANCE IMAGING SEQUENCES AND TECHNIQUE CONSIDERATIONS

MR imaging poses multiple challenges to imaging acutely injured patients. With a simple and robust

Disclosure: The authors have nothing to disclose.
[a] Department of Diagnostic and Interventional Imaging, University of Texas Health Science Center at Houston, 6431 Fannin Street, MSB 2.130B Houston, TX 77030, USA; [b] Department of Radiology, University of Texas Health Science Center at Houston, 6431 Fannin Street, MSB 2.130B Houston, TX 77030, USA
* Corresponding author.
E-mail address: Manickam.Kumaravel@uth.tmc.edu

1064-9689/16/$ – see front matter © 2016 Elsevier Inc. All rights reserved.

approach to imaging MSK trauma, relevant and clinically useful imaging can be produced. Based on the type of MR imaging magnet, variable sequences can be used. This article presents a brief summary of sequences used in our institution, which can further be generalized in any modern MR imaging magnet.

The standard MSK technique should include multiplanar proton density (PD) fat-saturation (FS) images, a single-plane T1-weighted sequence and a single-plane T2-weighted sequence. Fast-spin echo (FSE) imaging should be used to reduce imaging time while maintaining sufficient image quality and detail. In some cases (eg, injury to a nonjoint extremity) we begin by obtaining a large field of view coronal short-tau inversion recovery sequence (STIR) over the area of interest. Once the area of concern is identified, multiplanar PD axial, T2-weighted FS and T1-weighted images can be obtained. In addition, single-shot imaging could also be performed for rapid acquisition of images in a patient who cannot stay still. Arthrograms and contrast are unnecessary in MSK evaluation in the trauma setting.

Occult Scaphoid Fracture

Scaphoid fractures can present a diagnostic dilemma in the setting of posttraumatic wrist pain and normal radiographs. Up to 65% of scaphoid fractures are radiographically occult immediately following injury.[1] In general, wrist splinting with follow-up radiographs assessing for bony remodeling is the management of choice at most institutions for suspected occult scaphoid fractures. MR imaging has excellent sensitivity for fractures and can be used in the early posttraumatic setting to confidently exclude fracture and avoid unnecessary immobilization.[2–4]

MR imaging has been shown to be both more specific and more sensitive for radiographically occult scaphoid fractures compared with both CT and plain films, with sensitivity and specificity around 100%.[5] Small field of view acquisition using both FS T1-weighted and fat suppressed T2-weighted images of the wrist are sufficient for diagnosis. The coronal plane is the easiest plane in which to detect scaphoid injury because most fractures are oriented transverse or oblique to the long axis of the scaphoid. Coronal planes are preferred using STIR for screening or rapid evaluation. Trabecular disruption in the scaphoid manifests as linear T1 hypointensities and T2 hyperintensities without cortical disruption in nondisplaced fractures. Otherwise, bone edema, trabecular disruption, and cortical disruption may be present on MR imaging in radiographically occult scaphoid fractures (**Fig. 1**).

Occult Hip Fracture

Occult hip fractures in the setting of trauma or falls can be readily appreciated using MR imaging. Up to 46% to 54% of fractures of the hip and/or pelvis

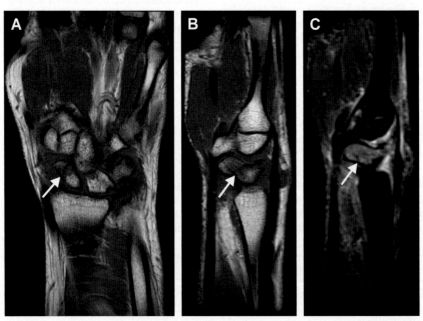

Fig. 1. Occult scaphoid fracture. (*A*) Coronal T1-weighted image shows linear hypointense fracture lines in the scaphoid waist. (*B*) In this case the fracture line is better seen on sagittal T1 images. (*C*) Sagittal T2 FS images show diffuse increased signal in the scaphoid consistent with bone edema and surrounding soft tissue edema.

are occult on initial radiographs.[6,7] Hip fractures have significant morbidity and prompt diagnosis is necessary to ensure the best outcomes.[8]

In addition to MR imaging having superior sensitivity for detection of hip fractures, it is also helpful in detecting unexpected fractures of the pelvis and soft tissue injury, which clinically can mimic hip fractures after trauma.

Similar to other sites of fracture, pelvic and hip fractures show linear T1 hypointensities and edema on T2-weighted images. STIR imaging provides increased sensitivity for detection of marrow and soft tissue edema. A small field of view used for hip imaging may exclude the sacrum, depending on the institution's protocol. In our opinion, a wider field of view that includes the ipsilateral sacrum provides both sufficient resolution and sufficient sensitivity for detection of ipsilateral bony abnormalities and significant soft tissue injuries in the setting of trauma (**Fig. 2**).

Traumatic Chondral and Osteochondral Injuries

Traumatic chondral injuries are most often occult on radiographs, but are superbly shown on MR imaging.[9] The Outerbridge grading system is preferred by our surgeons:

- Grade 0: normal
- Grade 1: softening, mildly increased T2-weighted signal without any significant loss of thickness
- Grade 2: defect less than 50% of cartilage surface
- Grade 3: defect greater than 50% of cartilage surface
- Grade 4: full-thickness defect, often with underlying bone edema

It is important to note the size, location, cartilage surface integrity (such as fraying), and grade of the lesion in the report. Multiplanar imaging is needed for all joints. Most joint surfaces extend along multiple planes and evaluation in the axial, sagittal, and coronal planes may be necessary to see the full extent of the articular surface. Also, careful evaluation of the joint space for chondral and osteochondral bodies (free-floating avulsed cartilage) is needed because these can lead to locking in the acute setting and eventually early onset osteoarthritis. In the presence of bone edema, careful inspection of the cartilage is needed (**Fig. 3**).

Osteochondral defects (OCDs) can be seen on radiographs during the initial trauma work-up, but surgeons prefer further characterization with MR imaging before repair. In particular, detail of the cartilage is not possible with radiography. It is important to identify lesions that have full-thickness cartilage injuries with fracture extending into the underlying bone as well. The most important information to report is the stability of the OCD, because this guides treatment. Findings on T2-weighted images suggestive of an unstable fracture are as follows[10] (**Fig. 4**):

- Increased signal tracking around the fragment
- A 5-mm focus of cystic change between the OCD and adjacent normal bone
- High-signal-intensity linear defect in overlying cartilage and/or 5-mm focal cartilage defect

Lisfranc Injury

Lisfranc injuries are associated with grave outcomes when missed. Approximately 50% of untreated Lisfranc ligamentous complex injuries go on to develop severe degenerative arthritis, plano-valgus deformity, and instability of the midfoot.[11,12]

Injury to the Lisfranc ligamentous complex commonly occurs with an associated fracture dislocation in high-velocity injuries, and can be readily discerned using plain film radiography. In low-velocity injury, subtle disruption of the ligamentous complex can be missed with weight-bearing radiography alone. Also, in the setting of polytrauma, injury to the Lisfranc ligamentous

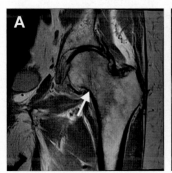
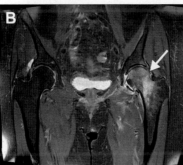

Fig. 2. Occult hip fracture. (*A*) Narrow field of view coronal T1-weighted image shows linear hypointensities. (*B*) Wide field of view coronal T2 FS image shows significant bone edema focused in the femoral neck. Edema is most commonly seen in the medial femoral neck in occult hip fractures.

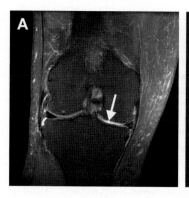
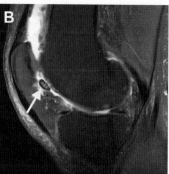

Fig. 3. Chondral injury. (*A*) Coronal PD FS image shows a full-thickness cartilage defect (grade 4) with mild underlying bone edema following trauma in the weight-bearing surface of the medial femoral condyle. (*B*) Sagittal PD FS in the same patient shows an osteochondral body along the anterior articular surface.

complex may be overlooked or the patient may not be able to participate in weight-bearing views, resulting in late diagnosis. The exquisite anatomic detail of this complex ligament can be readily appreciated using MR imaging, which is a helpful adjunct in the assessment and treatment planning of the foot.

The Lisfranc ligament complex consists of 3 ligament bundles connecting the medial cuneiform and the base of the second metatarsal. The complex consists of the dorsal, interosseous, and plantar bundles. Stability of the midfoot is primarily derived from the plantar and interosseous ligament bundles, and careful assessment of these structures is prudent.[11] Small-field-of-view, multiplanar MR images using T1-weighted non–fat-suppressed images and fluid-sensitive fat-suppressed images should be obtained. MR imaging shows T2 signal prolongation in an injured ligament with partial tearing or frank disruption of the ligament (**Fig. 5**). T1-weighted imaging helps detect occult fractures and pathologic widening of the space between the second metatarsal

base and the medial cuneiform and first metatarsal. Also, MR imaging can help show subtle dorsal displacement of the second metatarsal base caused by dorsal Lisfranc ligament disruption. Marrow edema can help direct attention to locate subtle ligament injury.

Patellar Dislocation, Transient Patellar Dislocation

Patellar dislocation can generally be established on physical examination and plain film radiography.[13] However, some investigators have found that greater than 50% of patellar dislocations are not diagnosed correctly initially.[14,15] Significant swelling and spontaneous reduction of the patella make clinical and radiographic evaluation difficult.[16,17] In the presence of hemarthrosis and suspected patellar dislocation, MR imaging is indicated to look for OCDs, fractures, and disruption of stabilizing soft tissue structures.

The evaluation of patellar dislocation with MR imaging can be used to assess for osteochondral

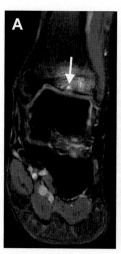
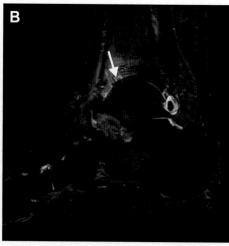

Fig. 4. Acute traumatic OCD. Coronal (*A*) and sagittal (*B*) T2 FS images of the ankle joint show a 6-mm cystic focus between a chondral lesion and adjacent bone, suggestive of unstable OCD. Also, note the extensive marrow edema about the lesion.

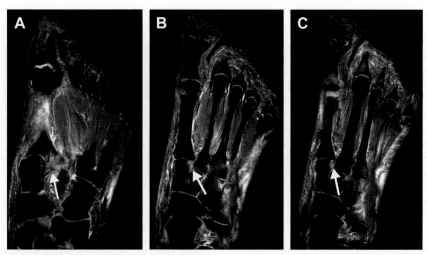

Fig. 5. Lisfranc injury occult on radiographs. (*A*) Axial PD FS image shows increased signal within partially torn fibers in the plantar Lisfranc ligament. (*B*) Axial PD FS image in the same patient shows increased signal and disruption of the interosseous Lisfranc ligament. (*C*) Axial PD FS image through the dorsum of the foot shows low-grade tear of the dorsal Lisfranc ligament.

lesions, which can be missed or underestimated using radiography alone. Cartilage injury occurs in up to 95% of first-time patellar dislocations and has important implications for management.[18] The size of the osteochondral injury helps the surgeon determine whether conservative or surgical management is appropriate. Although no strict criteria exist, lesions with subchondral bone greater than 9 mm are often fixated surgically and hence the size of the osteochondral lesion should always be reported.[13] The integrity of the medial patellar retinaculum and medial patellofemoral ligament should be carefully assessed in patellar dislocation. In a normally aligned patella on axial images, increased marrow signal on T2-weighted images in the medial aspect of the patella and lateral femoral condyle represent bone bruises and indicate lateral dislocation of the patella (**Fig. 6**).

Internal Derangement of the Knee

Internal derangement of the knee from trauma is best assessed using MR imaging and is by far the most common use of MR imaging in the moderate-velocity to high-velocity trauma setting. If clinical examination or mechanism is suggestive of soft tissue injury, an MR imaging scan can be obtained to assess the integrity of the internal knee structures. Quick treatment and recognition of injury helps in rapid return of function and prevention of long-term disability.

In low-velocity trauma, isolated injury to one of the knee stabilizers can be elucidated on history and physical examination, with MR imaging used to confirm the findings and determine severity. A mechanism of injury–based approach, as described by Hayes and colleagues[19] in 2000, is an excellent guide for evaluation of the knee on

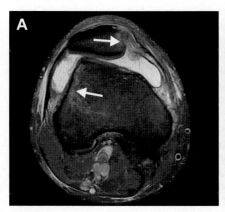
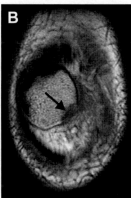

Fig. 6. Patellar dislocation. (*A*) Axial PD FS of the knee shows avulsion of the medial retinaculum at the patella with increased T2 signal and fraying. Also, bone edema is seen in the medial patella and lateral femur; the so-called Kissing contusions. The patella is displaced laterally and there is an associated effusion. (*B*) Coronal T1 image of the same patient shows bony avulsion of the medial inferior patella.

MR imaging in low-velocity trauma. However, in high-velocity trauma, damage to more than 1 supporting structure of the knee occurs because of multiple varying forces resulting in a complex injury pattern. In these situations, an understanding of the normal anatomy is paramount to describing the multitude of injuries often sustained in high-velocity trauma to the knee.

Radiographic abnormalities of the knee that suggest internal derangement include Segond fractures, knee dislocation, arcuate sign, lateral femoral notch sign, and many others. These radiographic findings need to be followed up with MR imaging, because internal derangement of soft tissue structures in the knee is highly likely.

On MR imaging, the anterior cruciate ligament (ACL) should be taut, with clear delineation of the anterolateral and posteromedial bundles. Traumatic injury to the ACL resulting in partial disruption may show increased T2-weighted signal and fraying of the ACL fibers. Sagittal PD or T2-weighted images are best to see the entirety of the ACL fibers. The coronal and axial planes are helpful for assessing the insertions of the ACL (the medial lateral femoral condyle and anterior tibial spine) and associated avulsion injuries. Indirect signs on MR imaging of ACL injury include[20]:

- Bone contusions of the lateral femoral condyle and posterior tibial plateau
- Increased sulcation of greater than 2 mm of the lateral femoral condyle
- Segond fracture
- So-called kissing contusions of the anterior tibia and femur
- Laxity of the posterior cruciate ligament (PCL)

Complete tears of the ACL are straightforward, and show significantly increased T2-weighted signal and no intact ACL fibers in the anatomic location of the ACL.

Injury to the PCL usually requires high-velocity trauma. This ligament is significantly stronger than its anterior counterpart and requires much more force to result in injury.[21] The so-called dashboard injury occurs when the anterior proximal tibia strikes an object during knee flexion with forces applied in anterior-posterior direction. Contusion of the anterior tibia (increased T2-weighted signal) should lead clinicians to suspect this mechanism and subsequent injury to the PCL. Injury to the PCL appears on MR imaging similar to injury to the ACL (**Fig. 7**):

- Increased T2-weighted signal
- Disruption of the obliquely oriented fibers
- With or without avulsed bone fragment at insertion or origin

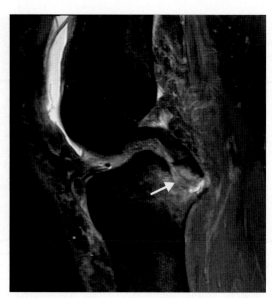

Fig. 7. PCL avulsion injury. Sagittal PD FS image shows heterogeneous increased signal at the tibial insertion of the PCL. Also, mild increased intrasubstance signal is seen in the PCL. Curvilinear low intensity at the base of the PCL represents avulsed bone fragment with edema at the bone donor site.

- With or without loss of continuity of fibers

Sagittal images using T2-weighting or PD images are the best to visualize the entire PCL and assess for disorder. Coronal oblique T2-weighted images also show the entirety of the ACL.

A comment on injury to the lateral collateral ligament (LCL) complex and medial collateral ligament (MCL) of the knee is required when discussing traumatic internal derangement of the knee. These structures are often abnormal with injury to the ACL and PCL. Understanding the anatomy is key to diagnosing injury on MR imaging. Similar to other soft tissues, injury manifests as increased T2-weighted signal in the structure of concern and disruption of normal anatomy, underscoring the need for a firm grasp on anatomy. The MCL originates from the medial femoral condyle and runs almost vertically, inserting on the medial tibia just posterior to the pes anserinus.[20,22] The MCL is separated into 2 bundles: deep and superficial. The deep bundle has attachments to the medial meniscus and the superficial bundle inserts on the medial proximal tibial metaphysis, separated by a bursa. Given its course, coronal MR images are easiest to use for evaluation of trauma, in particular the distal attachment (**Fig. 8**).

The LCL is more complex, because it consists of both a true ligament (fibular collateral) and contributions from tendons of the biceps femoris and

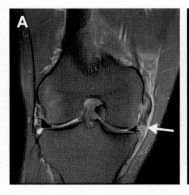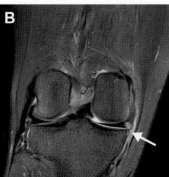

Fig. 8. MCL tear. (A) Coronal PD FS image shows increased signal and laxity of the proximal MCL fibers and deep MCL tear. (B) Coronal PD FS shows high-grade tear of the deep MCL with buckling of the MCL fibers deep to the meniscocapsular ligament.

the iliotibial band. The fibular collateral originates from the lateral femoral condyle and joins with the biceps femoris tendon distally to insert on the fibular head. The iliotibial band extends vertically along the lateral knee inserting on to Gerdy tubercle on the anterior tibia. Like the MCL, the LCL is best assessed on coronal T2-weighted images.

Posterolateral corner injuries deserve special attention. The components of this complex structure can be challenging to evaluate on MR imaging. Also, these types of injuries can be serious when missed, because these complex structures are the primary stabilizers of the knee.[19] The stabilizing posterolateral corner structures consist of:

- LCL: best seen on coronal images, although sagittal images are often helpful to see the fibular collateral ligament
- Popliteofibular ligament: extends from popliteus tendon to the fibular styloid process, and is best seen on coronal and sagittal images
- Popliteus muscle and tendon: best seen on coronal images
- Arcuate ligament: extends from the fibular styloid process to the posterior joint capsule and lateral femoral condyle, and is best interrogated on coronal and sagittal images

- Posterior joint capsule: best seen on axial images
- Fabellofibular ligament: if a fabella is present, then the ligament connects the fabella to the fibular styloid process and is best seen on coronal images, if at all

These structures normally have low signal intensity on all image sequences. When injured, thickening or intermediate to high signal intensity can be seen on fat-suppressed T2-weighted images (Fig. 9).[23] Also, complete disruption or tearing can be seen when these structures are injured. Marrow edema at origin and insertion sites of the aforementioned structures can indicate injury when the structure itself is difficult to identify. For example, the arcuate sign, which is an avulsion of the fibular head, can indicate posterolateral corner injury. Also, disruption of the lateral posterior joint capsule at the level of the joint space usually indicates arcuate ligament disruption.[23]

Sternoclavicular Joint Injury

Traumatic sternoclavicular dislocation is rare, accounting for approximately 3% of all joint injuries.[24,25] Anterior dislocation is by far the most common type followed by posterior dislocation.

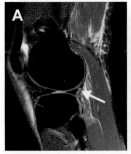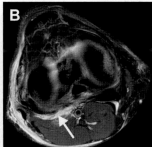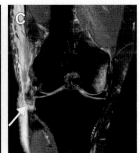

Fig. 9. Posterolateral corner injury. (A) Sagittal PD FS image shows increased signal and discontinuity of the distal popliteal fibular ligament just proximal to insertion on the fibular styloid. (B) Axial PD FS shows increased signal and tearing of the posterior lateral joint capsule, which suggests arcuate ligament injury. Also, increased signal seen in the lateral retinaculum, consistent with sprain (C) High-grade tear of the LCL and conjoined tendon.

Posterior dislocation can be serious because many vital structures lie just posterior to this joint (trachea, aorta, subclavian vessels, nerves, lungs) and recognition is critical for proper management.[26]

The sternoclavicular joint is composed of the medial head of the clavicle, first rib cartilage, anterior sternoclavicular ligament, interclavicular ligament, costoclavicular ligament, and articular disk.[26–28] These structures are easily evaluated using MR imaging. Axial and coronal planes provide the best view of this joint. T2-weighted signal abnormality, frank dislocation, or disruption of any of the aforementioned structures should be mentioned in the report (**Fig. 10**). Most importantly, MR imaging allows radiologists to assess for damage to adjacent vital structures (nerves, vessels, soft tissues) in posterior dislocations.

A special comment on young adults and children is needed. The epiphysis of the medial clavicle does not ossify until nearly 25 years of age.[29] When reviewing a potentially injured sternoclavicular joint in young adults, it is critical to note whether the injury is a true dislocation or a physeal injury.

Acromioclavicular Joint Injury

Acromioclavicular (AC) joint injury is classified using the Rockwood system at our institution. Historically, radiographs with weight-bearing views were the imaging method of choice, but MR imaging has been slowly replacing this modality as the preferred modality in evaluation of suspected AC joint injury. Distinguishing grade 2 from grade 3 injuries is challenging with radiographs alone and imaging can be confusing with effects of age and systemic disease processes.[30,31] Determining grade 2 versus 3 is critical, because a grade 2 injury is treated conservatively and a grade 3 injury

is treated surgically. MR imaging is superior in showing injury to this joint.

Imaging evaluation of the AC joint is best done in the coronal oblique and sagittal planes and should assess for:

- Widening of the AC joint
- Widening of the coracoclavicular (CC) distance
- Integrity of the superior and inferior AC ligaments
- Integrity of the conoid and trapezoid CC ligaments
- Position of the lateral clavicle relative to the acromion

Injury to ligaments shows increased T2-weighted signal or disruption. Edema and hemorrhage may be seen as secondary signs of AC joint injury.

Costochondral Injury

Costochondral injury is extremely difficult to identify on plain radiography and can easily be missed on CT images during the trauma work-up. Nondisplaced costochondral fractures are even more difficult to see on CT. Unexplained chest pain following trauma is often caused by these types of injuries and MR imaging is an effective method for evaluation of chest wall pain following trauma.[32] Coronal and axial T2 FS images are the best way to evaluate this region. Frank disruption or increased T2-weighted signal indicates injury (**Fig. 11**).

Tendon Injuries

Evaluation of tendon injury is generally done using MR imaging. The superior soft tissue contrast and detail provided by MR imaging allow precise characterization of tendon injury.[33,34] Also, MR imaging

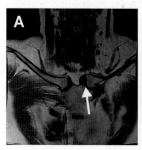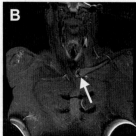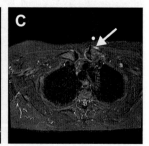

Fig. 10. Anterior sternoclavicular dislocation. (*A*) Coronal T1 shows slight superior subluxation of the left clavicle relative to the manubrium. (*B*) Coronal T2 FS shows increased signal tracking around the left sternoclavicular joint and articular disc injury. (*C*) Axial STIR images show anterior dislocation of the of the sternoclavicular joint with increased signal throughout the joint space.

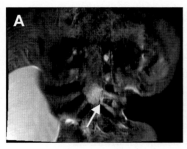

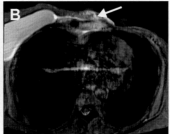

Fig. 11. Costochondral injury. (*A*) Coronal and (*B*) axial T2 FS images show increased signal at the costochondral junction with overlying soft tissue contusion and sternal contusion consistent with costochondral injury.

is superior to other modalities, like ultrasonography, in detecting disorder in adjacent structures. MR imaging is an invaluable tool for surgical planning and comment on the following is essential in the radiologist's report:

- Complete versus partial tear
- Amount of tendon retraction
- Quality of the remaining tendon fibers

Normal tendons appear as low-signal-intensity structures on all sequences. Disorders manifest as intrasubstance/adjacent increased signal on T2-weighted images, thickening, or discontinuity (partial or complete tear) (**Fig. 12**).

Muscle Injury

Muscle injury in trauma (sports-related trauma, high-velocity blunt trauma, penetrating injury) is extremely common. Sports-related muscle trauma is most likely to occur at the myotendinous junctions of muscles that cross 2 joints. These muscle strains show increased signal on T2-weighted images in and/or around the myotendinous complex, around the epimysium, and/or within the adjacent muscle[35] (**Fig. 13**). The presence of hematoma or disruption of fibers occurs in more severe sports-related injuries. The appearance of hematoma depends on the age of blood products; in the

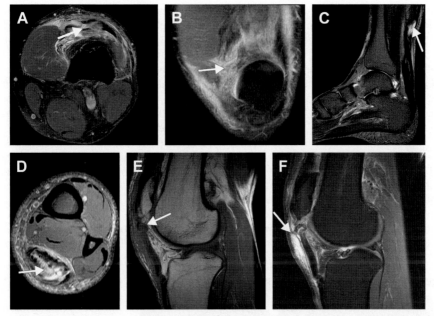

Fig. 12. Tendon injuries. (*A*) Axial and (*B*) coronal PD FS images show a complete tear of the vastus medialis tendon with retraction and thickening of the vastus medialis obliquus tendon at its insertion on the quadriceps tendon and significant surrounding soft tissue edema and hemorrhage. The medial quadriceps tendon shows a partial tear. Note the normal hypointense signal of the contralateral vastus lateralis tendon. Also note the laminar appearance of the quadriceps tendon. (*C*) Sagittal PD FS and (*D*) axial PD images show markedly increased signal with partial disruption of the Achilles tendon near the myotendinous junction. (*E*) Sagittal T1 and (*F*) sagittal PD FS of the knee show full-thickness tear with retraction of fibers of the proximal patellar tendon. T1-weighted images are used to assess for bone avulsion fragments.

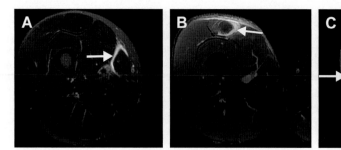

Fig. 13. Muscle strain. (*A*) Axial STIR image of the midthigh shows increased signal in the epimysium of the sartorius consistent with muscle strain. (*B*) Axial and (*C*) sagittal T2 FS images show the rectus femoris muscle peeling off the tendon at its myotendinous insertion with moderate retraction of the muscle consistent with high-grade muscle strain.

hyperacute setting blood may appear isointense on T1-weighted imaging and either bright or dark on T2-weighted imaging.

Blunt injury in high-velocity trauma, or a direct blow, results in intramuscular hematoma formation and/or disruption of muscle fibers at the site of impact. The hematoma appearance on MR imaging varies depending on the age of the blood products. Intramuscular hematomas may appear masslike, if severe (**Fig. 14**). Diffuse increased signal on T2-weighted images can be seen in the absence of a defined hematoma indicating edema of the muscle belly. Underlying bone contusions show diffuse increased marrow signal on T2-weighted images. Also, overlying soft tissue swelling should be seen in the setting of blunt trauma.

In the setting of penetrating injury to a muscle, MR imaging is generally not used because these patients go straight to the operating room for exploration.

Morel-Lavallée

The Morel-Lavallée lesion is a well-defined collection of lymph and blood products, most commonly seen in the anterolateral thigh, as a result of trauma. Violent shearing forces between subcutaneous fat and deep fascia overlying muscle disrupt the lymphatics and bridging vessels, filling a potential space superficial to the deep fascia.[36–38] Accumulation of hemolymph can occur rapidly, as in the case of arterial disruption, or slowly over weeks in the case of lymphatic and venous disruption.[36,39] Other anatomic sites in which this lesion has been described include knee, lumbar region, and scapula.[36,38,40]

The MR imaging features of Morel-Lavallée lesions are fairly specific. The anatomic location and fluid contents provide important clues. A well-defined fluid collection accumulating superficial to the deep fascia and below the subcutaneous fat in the setting of trauma should steer the diagnosis to Morel-Lavallée lesion. These lesions consist of blood and lymph. As such, the appearance on MR imaging is that of a fluid collection isointense or slightly increased on T1-weighted images with T2 prolongation (**Fig. 15**). Occasionally, a fluid-fluid level is seen showing the layering of blood sediment.[37] Fat lobules are occasionally seen within the fluid collection on imaging, and T2 FS techniques should be used to help with diagnosis. Noting whether a capsule is present is important because this usually precludes conservative management and necessitates surgery.[37]

SUMMARY

MR imaging use in the acute traumatic setting is increasing rapidly as the availability and speed of

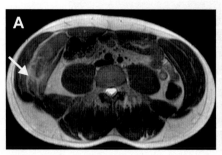
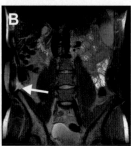

Fig. 14. Blunt muscle trauma: (*A*) Axial T2 and (*B*) coronal T2 FS shows avulsion of the internal oblique muscle fibers from the iliac bone, strain of the transverse abdominis, and adjacent hematoma.

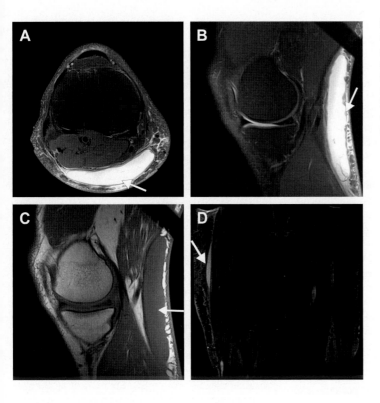

Fig. 15. Morel-Lavallée. (*A*) Axial and (*B*) sagittal PD FS images show a fluid collection superficial to deep fascia of the posterior knee. (*C*) Sagittal T1 image shows isointense collection consistent with a hemolymphoma. (*D*) Coronal STIR of the thigh shows the most common location of this shear injury.

MR imaging scanners increases. It is superior for evaluation of MSK soft tissue injury, compared with all other imaging modalities. Radiologists involved in emergency care, not just MSK-trained radiologists, should become comfortable interpreting basic MSK trauma on MR imaging as MR imaging becomes increasingly used in ER settings.

REFERENCES

1. Breitenseher MJ, Gaebler C. Trauma of the wrist. Eur J Radiol 1997;25:129–39.
2. Brydie A, Raby N. Early MRI in the management of clinical scaphoid fracture. Br J Radiol 2003;76: 296–300.
3. Nikken JJ, Oei EH, Ginai AZ, et al. Acute wrist trauma: value of a short dedicated extremity MR imaging examination in prediction of need for treatment. Radiology 2005;234:116–24.
4. Quinn SF, Belsole RJ, Greene TL, et al. Advanced imaging of the wrist. Radiographics 1989;9:229–46.
5. Memarsadeghi M, Breitenseher MJ, Schaefer-Prokop C, et al. Occult scaphoid fractures: comparison of multidetector CT and MR imaging–initial experience. Radiology 2006;240:169–76.
6. Bogost GA, Lizerbaum EK, Crues JV. MR imaging in evaluation of suspected hip fracture: frequency of unsuspected bone and soft tissue injuries. Radiology 1995;197:263–7.
7. Oka M, Monu JU. Prevalence and patterns of occult hip fractures and mimics revealed by MRI. AJR Am J Roentgenol 2004;182:283–8.
8. Rudman N, McIlmail D. Emergency department evaluation and treatment of hip and thigh injuries. Emerg Med Clin North Am 2000;18:29–66.
9. Brossmann J, Preidler KW, Daenen B, et al. Imaging of osseous and cartilaginous intraarticular bodies in the knee: comparison of MR imaging and MR arthrography with CT and CT arthrography in cadavers. Radiology 1996;200:509–17.
10. DeSmet AA, Ilahi OA, Graf BK. Reassessment of the MR criteria for stability of osteochondritis dissecans in the knee and ankle. Skeletal Radiol 1996;25:159–63.
11. Siddiqui NA, Galizia MS, Almusa E, et al. Evaluation of the tarsometatarsal joint using conventional radiography, CT and MR imaging. Radiographics 2014;34:514–31.
12. Philbin T, Rosenberg G, Sferra JJ. Complications of missed or untreated Lisfranc injuries. Foot Ankle Clin 2003;8:61–71.
13. Jain NP, Khan N, Fithian DC. A treatment algorithm for primary patellar dislocations. Sports Health 2011;3:170–4.
14. Keene JS. Diagnosis of undetected knee injuries: interpreting subtle clinical and radiologic findings. Postgrad Med 1989;85:153–63.
15. Casteleyn PP, Handelbeng F. Arthroscopy in the diagnosis of occult dislocation of the patella. Acta Orthop Belg 1989;55:381–3.

16. Hughston JC, Walsh WM, Puddu G. Patella subluxation and dislocation. In: Sledge CB, editor. Monographs in clinical orthopedics, vol. 5. Philadelphia: Saunders; 1984. p. 1–191.

17. Hughston JC. Patellar subluxation: a recent history. Clin Sports Med 1989;8:153–62.

18. Nomura E, Inoue M, Kurimura M. Chondral and osteochondral injuries associated with acute patellar dislocation. Arthroscopy 2003;19:717–21.

19. Hayes CW, Brigido MK, Jamadar DA, et al. Mechanism-based pattern approach to classification of complex injuries of the knee depicted at MR imaging. Radiographics 2000;20:S121–34.

20. Sanders TG, Miller MD. A systematic approach to magnetic resonance imaging interpretation of sports medicine injuries of the knee. Am J Sports Med 2005;33:131–48.

21. Race A, Amis AA. The mechanical properties of the two bundles of the human posterior cruciate ligament. J Biomech 1994;27:13–24.

22. Schweitzer MS, Tran D, Deely DM, et al. Medial collateral ligament injuries: evaluation of multiple signs, prevalence and location of associated bone bruises, and assessment with MR imaging. Radiology 1995;194:825–9.

23. Vinson EN, Major NM, Helms CA. The posterolateral corner of the knee. AJR Am J Roentgenol 2008;190:449–58.

24. Van Tongel A, De Wilde L. Sternoclavicular joint injuries: a literature review. Muscles Ligaments Tendons J 2012;1:100–5.

25. Groh GI, Wirth MA. Management of traumatic sternoclavicular joint injuries. J Am Acad Orthop Surg 2011;19:1–7.

26. Restrepo CS, Martinez S, Lemos DF, et al. Imaging appearances of the sternum and sternoclavicular joints. Radiographics 2009;29:839–59.

27. Stark P, Jaramillo D. CT of the sternum. AJR Am J Roentgenol 1986;147:72–7.

28. Goodman LR, Teplick SK, Kay H. Computed tomography of the normal sternum. AJR Am J Roentgenol 1983;141:219–23.

29. Webb PA, Suchey JM. Epiphyseal union of the anterior iliac crest and medial clavicle in a modern multiracial sample of American males and females. Am J Phys Anthropol 1985;68:457–66.

30. Alyas F, Curtis M, Speed C, et al. MR imaging appearances of acromioclavicular joint dislocation. Radiographics 2008;28:463–79.

31. Bossart PJ, Joyce SM, Manaster BJ, et al. Lack of efficacy of "weighted" radiographs in diagnosing acute acromioclavicular separation. Ann Emerg Med 1988;17:20–4.

32. Subhas N, Kline MJ, Moskal MJ, et al. MRI evaluation of costal cartilage injuries. AJR Am J Roentgenol 2008;191:129–32.

33. Clavero JA, Alomar X, Monill JM, et al. MR imaging of ligament and tendon injuries of the fingers. Radiographics 2002;22:237–56.

34. Hodgson RJ, O'Connor PJ, Grainger AJ. Tendon and ligament imaging. Br J Radiol 2012;85:1157–72.

35. May DA, Disler DG, Jones EA, et al. Abnormal signal intensity in skeletal muscle at MR imaging: patterns, pearls, and pitfalls. Radiographics 2000;20:S295–315.

36. Kottmeier SA, Wilson SC, Born CT, et al. Surgical management of soft tissue lesions associated with pelvic ring injury. Clin Orthop 1996;329:46–53.

37. Gilbert BC, Bui-Mansfield LT, Dejong S. MRI of a Morel-Lavallée lesion. AJR Am J Roentgenol 2004;182:1347–8.

38. Parra JA, Fernandez MA, Encinas B, et al. Morel-Lavallée effusions in the thigh. Skeletal Radiol 1997;26:239–41.

39. Hak DJ, Olson SA, Matta JM. Diagnosis and management of closed internal degloving injuries with pelvic and acetabular fractures: the Morel-Lavallée lesion. J Trauma 1997;42:1046–51.

40. Sawkwar AA, Swishcuk LE, Jadhav S. Morel-Lavallee seroma: a review of 2 cases in the lumbar region in the adolescent. Emerg Radiol 2011;18:495–8.

Magnetic Resonance Imaging of Abdominal and Pelvic Pain in the Pregnant Patient

CrossMark

Akshay D. Baheti, MD, DO[a],*, Refky Nicola, MS, DO[b],
Genevieve L. Bennett, MD[c], Ritu Bordia, MBBS, MPH[d],
Mariam Moshiri, MD[a], Douglas S. Katz, MD[d], Puneet Bhargava, MD[a]

KEYWORDS

- Pregnancy • Emergency • MR imaging • Acute abdomen • Appendicitis

KEY POINTS

- Evaluating the acute abdomen in pregnancy is complex because of altered physiology and the need to avoid radiation exposure.
- MR imaging is a safe and efficacious tool for accurate evaluation of the pregnant patient due to the lack of radiation exposure and its intrinsic high soft-tissue contrast.
- Developing dedicated protocols for evaluating the acute abdomen in pregnancy and institutional guidelines on issues including patient informed consent and IV contrast administration is important.
- Most acute abdominal and pelvic abnormalities can be diagnosed in a safe and timely manner using MR imaging.

Evaluation of the acute abdomen in a pregnant woman poses special challenges for both the radiologist and the referring physician for several reasons. The most appropriate imaging modality should be selected, balancing the risks of fetal radiation exposure with the potential benefits of establishing a prompt and accurate diagnosis. Imaging protocols vary from institution to institution, with a broad consensus slowly evolving over time. This review discusses the role of MR imaging in evaluating the common nonfetal causes of acute abdominal and pelvic abnormalities in the pregnant woman.

POTENTIAL RISKS OF RADIATION EXPOSURE TO THE FETUS

The potential effects of radiation exposure to the fetus have been discussed extensively in the literature.[1] As always, the most important principle in imaging the pregnant patient is that of ALARA (as low as reasonably achievable). The potential clinical benefits must be considered against the potential risk of radiation exposure when selecting the appropriate imaging modality. According to the most recent guidelines from the American College of Radiology (ACR), the risk of radiation-induced

---

The authors have nothing to disclose.
[a] Department of Radiology, University of Washington, 1959 NE Pacific Street, Room BB308, Box 357115, Seattle, WA 98195, USA; [b] Department of Radiology, University of Rochester Medical Center, 601 Elmwood Avenue, Box 648, Rochester, NY 14642, USA; [c] Department of Radiology, New York University School of Medicine, 660 First Avenue, New York, NY 10016, USA; [d] Section of Neuroradiology, Department of Radiology, Winthrop-University Hospital, 259 First Street, Mineola, NY 11501, USA
* Corresponding author.
E-mail address: akshaybaheti@gmail.com

Magn Reson Imaging Clin N Am 24 (2016) 403–417
http://dx.doi.org/10.1016/j.mric.2015.11.007
1064-9689/16/$ – see front matter © 2016 Elsevier Inc. All rights reserved.

deterministic effects are thought to be minimal for exposure less than the 50 mGy threshold (5 rad).[1]

The average radiation exposure of a single abdominal and pelvic computed tomographic (CT) examination performed with current equipment using an appropriate protocol should be much less than the 50-mGy threshold.[2,3] However, if ionizing radiation can be completely avoided, and diagnostic accuracy can be maintained at a high level, then the use of imaging modalities that do not impart ionizing radiation to the fetus, particularly in the earlier stages of gestation, would be preferable.

SAFETY OF MR IMAGING IN PREGNANCY

Because of the absence of exposure to ionizing radiation, its multiplanar imaging capabilities, and excellent imaging quality and soft-issue contrast, MR imaging has been shown to be an excellent option for imaging the pregnant patient with acute abdominal and pelvic disorders. The primary concerns for fetal exposure to MR imaging are the heating effects of the radiofrequency pulses and the effects of acoustic noise on the fetus.[4] Higher strengths of the magnetic field, use of a higher flip angle, an increased number of radiofrequency pulses, and decreased spacing between them, are all associated with a higher specific absorption rate, leading to potentially higher fetal tissue heating.[5] Sequences including single-shot fast spin-echo (SSFSE) are single acquisition echo-train spin-echo sequences and use 180° refocusing pulses. They are associated with higher fetal heating than gradient-echo sequences, which do not use the refocusing pulse.[2,5] Tissue heating is however maximum at the maternal body surface and decreases near the center of the body, making fetal thermal damage less likely. To the authors' knowledge, there is no evidence of adverse fetal heating with a 1.5-T or lower field strength magnet.[2,5,6] Similarly, exposure to acoustic noise has not been proven to adversely affect fetal hearing, because the noise gets attenuated while traveling through the amniotic fluid and gets delivered to the fetus at less than 30 dB.[7–10]

A few animal studies have raised the possibility of adverse effects of noncontrast MR imaging (ranging from 0.35 T to 1.5 T) on mice and chick embryos, whereas another study (4.7-T strength) found no significant adverse effects.[11–14] The duration of exposure of the embryos to MR imaging in these studies ranged from 6 to 48 hours, which does not parallel the situation in clinical practice. The applicability of these findings to the human embryo is somewhat controversial. Overall, MR imaging has been used safely for imaging obstetric patients for more than the past 2 decades, without any documented adverse fetal effects.[15] The International Commission on Non-Ionizing Radiation Protection, in its statement on MR imaging in pregnancy, published in 2004 and updated in 2009, stated that "there is no clear evidence that exposure to static or low frequency magnetic fields can adversely affect pregnancy outcome," but concluded that the overall evidence to provide unequivocal guidelines is insufficient. It recommended that MR imaging should be performed in pregnancy only after a critical risk-benefit analysis, particularly in the first trimester, and that imaging time should be minimized.[16,17] The ACR guidelines on imaging patients in pregnancy do not recommend any special consideration for first trimester MR imaging, given the absence of documented adverse effects.[18]

According to the ACR guidelines, MR imaging can be performed in any stage of pregnancy if, in the medical opinion of a level 2 MR imaging personnel-designated attending radiologist, the examination is indicated after considering the risk-benefit ratio. The following should be documented in the radiology report or in the patient's medical records after conferring with the referring physician:

i. The information was not/cannot be obtained by using ultrasound (US);
ii. The information obtained from the examination will potentially directly benefit maternal or fetal care during the pregnancy;
iii. The referring physician does not think it is wise to wait until after the patient delivers to obtain the MR imaging.

SAFETY OF INTRAVENOUS GADOLINIUM IN PREGNANCY

Intravenous (IV) gadolinium in pregnancy is considered a category C drug, with teratogenic effects having been demonstrated in animals without any definite effects on human fetuses.[19,20] Because IV gadolinium crosses the placenta and remains in the amniotic fluid indefinitely, being recycled by the fetal kidneys, there is a theoretic risk of free gadolinium ions dissociating from the chelate and having an adverse effect on fetal development.[3,18,19] According to the ACR guidelines for imaging pregnant patients, IV gadolinium should not be routinely used in pregnancy.[18] Any decision to administer IV gadolinium in pregnancy should be made only after carefully balancing the risk and potential benefit and should be considered only in very select situations. The authors' practices almost never perform IV contrast-enhanced MR imaging in pregnant patients, cautiously using it only when absolutely necessary for the diagnosis, as in staging of malignancies, for example. Whenever unavoidable, a decision to administer IV gadolinium should be made only after close consultation with the referring physician(s) and with the patient. The ACR recommends obtaining written informed consent from pregnant patients before an MRI examination.[21]

STATUS OF ACADEMIC RADIOLOGY PRACTICES IN ABDOMINAL IMAGING OF PREGNANT PATIENTS

In a survey of 85 academic abdominal imaging divisions across the United States published in 2007, 74% had a written departmental policy regarding the use of MR imaging in pregnancy.[22] Over 90% of respondents performed CT and MR imaging in pregnancy, depending on the patient's needs. CT was preferred over MR imaging in the setting of trauma in all 3 trimesters, and for evaluating suspected appendicitis, abscess, or renal calculus in the second and third trimesters. MR imaging was preferred over CT for diagnosing appendicitis and abscess in the first trimester.[22] A more recent albeit smaller survey of 45 radiologists on the same topic also included nonacademic radiologists in it (48% in academic practice, 19% in community hospitals having residents, and the rest in nonspecialty/subspecialty private practice).[23] Forty-three percent of the respondents had a written policy on imaging in pregnancy, and 72% had dedicated low-radiation-dose CT protocols for imaging pregnant patients. Forty-eight percent preferred noncontrast CT, whereas 45% preferred MR imaging to evaluate suspected renal calculi after an indeterminate US examination. No specific questions were asked

on appendicitis, but MR imaging was preferred over CT in evaluating generalized abdominal pain and suspected inflammatory bowel disease (IBD).[23] The authors currently consider MR imaging to be an invaluable tool for evaluating abdominal pain in pregnancy and think that it should be the preferred modality along with US in all settings except trauma, where CT has substantial operational advantages.

MR IMAGING PROTOCOL

Many practices have dedicated MR protocols for imaging the abdomen and pelvis in pregnancy, using sequences that minimize motion artifacts due to respiration, peristalsis, and fetal movements.[22] At the authors' institutions, they use single-shot fast-spin echo (SSFSE/HASTE [half-Fourier acquisition single-shot turbo-spin echo]) and T2-weighted (T2W) fat-saturated sequences in all three planes, along with axial gradient-echo T1-weighted in-phase and out-of-phase sequences in all patients (Table 1). A large field of view is generally used, but focused smaller field-of-view images can be obtained if necessary. Typically, the examination time is optimized and kept to a minimum. A 2009 study demonstrated MR imaging without oral contrast to be efficacious for diagnosis of the causes of acute pelvic pain in both pregnant and nonpregnant women, which is consistent with the authors' own experience.[24] Oral contrast is not given before the MR imaging in the authors' practices.

GENERAL PRINCIPLES OF IMAGING PREGNANT PATIENTS WITH ABDOMINAL AND PELVIC PAIN

Evaluation of abdominal pain during pregnancy is more challenging because of multiple reasons. Physiologic changes during pregnancy can mimic

Table 1
1.5-T MR imaging protocol to image pregnant patients

Plane	Sequence	Breath-Hold	TR (ms)	TE (ms)	Slice Thickness (mm)	Slice Spacing	SAR	b-value
Ax/Cor (large FOV)	SSFSE	Yes	580	90	5	6	3	—
Ax/Cor/Sag (focused)	SSFSE	Yes	577	91	4–5	5.5	2	—
Ax/Cor/Sag	SSFSE FS	Yes	550	90	5	6	2	—
Ax	In- and out-of-phase	Yes	4.6/2.3	119	7	8	1.9	—
Ax/Cor	DWI/ADC (sos)	Yes	6283	64	6	7	0.9	0, 400, 800
Ax/Cor/Sag	Pre- and post-contrast T1FS (sos)	Yes	4.4	2.2	4.4	2.2	0.4	—

Abbreviations: Ax, axial; Cor, coronal; Sag, sagittal; sos, as required.

various abnormalities and create diagnostic uncertainty (as, for example, nausea and vomiting in early pregnancy). Furthermore, the uterus usually becomes an abdominal organ after 12 weeks, making it difficult to localize pain on physical examination and concealing or delaying various clinical signs and symptoms, making the role of imaging critical for prompt and accurate diagnosis.[19,25,26] The most important role of imaging is to differentiate between an urgent surgical and nonsurgical condition. Initial imaging of suspected obstetric causes of abdominal or pelvic pain is usually performed with sonography. US is also usually the first imaging examination performed for evaluating suspected nonobstetric causes of acute abdominal or pelvic pain, with MR imaging increasingly performed as a second-line imaging examination when the sonographic examinations are equivocal or nondiagnostic (which is frequently the case in pregnancy). Many studies in the literature have shown that MR imaging is useful for the diagnosis of pregnant patients presenting with abdominal pain.[25,27–30] A study of 118 pregnant patients (mean gestational age 20.6 weeks) presenting with acute abdominal or pelvic pain found MR imaging to have a sensitivity, specificity, positive predictive value, and negative predictive value for diagnoses requiring surgery or an interventional radiology procedure of 89%, 95%, 76%, and 98%, respectively.[25]

The most common causes of abdominal pain in pregnancy are listed in **Table 2**.[19,25,26,31] In this article, the authors discuss the role of MR imaging in evaluating the most common entities presenting with an acute abdominal and/or pelvic condition in pregnancy.

APPENDICITIS

Acute appendicitis is the most common nonobstetric surgical cause of abdominal pain during pregnancy. The incidence is estimated at 1 in 800 to 1 in 1700 pregnancies.[19,32–34] The clinical diagnosis of appendicitis in pregnancy is based on the classic triad of right lower quadrant pain, fever, and leukocytosis. Acute appendicitis is relatively difficult to diagnose during pregnancy for several reasons. The gravid uterus can mask underlying tenderness. The appendix is also often displaced from the right lower quadrant in the third trimester, and mild leukocytosis can frequently be physiologic during pregnancy.[31,32,35] Furthermore, appendicitis is more morbid during pregnancy because there is a higher rate of perforation and associated complications, which can also result in premature labor, fetal morbidity, and mortality.[31,32,36] Pregnancy-related complications are higher in pregnant women with perforated appendicitis compared with those with nonperforated appendicitis. A retrospective review of 778 pregnancies

Table 2
Differential diagnosis for nonobstetric causes of acute abdominal pain in pregnancy and the recommended imaging modalities

Site	Preferred Imaging Modalities for Diagnosis
Upper abdominal pain	
Gallbladder disease	US > MR imaging
Hepatitis	US > MR imaging
Pancreatitis	US/MR imaging > CT
Bowel obstruction	US/MR imaging > CT
Perforated ulcer	Abdominal radiographs > CT
Lower abdominal pain	
Appendicitis	US > MR imaging > CT
Nephrolithiasis	US > MR imaging/CT
Inflammatory bowel disease	MR imaging > CT
Gynecologic causes (ovarian torsion, complicated adnexal cysts, degenerating fibroid, pelvic inflammatory disease)	US > MR imaging
Diverticulitis	MR imaging > CT
Trauma	US > CT (MR imaging may be used in follow-up imaging)
Oncologic causes	CT/MR imaging

Data from Refs.[5,19,35,80]

requiring appendectomy found an increased rate of preterm delivery, low birth weight, still births, and neonatal mortality.[36] Another study of 3133 pregnant patients who underwent appendectomy found both complicated appendicitis and negative appendectomy to be associated with a significantly higher rate of fetal demise.[37] Thus, risk of delay in diagnosis must be balanced against the risk of negative laparotomy, making appropriate and timely imaging extremely important.

Role of Ultrasound

Graded-compression US is the preferred initial imaging modality for evaluating patients with suspected appendicitis as per the ACR Appropriateness Criteria due to its safety, availability, and low cost, although it has major limitations, particularly in the later stages of pregnancy. In addition, US is also helpful for the identification of alternate diagnoses, although the accuracy is less than that for MR imaging or CT.[31,32,38] The imaging criteria for appendicitis are the same as in nonpregnant patients. These imaging criteria include a dilated (>6 mm) thickened, tubular blind-ending, noncompressible structure, associated with inflammation of the adjacent fat. Associated appendicoliths may be identified.[3,19,32]

However, the limitations of US include its operator-dependence, inconsistent visualization of the appendix due to overlying bowel gas and the overlying uterus, and variability with patient body habitus and advanced gestational age, among other reasons,[19] explaining the relatively poor sensitivity and specificity reported in the more recent literature for US for appendicitis in pregnancy. An early study of 42 patients, published in 1992, found US to be 100% sensitive and 96% specific in the diagnosis of appendicitis in pregnancy.[39] However, these results were in Asian women in the earlier stages of gestation, and multiple more recent studies have reported a much lower sensitivity, ranging from 20% to 36%.[26,29,40–43]

Role of MR Imaging

MR imaging is the preferred second-line imaging modality in indeterminate cases of appendicitis, as per the ACR Appropriateness Criteria.[38] Multiple recent studies have shown MR imaging to have a higher sensitivity and specificity for the diagnosis compared with US, besides simultaneously evaluating other potential causes of pain.[25,27–30] A meta-analysis of 6 studies described the pooled sensitivity, specificity, and positive and negative predictive values to be 0.91 (95% confidence interval [CI], 0.54–

0.99), 0.98 (95% CI, 0.87–0.99), 0.86 (95% CI, 0.38–0.98), and 0.99 (95% CI, 0.93–0.99), respectively.[44]

Protocol

SSFSE sequences in all 3 planes are the most useful for identifying the appendix, particularly the coronal and right lower quadrant sagittal planes. Fat suppression is helpful to increase the conspicuity of inflammatory changes. A few publications have advocated using negative oral contrast to increase diagnostic confidence, giving 300 to 450 mL of oral iron oxides combined with 300 mL of barium sulfate 1 to 1.5 hours before the MR examination.[26,43] However, multiple other reports have noted similar sensitivity and specificity without administering oral contrast.[27,28,40] The authors' practices do not give oral contrast. Two additional sequences may be used for the MR imaging appendicitis protocol. Adjacent vessels, particularly the gonadal vein and its tributaries, can mimic the appendix on SSFSE images, especially in the later stages of gestation. A transverse 2-dimensional time-of-flight (TOF) gradient-echo sequence can be used to differentiate between the two.[26,43] Diffusion-weighted imaging (DWI) sequences are not universally used, but can be potentially useful to improve conspicuity. A recent study of 117 pregnant patients with clinically suspected acute appendicitis (compared with 50 control patients) found DWI to increase the conspicuity of the inflamed appendix. Quantitative evaluation of the DW signal intensity and apparent diffusion coefficient (ADC) values revealed a significant difference between the normal and inflamed appendix ($P<.001$), with the best discriminatory parameter being the signal intensity ratio on b = 500 value.[45] However, more studies are needed to validate this and compare its utility beyond fat-suppressed T2W images.

Normal appearance of the appendix on MR imaging

The normal appendix appears as a tubular, blind-ending structure arising from the cecum, containing air or oral contrast (if administered).[26,30,43] Oral contrast causes blooming on the in-phase and TOF images, also helping to differentiate the appendix from vessels. The normal appendix is 6 mm or less in diameter.[26,30,43]

MR imaging features of appendicitis

The characteristic MR imaging appearance of acute appendicitis is a fluid-filled appendix, measuring 7 mm or greater in diameter, with associated periappendiceal inflammation (**Figs. 1 and 2**). Other MR imaging findings include appendiceal wall thickness greater than 2 mm, T2

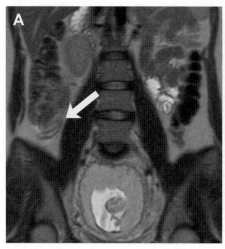
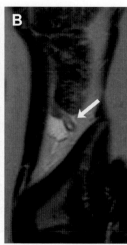

Fig. 1. A 32-year-old 14-week pregnant patient with right lower quadrant pain. Coronal (A) and sagittal (B) SSFSE MR images reveal a thick-walled appendix (arrows) with intraluminal fluid with mild periappendiceal T2 hyperintense signal consistent with inflammation. Note the sagittal SSFSE image demonstrating a dilated tubular inflamed appendix.

hyperintense appearance of the appendiceal lumen due to fluid or edema, and the absence of blooming.[3,26,30,32,35,43] Periappendiceal fat stranding and fluid are often best appreciated on the fat-suppressed sequence.[26] An appendicolith (or appendicoliths) may also be seen and appears hypointense on all sequences.[26,43] An associated phlegmon may be visualized as a heterogeneous T2 intermediate to hyperintense mass. Associated abscess formation would appear as a well-defined T2 hyperintense fluid collection. An air pocket within the abscess would demonstrate blooming on the in-phase and TOF images.[26,33,43]

An appendix between 6 and 7 mm in diameter, without luminal air or contrast, should be considered indeterminate for appendicitis. The presence of ancillary findings of inflammation can help in confirming the diagnosis in these cases. If these are also absent, the MR imaging findings should be reported as indeterminate for appendicitis.

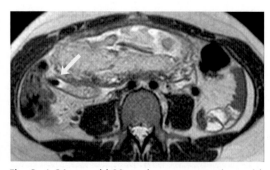

Fig. 2. A 34-year-old 20-week pregnant patient with right lower quadrant pain and vomiting. Axial T2-weighted single-shot fast spin-echo (T2-SSFSE) image shows an inflamed appendix with periappendiceal edema and fat stranding, with a T2 hypointense appendicolith noted near its base (arrow).

Low-radiation-dose contrast-enhanced CT may be performed following indeterminate MR imaging examinations, or when an MR imaging is unavailable and US is indeterminate.[3,19,38]

NEPHROLITHIASIS AND PYELONEPHRITIS

Urolithiasis is the most common nonobstetric cause for hospitalization in pregnancy.[31] Urinary tract infections (UTIs) are also more common in pregnancy, due to increased urinary stasis and vesicoureteral reflux. 48-80% of ureteral calculi pass spontaneously with conservative management, but those that do not can cause obstruction and further urinary stasis, leading to UTI and potential complications.[3,19,32,46] Accurately diagnosing urolithiasis can be relatively challenging in pregnancy, due to physiologic hydronephrosis that can be present in upwards of 60% to 94% of patients.[32] It occurs in the second and third trimesters and is attributed to mass effect caused by the gravid uterus as well as by hormone-related smooth muscle relaxation. The right side is affected in 80% to 90% of pregnant patients, with the left side less commonly affected.[32,35]

Role of Ultrasound

US is the recommended initial imaging modality for evaluating patients with suspected urolithiasis. Its sensitivity for the detection of calculi in the ureters and kidneys has been variable in the literature, ranging from 34% to 95%.[31,32] Gray-scale US evaluation, along with evaluation of ureteral jets and renal arterial resistive indices (RIs), is performed.[31,32,47,48] The absence of ureteral jets may be seen in up to 15% of asymptomatic pregnant women and is not specific for obstruction.[49]

The RIs of renal arteries of pregnant patients with only physiologic hydronephrosis is not usually elevated. In contrast, after the onset of acute obstruction, the RI can increase within 6 hours, with a difference of 0.04 or more between the symptomatic kidney compared with the asymptomatic kidney, or an RI > 0.7, indicating obstruction.[48] In a review of 262 pregnant patients with suspected urolithiasis, the accuracy of US increased from 56% to 72% when RI and ureteral jet analysis were performed.[47] The identification of twinkling artifacts can be useful on sonography for more accurate diagnosis of renal calculi. Transvaginal scanning may be helpful in identifying a distal ureteral calculus.[50]

Role of MR Urography

Physiologic hydronephrosis of pregnancy can frequently be differentiated from an obstructing ureteral calculus, as dilatation of the renal collecting system and more proximal ureter with associated smooth tapering of the mid and distal ureter (**Fig. 3**). Dilatation distal to the sacral promontory is much more suspicious for an obstructive process above and beyond the physiologic hydronephrosis of pregnancy.[26,32,35,51] A ureteral calculus can be visualized as a T2 hypointense filling defect with abrupt narrowing of the ureter distal to it (see **Fig. 3**). Secondary signs may be seen due to back-pressure changes, including renal enlargement and perirenal edema. These changes are better appreciated on fat-suppressed images.[26,32,35] Renal MR imaging may also depict pyelonephritis, which appears as heterogeneous edematous changes in the kidneys on heavily T2W images as well as on DWIs as areas with restricted diffusion (**Fig. 4**). Noncontrast CT as well as sonography is relatively less sensitive for depicting these findings in pyelonephritis.[52,53] Renal and perirenal abscesses may also develop in complicated pyelonephritis, which are visualized as T2 hyperintense collections.[52,53] The biggest disadvantage of MR imaging is its limited ability to depict small calculi, particularly in the kidneys, but also in the ureters. A study of 64 patients found that MR imaging depicted only 72% on calculi seen on CT, but was more sensitive for the demonstration of perirenal edema and hydroureter.[54]

Role of Computed Tomography

CT currently may be preferred over MR imaging for assessment of known or suspected urolithiasis, given the limitations of current MR imaging techniques for accurate depiction of ureteral and renal calculi. The radiation exposure from low-radiation-dose noncontrast CT using modern dose reduction algorithms has been reported to be relatively small, with exposures as low as 1.1 mSv having been reported, without any significant decrease in accuracy.[55,56]

Considering the generally semiurgent as opposed to emergency nature of urolithiasis in pregnancy and the moderately good sensitivity of US and MR imaging, the authors think that MR imaging should be performed before resorting to a CT. A recent prospective study of 2759 patients (pregnant patients were excluded) randomized to initial US and initial CT found no significant difference in complications, adverse events, pain scores, return emergency visits, or hospitalizations between the 2 imaging modalities, again giving credence to the policy of using CT as a secondary resort.[57]

GYNECOLOGIC AND OBSTETRIC DISORDERS

Pelvic pain can occur secondary to various ovarian and uterine disorders, including simple and

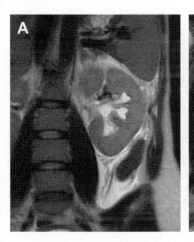
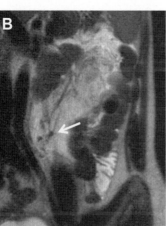

Fig. 3. A 30-year-old 10-week pregnant patient with left flank pain. US (not shown) showed mild left hydronephrosis and proximal hydroureter without an obvious calculus, and MR imaging was performed for further evaluation. T2W SSFSE coronal images (*A, B*) demonstrate a 6-mm mid ureteric calculus (*arrow*) causing mild proximal hydronephrosis and hydroureter. The patient was managed conservatively and passed the calculus spontaneously.

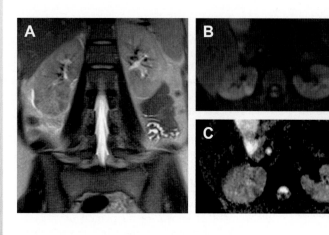

Fig. 4. A 32-year-old 21-week pregnant patient with right flank pain and leukocytosis. UTI was suspected. US (images not shown) did not reveal hydronephrosis or calculi, and MR imaging was performed for further evaluation. Coronal T2W (*A*) and axial DWI and ADC images (*B, C*) of the kidneys show mild bilateral parenchymal heterogeneity with multiple wedge-shaped areas of restricted diffusion and low ADC values (more on the right side), consistent with bilateral pyelonephritis. The patient responded well to antibiotics.

complicated ovarian cysts, ovarian torsion, pelvic inflammatory disease, benign or malignant adnexal tumors, particularly dermoids, and uterine fibroids (which may also undergo degeneration during pregnancy) (**Figs. 5** and **6**).[26,33,35] After initial US, MR imaging is the imaging procedure of choice for further evaluation of these conditions. The MR imaging features are similar to those seen in nonpregnant patients.[26,33,35] For example, hemorrhagic ovarian cysts appear hyperintense on T1-weighted images (T1WI), ovarian dermoids demonstrate fat intensity on T1WI, which becomes suppressed on fat-saturated images (see **Fig. 5**), and cystic ovarian neoplasms appear as complex heterogeneous solid/cystic lesions.[5,26,33,35] Unlike the classic T2 hypointense appearance of a routine fibroid, a degenerating fibroid can appear hyperintense on T2WI due to edema and/or necrosis (see **Fig. 6**).[5,26,33,35]

MR imaging can also be used as a useful adjunct to an indeterminate US examination for other nonfetal obstetric indications, including for the evaluation of known or suspected placenta accreta, increta, and percreta, atypical sites of

implantation, particularly cesarean section scar and cervical implantation, for known or suspected cesarean scar dehiscence, and for the evaluation of pregnancies occurring in a congenitally malformed uterus or in abdominal pregnancy (**Figs. 7–9**).[58–60] MR imaging is highly sensitive for evaluating abnormal placentation, when suspicious findings are seen on US. Apart from direct visualization of placental invasion, other signs on MR imaging include visualization of irregular T2 hypointense bands (secondary to fibrin deposition), and tortuous and dilated flow voids located deep within the placenta (indicating anomalous vascular lacunae).[58] Uterine scar dehiscence, most commonly seen in patients with cesarean section scars, can also be well assessed on MR imaging. MR imaging depicts the myometrial thinning and scar thickness better, along with demonstrating herniation of placental membranes. MR imaging may also demonstrate more obvious abnormalities including hematomas and hemoperitoneum, although such patients will generally be diagnosed on US and go directly for surgery if necessary.[61,62] Similarly, MR imaging can best

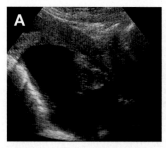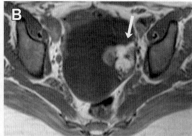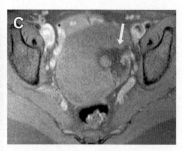

Fig. 5. A 29-year-old 15-week pregnant patient with mild pelvic pain. US (*A*) showed a cystic adnexal lesion, with isoechoic to mildly hyperechoic solid components without shadowing, which did not demonstrate any vascularity on Doppler images (not shown). MR imaging was performed for further evaluation, which revealed a T1 hyperintense component within the cyst (*B*), which lost signal on the T1W fast spin-echo image (*C*) (*arrows*), confirming the presence of fat in a dermoid.

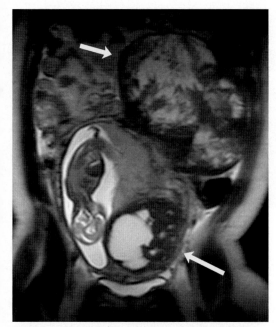

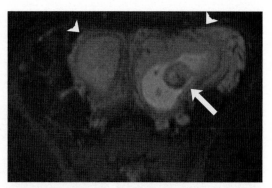

Fig. 8. A 30-year-old 14-week pregnant patient with uterine didelphys. Axial T2FS MR image shows the 2 horns of the uterus (*arrowheads*), with a fetus in the left horn (*arrow*).

Fig. 6. A 34-year-old 19-week pregnant patient with moderately severe pelvic pain. Coronal SSFSE image reveals a large heterogeneous exophytic uterine mass with multiple T2 hyperintense areas within it, representing a degenerating subserosal fibroid (*short arrow*). Note another intramural degenerating fibroid involving the lower segment of the uterus (*long arrow*).

depict the spectrum of Mullerian duct anomalies and relative fetal orientation and help differentiate between an ectopic versus implantation in a malformed uterus, helping guide clinicians in appropriate management.[63]

BILIARY TRACT DISORDERS

Acute cholecystitis is the second most common nonobstetric reason for surgery during pregnancy, with potential complications including choledocholithiasis and obstructive jaundice, pancreatitis, and peritonitis, which are associated with higher maternal and fetal mortality.[32,64,65] US is the imaging examination of choice. MR cholangiopancreatography (MRCP) has a higher sensitivity and specificity than US for the detection of biliary disorders and associated complications and is imaging examination of choice following initial US (**Fig. 10**).[21,31,32,66,67] A small study of 18 patients concluded that patients with biliary dilatation on US without a definite cause should be further evaluated with MRCP, to avoid unnecessary endoscopic retrograde cholangiopancreatography (ERCP), because more information was provided compared with initial sonography.[66] US revealed possible biliary dilatation in 8 of 18 patients in the study without depicting the cause. MRI correctly revealed the cause of four of these, and helped to exclude obstruction in the other four, who were successfully managed medically. All the patients without evidence of obstruction on MRCP in the study were successfully managed medically.[66] ERCP and/or surgery may be necessary for management after a definitive diagnosis, with the fetal radiation exposure during ERCP being within safe limits if performed by experienced operators.[68] As on sonography, the MR findings of cholecystitis include cholelithiasis, wall thickening

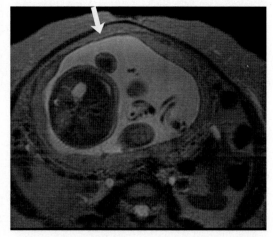

Fig. 7. A 32-year-old 27-week asymptomatic pregnant patient with history of cesarean section, with a US suggestive of possible uterine dehiscence (image not shown). Axial SSFSE MR image demonstrates a large anterior area of dehiscence (*arrow*) without herniation of the amniotic layers or the fetus through it.

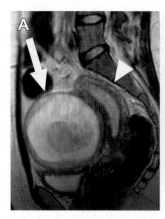
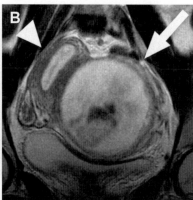

Fig. 9. A 27-year-old 27-week pregnant patient presenting with abdominal pain. Sagittal and coronal SSFSE MR images (*A*, *B*) show an intra-abdominal gestational sac (*arrows*) with the uterus seen separately (*arrowheads*), representing an abdominal ectopic pregnancy.

greater than 3 mm, wall edema, and surrounding inflammation, the latter of which is best seen on the fat-saturated images. Associated acute pancreatitis can be visualized as loss of the normal T1-hyperintense pancreatic signal and peripancreatic inflammation and fluid collections (**Fig. 11**).[32,35]

EVALUATION OF OTHER BOWEL DISORDERS

The most common bowel disorders encountered in pregnancy are IBD and small bowel obstruction. US may be used for initial evaluation of pregnant patients presenting with abdominal pain and suspected obstruction and can demonstrate the presence or absence of obstruction.[69,70] The authors'

practices perform MR imaging to evaluate known or suspected small bowel obstruction in pregnancy, because MR imaging can adequately show the site, severity, and potential cause of obstruction in most patients.[70,71]

Half the patients with IBD are diagnosed before the age of 35 years. Although somewhat controversial, the frequency of flare-ups does not appear to increase during pregnancy, although the

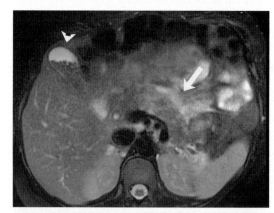

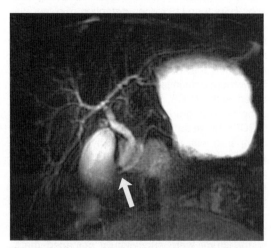

Fig. 10. A 26-year-old 17-week pregnant patient with right upper quadrant pain. US (image not shown) demonstrated cholelithiasis. The distal common bile duct (CBD) was not well visualized due to bowel gas. Coronal MRCP image demonstrates a distal CBD T2 hypointense calculus (*arrow*) with mild dilatation of the bile ducts.

Fig. 11. A 33-year-old 22-week pregnant patient with epigastric pain and a US suggestive of cholelithiasis without cholecystitis (image not shown). The patient's serum lipase was raised (512 U/L), and a clinical diagnosis of gallstone-induced pancreatitis was made. A noncontrast MR imaging was performed to confirm the diagnosis and to evaluate for possible associated complications. Axial T2FS image shows the pancreas to be mildly hyperintense with subtle peripancreatic fluid (*arrow*), along with cholelithiasis (*arrowhead*). Although the presence of necrotizing pancreatitis could not be excluded given the absence of IV contrast, the overall MR imaging findings were more consistent with mild interstitial edematous pancreatitis, with no associated peripancreatic collection. There was no choledocholithiasis on the associated MRCP images (not shown). The patient did well with conservative management.

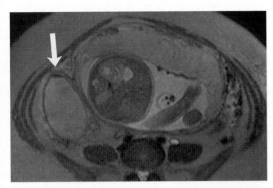

Fig. 12. A 29-year-old 28-week pregnant patient with Crohn disease, with acute right lower quadrant pain. Axial MR SSFSE image shows a well-defined collection in the right lower quadrant, containing a T2-hypointense focus of gas (*arrow*), representing an abscess communicating with the bowel. The adjacent terminal ileum appears T2 hyperintense and inflamed.

administer it in pregnant patients. MR findings of Crohn disease include mural thickening and edema, adjacent fat stranding, and complications of stricture, obstruction, abscess, and sinus tract/fistula formation (**Figs. 12 and 13**).[26,35]

OTHER CAUSES

Abdominal pain can occur because of a myriad number of causes. Depending on the clinical scenario, MR imaging is a helpful problem-solving tool. For example, it can be potentially used instead of CT in evaluating patients with suspected subacute intestinal obstruction or diverticulitis, pregnancy-associated liver disease (hemolysis, elevated liver enzymes and low platelets [HELLP] syndrome or acute fatty liver of pregnancy), pregnancy-associated desmoid, or in excluding or following fluid collections in a postoperative setting (**Fig. 14**).

severity of the flare-ups, when they occur, may be somewhat worse than in nonpregnant women.[72] The main clinical question is the current state of disease activity, and to decide between careful observation, medical management, or surgery.[72] Noncontrast MR imaging is the modality of choice to image IBD in pregnancy in both the acute and the nonacute settings as per the ACR Appropriateness Criteria.[73] In the emergency setting, particularly if there is a degree of bowel obstruction or if there is severe pain, pregnant patients may not be able to tolerate the relatively large volume of oral contrast required for optimized MR enterography, and in that situation, routine MR without oral contrast can be performed. Approximately 1000 mL of neutral enteric contrast is otherwise administered for MR enterography, if tolerated.[73] Cine images are also obtained in the coronal plane to evaluate the bowel. Glucagon is a class B drug in pregnancy, and its use to decrease artifacts related to bowel peristalsis is considered safe.[74] However, the authors still prefer to not routinely

ROLE OF MR IMAGING IN TRAUMA

Maternal death in trauma almost always results in fetal death, and hence, the major focus in such cases is on saving the mother.[75,76] Focused abdominal sonography for trauma followed by contrast-enhanced CT is the current standard of care in imaging pregnant patients with acute trauma, because a single CT examination should be less than the suggested threshold of 50 mGy exposure and would provide the maximum amount of information in the shortest time.[75–77] Unfortunately, most radiology practices, to the authors' knowledge, do not have dedicated CT protocols using low-dose scans in pregnant patients, and the need for rapid diagnosis makes last-minute improvisation difficult. Ideally, because trauma patients may require follow-up CT examinations, there should be a means in place for calculating radiation exposure through a physicist and/or a monitoring device, to calculate exposure and potential cumulative risk.[75–77] It is

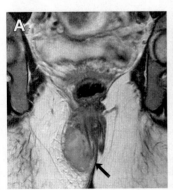
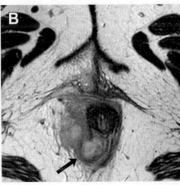

Fig. 13. A 31-year-old 28-week pregnant patient with known Crohn disease and severe perineal pain. Coronal and axial SSFSE MR images (*A, B*) show a transsphincteric fistula with an associated abscess (*arrows*).

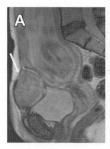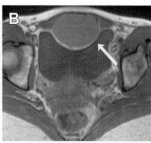

Fig. 14. A 32-year-old 19-week pregnant patient with a gradually progressive painless lump in the lower abdomen. Sagittal SSFSE (*A*) and axial T1WI MR images (*B*) show a well-defined 6.8 × 4.4-cm T2 hyperintense and mildly T1 hyperintense (relative to muscle) anterior abdominal wall mass (*arrows*), representing a soft-tissue neoplasm. The possibility of a pregnancy-associated desmoid was raised in the given clinical setting, which was proven on pathology.

important to note that pregnant patients are more likely to have severe abdominal injuries compared with chest and head injuries. Unfortunately, a common cause of abdominal/pelvic trauma in pregnancy is nonaccidental, that is, assault from the patient's significant other.[77,78]

MR imaging is rarely performed in the acute trauma setting at the present time, because it requires more time, removes the patient from the emergency team, creates difficulty in patient monitoring, and carries the minor risks of gadolinium administration.[75,77] However, MR imaging does have a potential role in the follow-up imaging of such patients, to prevent cumulative ionizing radiation exposure. For example, MR imaging is preferred for evaluating suspected ileus and following-up collections, as well as suspected pancreatic ductal injuries.[75] MR imaging can also

be potentially used in excluding suspected fractures or solid organ injuries, in stable patients with negative US, and a relatively low pretest probability, although the authors are unaware of any study that has evaluated such patients. At the time of this writing, there are no original data on the utility of MR imaging in imaging trauma in pregnancy.

EVALUATION OF MALIGNANCY

Patients with known or suspected malignancy may potentially require more than one imaging examination during the course of their pregnancy, most commonly for staging a newly detected cancer, and the latter scenario may occasionally occur on a relatively urgent basis, particularly given the patient's pregnancy status and the need for rapid and accurate diagnosis and staging. For example, cervical cancer can be detected on a Papanicolaou test when a pregnant patient is initially evaluated. Comprehensive patient counseling is essential, and based on patient preference, the particular malignancy and its staging and needed treatment, and the desire to continue the pregnancy, a detailed workup with either contrast-enhanced CT of the chest, abdomen, and pelvis, or with a CT of the chest with a noncontrast MR imaging of the abdomen and pelvis can be performed, depending on the particular situation. Contrast may be given if indicated for the MR imaging, but should be considered on a case-by-case basis (**Fig. 15**).

Patients may also need restaging/surveillance scans, on a more subacute basis. These imaging examinations can often be postponed until after pregnancy, or to the third trimester, depending on the patient's clinical status and preference. An MR imaging examination is a useful substitute

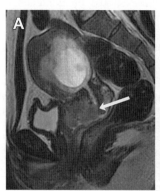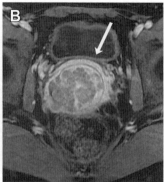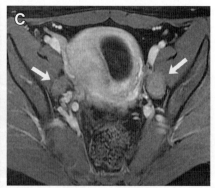

Fig. 15. A 34-year-old 9-week pregnant patient with a Papanicolaou test positive for malignant cells. An IV contrast-enhanced staging MR imaging was performed. Sagittal SSFSE (*A*) and axial post-contrast T1W images (*B, C*) show an exophytic T2 hyperintense, hypoenhancing mass, arising from the anterior cervical wall, without definite bladder invasion (*arrows*), which is consistent with T3 stage disease. Bilateral enlarged internal iliac nodes (*arrows*) are present (*C*), which are highly suspicious for metastatic disease.

for CT for follow-up and avoids additional ionizing radiation exposure to the fetus. In a study of 12 pregnant patients with cervical carcinoma, noncontrast MR imaging was found to be extremely useful in planning and following-up therapy.[79]

SUMMARY

In conclusion, noncontrast MR imaging of the abdomen and/or pelvis is an extremely useful imaging modality for the evaluation of multiple clinical conditions and scenarios in the pregnant patient, particularly for imaging of acute and subacute abdominal pain following inconclusive or indeterminate sonography, and should be liberally used in most clinical scenarios to minimize ionizing radiation exposure. Preparedness with dedicated protocols and appropriate patient counseling is necessary. The acceptability and utility of MR imaging are expected to further increase in the near future, as a greater number of radiologists become more comfortable with performing and interpreting abdominal and pelvic MR imaging in pregnant patients.

REFERENCES

1. American College of Radiology. ACR–SPR practice parameter for imaging pregnant or potentially pregnant adolescents and women with ionizing radiation. Amended 2014 (Resolution 39). Available at: http://www.acr.org/~/media/9e2ed55531fc4b4fa53ef3b6d3b25df8.pdf. Accessed September 10, 2014.
2. Wang PI, Chong ST, Kielar AZ, et al. Imaging of pregnant and lactating patients: part 1, evidence-based review and recommendations. AJR Am J Roentgenol 2012;198(4):778–84.
3. Wieseler KM, Bhargava P, Kanal KM, et al. Imaging in pregnant patients: examination appropriateness. Radiographics 2010;30(5):1215–29 [discussion: 1230–3].
4. De Wilde JP, Rivers AW, Price DL. A review of the current use of magnetic resonance imaging in pregnancy and safety implications for the fetus. Prog Biophys Mol Biol 2005;87(2–3):335–53.
5. Leyendecker JR, Gorengaut V, Brown JJ. MR imaging of maternal diseases of the abdomen and pelvis during pregnancy and the immediate postpartum period. Radiographics 2004;24(5):1301–16.
6. Levine D, Zuo C, Faro CB, et al. Potential heating effect in the gravid uterus during MR HASTE imaging. J Magn Reson Imaging 2001;13(6):856–61.
7. Reeves MJ, Brandreth M, Whitby EH, et al. Neonatal cochlear function: measurement after exposure to acoustic noise during in utero MR imaging. Radiology 2010;257(3):802–9.
8. Kok RD, de Vries MM, Heerschap A, et al. Absence of harmful effects of magnetic resonance exposure at 1.5 T in utero during the third trimester of pregnancy: a follow-up study. Magn Reson Imaging 2004;22(6):851–4.
9. Glover P, Hykin J, Gowland P, et al. An assessment of the intrauterine sound intensity level during obstetric echo-planar magnetic resonance imaging. Br J Radiol 1995;68(814):1090–4.
10. Coakley FV, Glenn OA, Qayyum A, et al. Fetal MRI: a developing technique for the developing patient. AJR Am J Roentgenol 2004;182(1):243–52.
11. Heinrichs WL, Fong P, Flannery M, et al. Midgestational exposure of pregnant BALB/c mice to magnetic resonance imaging conditions. Magn Reson Imaging 1988;6(3):305–13.
12. Yip YP, Capriotti C, Talagala SL, et al. Effects of MR exposure at 1.5 T on early embryonic development of the chick. J Magn Reson Imaging 1994;4(5):742–8.
13. Okazaki R, Ootsuyama A, Uchida S, et al. Effects of a 4.7 T static magnetic field on fetal development in ICR mice. J Radiat Res 2001;42(3):273–83.
14. Ryan BM, Symanski RR, Pomeranz LE, et al. Multigeneration reproductive toxicity assessment of 60-Hz magnetic fields using a continuous breeding protocol in rats. Teratology 1999;59(3):156–62.
15. Shellock FG, Crues JV. MR procedures: biologic effects, safety, and patient care. Radiology 2004;232(3):635–52.
16. International Commission on Non-Ionizing Radiation Protection. Amendment to the ICNIRP "Statement on medical magnetic resonance (MR) procedures: protection of patients". Health Phys 2009;97(3):259–61.
17. International Commission on Non-Ionizing Radiation Protection. Medical magnetic resonance (MR) procedures: protection of patients. Health Phys 2004;87(2):197–216.
18. Expert Panel on MR Safety, Kanal E, Barkovich AJ, et al. ACR guidance document on MR safe practices: 2013. J Magn Reson Imaging 2013;37(3):501–30.
19. Patel SJ, Reede DL, Katz DS, et al. Imaging the pregnant patient for nonobstetric conditions: algorithms and radiation dose considerations. Radiographics 2007;27(6):1705–22.
20. Katzberg RW, McGahan JP. Science to practice: will Gadolinium–enhanced MR imaging be useful in assessment of at-risk pregnancies? Radiology 2011;258(2):325–6.
21. Kanal E, Barkovich AJ, Bell C, et al. ACR guidance document for safe MR practices: 2007. AJR Am J Roentgenol 2007;188(6):1447–74.
22. Jaffe TA, Miller CM, Merkle EM. Practice patterns in imaging of the pregnant patient with abdominal pain: a survey of academic centers. AJR Am J Roentgenol 2007;189(5):1128–34.

23. Shamitoff A, Lamba R, Bennett GL, et al. Practice patterns in imaging of the abdomen and pelvis of the pregnant patient: a survey from the 2012 Radiological Society of North America Annual Meeting controversies session. Ultrasound Q 2015;31(1):2–4.

24. Singh AK, Desai H, Novelline RA. Emergency MRI of acute pelvic pain: MR protocol with no oral contrast. Emerg Radiol 2009;16(2):133–41.

25. Oto A, Ernst RD, Ghulmiyyah LM, et al. MR imaging in the triage of pregnant patients with acute abdominal and pelvic pain. Abdom Imaging 2009;34(2):243–50.

26. Pedrosa I, Zeikus EA, Levine D, et al. MR imaging of acute right lower quadrant pain in pregnant and nonpregnant patients. Radiographics 2007;27(3):721–43 [discussion: 743–53].

27. Cobben LP, Groot I, Haans L, et al. MRI for clinically suspected appendicitis during pregnancy. AJR Am J Roentgenol 2004;183(3):671–5.

28. Oto A, Ernst RD, Shah R, et al. Right-lower-quadrant pain and suspected appendicitis in pregnant women: evaluation with MR imaging–initial experience. Radiology 2005;234(2):445–51.

29. Pedrosa I, Lafornara M, Pandharipande PV, et al. Pregnant patients suspected of having acute appendicitis: effect of MR imaging on negative laparotomy rate and appendiceal perforation rate. Radiology 2009;250(3):749–57.

30. Pedrosa I, Levine D, Eyvazzadeh AD, et al. MR imaging evaluation of acute appendicitis in pregnancy. Radiology 2006;238(3):891–9.

31. Katz DS, Klein MA, Ganson G, et al. Imaging of abdominal pain in pregnancy. Radiol Clin North Am 2012;50(1):149–71.

32. Wang PI, Chong ST, Kielar AZ, et al. Imaging of pregnant and lactating patients: part 2, evidence-based review and recommendations. AJR Am J Roentgenol 2012;198(4):785–92.

33. Beddy P, Keogan MT, Sala E, et al. Magnetic resonance imaging for the evaluation of acute abdominal pain in pregnancy. Semin Ultrasound CT MR 2010;31(5):433–41.

34. Andersen B, Nielsen TF. Appendicitis in pregnancy: diagnosis, management and complications. Acta Obstet Gynecol Scand 1999;78(9):758–62.

35. Spalluto LB, Woodfield CA, DeBenedectis CM, et al. MR imaging evaluation of abdominal pain during pregnancy: appendicitis and other nonobstetric causes. Radiographics 2012;32(2):317–34.

36. Mazze RI, Kallen B. Appendectomy during pregnancy: a Swedish registry study of 778 cases. Obstet Gynecol 1991;77(6):835–40.

37. McGory ML, Zingmond DS, Tillou A, et al. Negative appendectomy in pregnant women is associated with a substantial risk of fetal loss. J Am Coll Surg 2007;205(4):534–40.

38. American College of Radiology ACR Appropriateness Criteria; last reviewed 2013. Available at: http://www.acr.org/~/media/7425a3e08975451eab571a316db4ca1b.pdf. Accessed September 30, 1014.

39. Lim HK, Bae SH, Seo GS. Diagnosis of acute appendicitis in pregnant women: value of sonography. AJR Am J Roentgenol 1992;159(3):539–42.

40. Israel GM, Malguria N, McCarthy S, et al. MRI vs. ultrasound for suspected appendicitis during pregnancy. J Magn Reson Imaging 2008;28(2):428–33.

41. Kim YS, Kim Y, Cho OK, et al. Sonography for right lower quadrant pain. J Clin Ultrasound 2001;29(3):157–85.

42. Poortman P, Lohle PN, Schoemaker CM, et al. Comparison of CT and sonography in the diagnosis of acute appendicitis: a blinded prospective study. AJR Am J Roentgenol 2003;181(5):1355–9.

43. Dewhurst C, Beddy P, Pedrosa I. MRI evaluation of acute appendicitis in pregnancy. J Magn Reson Imaging 2013;37(3):566–75.

44. Long SS, Long C, Lai H, et al. Imaging strategies for right lower quadrant pain in pregnancy. AJR Am J Roentgenol 2011;196(1):4–12.

45. Inci E, Kilickesmez O, Hocaoglu E, et al. Utility of diffusion-weighted imaging in the diagnosis of acute appendicitis. Eur Radiol 2011;21(4):768–75.

46. Semins MJ, Matlaga BR. Management of urolithiasis in pregnancy. Int J Womens Health 2013;5:599–604.

47. Andreoiu M, MacMahon R. Renal colic in pregnancy: lithiasis or physiological hydronephrosis? Urology 2009;74(4):757–61.

48. Shokeir AA, Mahran MR, Abdulmaaboud M. Renal colic in pregnant women: role of renal resistive index. Urology 2000;55(3):344–7.

49. Wachsberg RH. Unilateral absence of ureteral jets in the third trimester of pregnancy: pitfall in color Doppler US diagnosis of urinary obstruction. Radiology 1998;209(1):279–81.

50. Shabana W, Bude RO, Rubin JM. Comparison between color Doppler twinkling artifact and acoustic shadowing for renal calculus detection: an in vitro study. Ultrasound Med Biol 2009;35(2):339–50.

51. Roy C, Saussine C, Jahn C, et al. Fast imaging MR assessment of ureterohydronephrosis during pregnancy. Magn Reson Imaging 1995;13(6):767–72.

52. Aoyagi J, Odaka J, Kuroiwa Y, et al. Utility of non-enhanced magnetic resonance imaging to detect acute pyelonephritis. Pediatr Int 2014;56(3):e4–6.

53. Craig WD, Wagner BJ, Travis MD. Pyelonephritis: radiologic-pathologic review. Radiographics 2008;28(1):255–77 [quiz: 327–8].

54. Regan F, Kuszyk B, Bohlman ME, et al. Acute ureteric calculus obstruction: unenhanced spiral CT versus HASTE MR urography and abdominal radiograph. Br J Radiol 2005;78(930):506–11.

55. Sung MK, Singh S, Kalra MK. Current status of low dose multi-detector CT in the urinary tract. World J Radiol 2011;3(11):256–65.

56. Eisner B. Imaging calculi in pregnancy–is the future ultra low dose computerized tomography with iterative reconstruction technique? J Urol 2012;188(1): 12–3.

57. Smith-Bindman R, Aubin C, Bailitz J, et al. Ultrasonography versus computed tomography for suspected nephrolithiasis. N Engl J Med 2014; 371(12):1100–10.

58. Derman AY, Nikac V, Haberman S, et al. MRI of placenta accreta: a new imaging perspective. AJR Am J Roentgenol 2011;197(6):1514–21.

59. Kani KK, Lee JH, Dighe M, et al. Gestational trophoblastic disease: multimodality imaging assessment with special emphasis on spectrum of abnormalities and value of imaging in staging and management of disease. Curr Probl Diagn Radiol 2012;41(1):1–10.

60. Lim AK, Patel D, Patel N, et al. Pelvic imaging in gestational trophoblastic neoplasia. J Reprod Med 2008;53(8):575–8.

61. Mahajan D, Kang M, Sandhu MS, et al. Rare complications of cesarean scar. Indian J Radiol Imaging 2013;23(3):258–61.

62. Maldjian C, Milestone B, Schnall M, et al. MR appearance of uterine dehiscence in the post-cesarean section patient. J Comput Assist Tomogr 1998;22(5):738–41.

63. Robbins JB, Parry JP, Guite KM, et al. MRI of pregnancy-related issues: mullerian duct anomalies. AJR Am J Roentgenol 2012;198(2):302–10.

64. Lu EJ, Curet MJ, El-Sayed YY, et al. Medical versus surgical management of biliary tract disease in pregnancy. Am J Surg 2004;188(6):755–9.

65. Mendez-Sanchez N, Chavez-Tapia NC, Uribe M. Pregnancy and gallbladder disease. Ann Hepatol 2006;5(3):227–30.

66. Oto A, Ernst R, Ghulmiyyah L, et al. The role of MR cholangiopancreatography in the evaluation of pregnant patients with acute pancreaticobiliary disease. Br J Radiol 2009;82(976):279–85.

67. Shanmugam V, Beattie GC, Yule SR, et al. Is magnetic resonance cholangiopancreatography the new gold standard in biliary imaging? Br J Radiol 2005;78(934):888–93.

68. Kahaleh M, Hartwell GD, Arseneau KO, et al. Safety and efficacy of ERCP in pregnancy. Gastrointest Endosc 2004;60(2):287–92.

69. Hefny AF, Corr P, Abu-Zidan FM. The role of ultrasound in the management of intestinal obstruction. J Emerg Trauma Shock 2012;5(1):84–6.

70. Silva AC, Pimenta M, Guimaraes LS. Small bowel obstruction: what to look for. Radiographics 2009; 29(2):423–39.

71. McKenna DA, Meehan CP, Alhajeri AN, et al. The use of MRI to demonstrate small bowel obstruction during pregnancy. Br J Radiol 2007;80(949):e11–4.

72. Ferguson CB, Mahsud-Dornan S, Patterson RN. Inflammatory bowel disease in pregnancy. BMJ 2008;337:a427.

73. American College of Radiology. ACR Appropriateness Criteria; last reviewed 2014. Available at: https://acsearch.acr.org/docs/69470/Narrative. Accessed June 10, 2015.

74. Rayburn W, Piehl E, Sanfield J, et al. Reversing severe hypoglycemia during pregnancy with glucagon therapy. Am J Perinatol 1987;4(3):259–61.

75. Sadro C, Bernstein MP, Kanal KM. Imaging of trauma: part 2, abdominal trauma and pregnancy–a radiologist's guide to doing what is best for the mother and baby. AJR Am J Roentgenol 2012; 199(6):1207–19.

76. Lowdermilk C, Gavant ML, Qaisi W, et al. Screening helical CT for evaluation of blunt traumatic injury in the pregnant patient. Radiographics 1999;19 Spec No:S243–55 [discussion: S256–8].

77. Raptis CA, Mellnick VM, Raptis DA, et al. Imaging of trauma in the pregnant patient. Radiographics 2014; 34(3):748–63.

78. Shah KH, Simons RK, Holbrook T, et al. Trauma in pregnancy: maternal and fetal outcomes. J Trauma 1998;45(1):83–6.

79. Balleyguier C, Fournet C, Ben Hassen W, et al. Management of cervical cancer detected during pregnancy: role of magnetic resonance imaging. Clin Imaging 2013;37(1):70–6.

80. Masselli G, Brunelli R, Casciani E, et al. Acute abdominal and pelvic pain in pregnancy: MR imaging as a valuable adjunct to ultrasound? Abdom Imaging 2011;36(5):596–603.

Magnetic Resonance of Pelvic and Gastrointestinal Emergencies

Sirote Wongwaisayawan, MD[a], Rathachai Kaewlai, MD[a],
Matthew Dattwyler, MD[b], Hani H. Abujudeh, MD[b],
Ajay K. Singh, MD[b],*

KEY WORDS

- Magnetic resonance imaging • Pelvic emergencies • Gastrointestinal emergencies
- Degenerating leiomyoma • Ovarian torsion • Pelvic inflammatory disease • Testicular torsion
- Acute appendicitis

KEY POINTS

- Magnetic resonance (MR) imaging of the abdomen and pelvis is playing an increasing role in the emergency setting, both in primary diagnosis and as a problem-solving modality.
- MR imaging is especially useful in patients in whom exposure to ionizing radiation is a concern, including patients who are pregnant, children, and patients with chronic diseases that necessitate multiple scans, such as Crohn disease.
- MR sequences should be tailored to the patient's specific clinical presentation with the aim of minimizing scan time while maximizing diagnostic accuracy.

INTRODUCTION

Magnetic resonance (MR) imaging is an established imaging method for the evaluation of many abdominal and pelvic diseases. The ability to distinguish different types of soft tissues based on their intrinsic signal intensity, multiplanar capability, and the identification of pathology without exposing patients to radiation are the major advantages of MR imaging. Although imaging of the gastrointestinal (GI) tract can be a challenge for MR imaging because of peristalsis, fast MR techniques allow accurate depiction of many acute GI conditions. MR imaging can provide clear, valuable information for clinical management in patients with acute pelvic pain, acute scrotum, and suspected appendicitis. In addition to these conditions, acute pancreaticobiliary diseases, such as

acute cholecystitis, cholelithiasis, choledocholithiasis, cholangitis, and pancreatitis also can be depicted with MR imaging and MR cholangiopancreatography (MRCP), which are discussed in the article (See Bates DDB, LeBedis CA, Soto J, et al: Use of MR in Pancreaticobiliary Emergencies, in this issue). In this article, the authors discuss MR imaging protocols and findings of acute pelvic, scrotal, and GI pathologies.

NORMAL ANATOMY AND IMAGING TECHNIQUES

Female pelvic structures (uterus, cervix, vagina, ovary, and adnexa) are readily demonstrated on MR imaging. T2-weighted imaging is the mainstay sequence for differentiation of zonal anatomy of the uterus. Three distinct zones (**Fig. 1**) of the

The authors have nothing to disclose.
[a] Department of Diagnostic and Therapeutic Radiology, Faculty of Medicine, Ramathibodi Hospital, Mahidol University, 270 Rama VI Road, Ratchatewi, Bangkok 10400, Thailand; [b] Department of Radiology, Massachusetts General Hospital, Boston, MA, USA
* Corresponding author. 2 Avery Street, #32H, Boston, MA 02111.
E-mail address: asingh1@partners.org

Magn Reson Imaging Clin N Am 24 (2016) 419–431
http://dx.doi.org/10.1016/j.mric.2015.11.008
1064-9689/16/$ – see front matter © 2016 Elsevier Inc. All rights reserved.

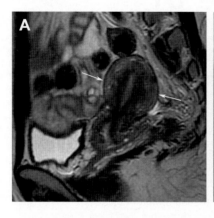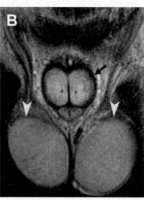

Fig. 1. Normal anatomy. (*A*) Sagittal T2-weighted MR image of the female pelvis shows a uterus in an anteflexed position (*arrows*) with 3 distinct layers of innermost endometrium (high signal intensity), junctional zone (low signal intensity), and outermost myometrium (intermediate signal intensity). Zonal anatomy also can be observed in the uterine cervix with central hyperintense endocervical mucosa, middle hypointense zone, and outer intermediate signal intensity. The vagina has a thin, smooth fibromuscular wall of hypointensity with central hyperintense mucosa. (*B*) Coronal T2-weighted MR image of the testicles (*arrowheads*) demonstrates homogeneous slightly hyperintense signal of the testicular parenchyma. A thin, hypointense stripe surrounding the testicles represents tunica albuginea and the visceral layer of tunica vaginalis. Paired corpora cavernosa and a corpus spongiosum of the penis is seen (*arrow*).

premenopausal uterus include an innermost layer of uterine endometrium, middle layer (junctional zone), and outermost layer. The innermost high T2 signal intensity represents the endometrium with varying thickness depending on age and menstrual cycle. Generally, an endometrial thickness of less than 10 mm is considered normal in reproductive-age women, whereas thickness of less than 5 mm is considered normal in postmenopausal women.[1] The middle layer is the junctional zone, which represents the inner myometrium. The junctional zone has low signal intensity relative to the adjacent outermost layer. The outermost layer is the myometrium, which has intermediate signal intensity on T2-weighted images. The uterine cervix also demonstrates zonal anatomy on T2-weighted images: central hyperintense zone of endocervical mucosa, middle hypointense zone of fibromuscular stroma, and outer intermediate signal intensity of loose stroma. This zonal anatomy is indistinct in the postmenopausal uterus, in which the junctional zone may not be visualized. On T1-weighted images, the uterus is isointense to the muscle and zonal anatomy is not appreciated. The normal ovarian stroma has intermediate signal intensity on T1-weighted images. On T2-weighted images, ovarian follicles demonstrate very high signal intensity. The ovarian medulla usually has higher signal intensity than the ovarian cortex. The vagina also demonstrates zonal anatomy on T2-weighted images: central hyperintense signal of mucosa and intraluminal fluid, middle hypointense zone of submucosal and muscularis layer, and outer hyperintense zone of adventitial layer and vascular plexus.[1]

The testicles lie within each hemiscrotum and are suspended by the spermatic cords. They have homogeneously intermediate signal intensity on T1-weighted images and are slightly hyperintense on T2-weighed images. Normal testicles show slow and steady contrast enhancement after gadolinium administration.[2] The surrounding tunica albuginea and the visceral layer of tunica vaginalis are seen as a thin stripe of low signal intensity on both T1-weighted and T2-weighted images due to their fibrous component (see **Fig. 1**). The epididymes are located along the superolateral aspect of the testicle and consist of head, body, and tail. The epididymal tail continues as the vas deferens to the spermatic cord. The epididymis has signal intensity similar to the testicular parenchyma on T1-weighted images and lower signal intensity than that of testicular parenchyma on T2-weighted images.

Distended bowel loops contain T2 hyperintense fluid, which serves as a natural contrast medium. The normal bowel wall is barely visible when the bowel loops are distended. Its thickness is up to 1 to 2 mm for small bowel and 3 mm for the large bowel. The small bowel diameter is usually less than 2.5 cm in diameter.[3] The appendix is a blind-ended tubular structure arising from the cecum with T1 hypointensity and T2 hyperintensity. Its wall thickness is less than 2 mm and the total axial diameter is usually less than 6 mm. Air bubbles within the lumen may be depicted. When fat suppression technique is applied adequately, the periappendiceal tissues appear hypointense.

IMAGING PROTOCOLS

MR imaging in the emergency setting requires the use of streamlined protocols to minimize imaging time while maintaining diagnostic accuracy for the most commonly encountered abdominopelvic pathologies. For the evaluation of lower abdominal and pelvic pain, our protocol begins with multiplanar T2 single-shot fast spin-echo (SSFSE) sequence to identify pathology and establish the best plane for additional imaging. This is followed by axial T2 fast-spin echo and axial short tau inversion recovery (STIR) sequences to highlight pathologies. In patients who are not pregnant, fat-saturated T1-weighted precontrast and postcontrast images are obtained (**Table 1**). Ideally acquisition will be monitored by the interpreting radiologist to adjust imaging planes and prescribe additional sequences as necessary for problem solving.

For evaluation of pancreaticobiliary pathology, our protocol includes coronal balanced steady-state gradient echo (FIESTA), coronal T2 SSFSE, axial fat-saturated T2, axial 3-point Dixon, dynamic contrast-enhanced fat-saturated T1 (pre-, 25, 35, 70, 180, and 240 seconds), and 3-dimensional MRCP.

PELVIC EMERGENCIES
Degenerating Leiomyoma

Uterine leiomyomas are the most common pelvic tumor in women, with a prevalence of 20% to 30% in women older than 30 years.[4] Abnormal menstrual bleeding, pelvic pain, or pressure-related symptoms can occur depending on number, size, and location of leiomyoma. Pain can occur in up to 30% of patients, and is usually a result of acute degeneration.[5] Large leiomyomas may outgrow their blood supply, leading to ischemia and necrosis. There are many types of degenerating leiomyoma: hyaline, calcific, cystic, myxoid,

fatty, and red degeneration. The most common type is hyaline degeneration, which accounts for up to 60% of degenerating leiomyomas.[6]

Because of its high soft tissue contrast, MR imaging is an excellent modality for detection of leiomyoma and related complications. Nondegenerating leiomyomata appear well-circumscribed, homogeneously hypointense on T2-weighted images when compared with the outer myometrium.[5] Several types of leiomyoma degeneration can be suggested based on MR appearances with an overall accuracy of 69%[5-9] (**Fig. 2**). Hyaline and calcific degenerations show low signal intensity or cobblestone appearance on T2-weighted images. Red degeneration represents hemorrhagic infarction secondary to obstructing venous return. It appears as T1 hyperintensity on the periphery of the leiomyoma or diffusely throughout the entire leiomyoma, and variable signal intensity on T2-weighed images. Sometimes, low T2 signal intensity rim can be seen. Myoma with myxoid degeneration will appear very hyperintense on T2-weighted images and enhances after gadolinium administration. Cystic degeneration also demonstrates high T2 signal intensity, but the cystic components do not enhance following gadolinium administration. MR imaging has good performance in diagnosis of hemorrhagic and cystic degeneration, with reported sensitivity of 100% and 80% and specificity of 86% and 98%, respectively.[7]

Twisted Pedunculated Leiomyoma

Acute torsion of a pedunculated leiomyoma is a very rare complication of leiomyoma. A leiomyoma may twist around its stalk, resulting in sudden onset of pain due to venous congestion and then

Table 1
Abdominopelvic emergency magnetic resonance imaging protocols

Acute Appendicitis	Acute Appendicitis (Pregnant)	Pancreaticobiliary Pathology
Axial, coronal, and sagittal T2 SSFSE	Axial, coronal, and sagittal T2 SSFSE	Coronal balanced steady state gradient echo
Axial T2 FSE	Axial T2 FSE	Coronal T2 SSFSE
Axial STIR	Axial STIR	Axial fat-saturated T2
Axial T1 fat-saturated precontrast and postcontrast	—	Axial 3-point Dixon
—	—	Dynamic contrast-enhanced fat-saturated T1 (pre-, 25, 35, 70, 180, and 240 s)
—	—	3D MRCP

Abbreviations: FSE, fast spin echo; MRCP, magnetic resonance cholangiopancreatography; SSFSE, single-shot fast spin-echo; STIR, short tau inversion recovery.

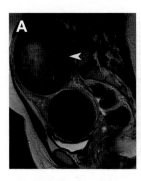
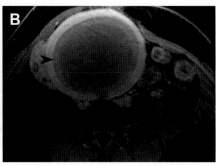

Fig. 2. Fibroid degeneration. (*A, B*) Sagittal T2-weighted (*A*) and axial contrast-enhanced, fat-suppressed T1-weighted (*B*) MR images of the pelvis show 2 large uterine leiomyomas (*arrowheads*) distorting the uterine contour and endometrial lining. The superior one demonstrates heterogeneous T2 signal intensity with lack of central enhancement, suggesting degeneration.

arterial compromise. The size of the myoma itself serves as a key factor for irreversible torsion. The larger size of the leiomyoma, the more difficult for spontaneous detorsion.[10] Clinical signs, symptoms, and ultrasound findings often mimic those of ovarian torsion[6] and depend on the degree of torsion.[11] MR imaging can demonstrate the pedunculated leiomyoma adjacent to the uterus, its stalk extending from the mass to the uterus and a separate, normal ipsilateral ovary. The presence of "bridging vascular sign" or curvilinear/tortuous vascular structures between the uterus and the mass suggest a uterine origin of the mass.[12] A separate, ipsilateral ovary is helpful to exclude an ovarian torsion. The lack of internal enhancement of leiomyoma helps suggest infarction secondary to a twist (**Fig. 3**).

Pelvic Inflammatory Disease/Tubo-ovarian Abscess

Pelvic inflammatory disease (PID) is a spectrum of upper genital tract infection in women, including endometritis, salpingitis, tubo-ovarian abscess (TOA) and/or pelvic peritonitis.[13] It usually affects young sexually active women as a result of ascending spread of microorganisms from the lower genital tract.[13,14] Currently, the diagnosis remains a challenge because signs and symptoms (lower abdominal or pelvic pain, deep

dyspareunia, abnormal bleeding, and abnormal vaginal or cervical discharge) are nonspecific, and present in only approximately 20% of patients.[13,15] TOA is a severe form of the acute PID that causes significant morbidity and occasional mortality. Transvaginal ultrasound is generally recommended as the first-line imaging modality, whereas MR imaging is a problem-solving tool for difficult cases. Computed tomography (CT) is usually reserved in patients with peritonitis and for guidance of interventional treatment. MR imaging is more specific and more accurate for identification and characterization of complex uterine and adnexal lesions than ultrasound. A direct comparison between MR imaging and transvaginal ultrasound shows that MR imaging has sensitivity, specificity, and accuracy of 95%, 89%, and 93%, respectively. In this study, ultrasound demonstrates sensitivity, specificity, and accuracy of 81%, 78%, and 80%, respectively.[16]

Fallopian tubes distended with pus can be clearly demonstrated on MR imaging (**Fig. 4**) as a sausagelike structure in the parauterine regions with content of varying signal intensity. Although fluid is generally T1 hypointense and T2 hyperintense, pus may exhibit complex signal intensity on both T1-weighted and T2-weighted images.[17] T1 hyperintensity and heterogeneous T2 signal intensity may be expected secondary to internal

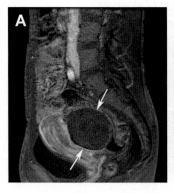
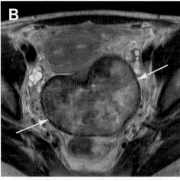

Fig. 3. Fibroid torsion. (*A, B*) Sagittal contrast-enhanced, fat-suppressed T1-weighted (*A*) and axial T2-weighted (*B*) MR images show a torsed pedunculated subserosal myoma (*arrows*) that demonstrates heterogeneous isointense to hyperintense T2 signal with hypointense T2 rim and shows no enhancement after contrast administration. Zonal anatomy of the uterine corpus is also observed on axial T2-weighted MR image.

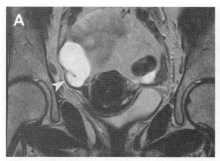
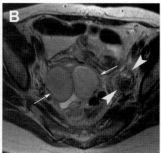
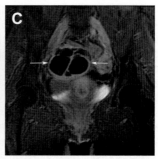

Fig. 4. Hydrosalpinx and tubo-ovarian abscess. (*A*) Coronal T2-weighted MR image of the pelvis demonstrates a dilated, tortuous, right fallopian tube filled with T2 hyperintense content, representing hydrosalpinx (*arrowhead*). (*B, C*) Axial T2-weighted (*B*) and coronal contrast-enhanced, fat-suppressed T1-weighted (*C*) MR images of another patient show a multiloculated cystic lesion at right adnexa (*arrows*) that demonstrates homogeneous hypointense T2 signal and peripheral rim enhancement after contrast administration. A normal-appearing left ovary *arrowheads* is also observed on axial T2-weighted MR image.

debris or hemorrhage. TOA can be seen as a multilocular cystic structure or an ill-defined heterogeneous mass with cystic and solid components. It often shows various signal intensity on both T1-weighted and T2-weighted images with enhancement of the walls, septae, and solid portions. Edematous change of surrounding pelvic soft tissue is usually present and seen as increased signal intensity on T2-weighted images. MR imaging has sensitivity ranging from 90% to 95% and specificity ranging from 89% to 93% for the diagnosis of acute PID.[8,18] Presence of surrounding pelvic soft tissue edema, and thick/smooth and enhanced septa of the mass combining with a correct clinical context can help accurately differentiate acute PID/TOA from ovarian tumors.

Ovarian Torsion

Torsion of the ovary, either complete or incomplete, around its ligamentous support often results in compromised blood supply to the ovary. When this occurs, venous blood flow becomes obstructed, leading to ovarian stromal congestion, edema, and eventually arterial ischemia with necrosis. Ovarian torsion usually affects premenopausal women, especially those who have underlying adnexal mass. In fact, up to 81% of ovarian torsion occur on preexisting adnexal lesions such as functional cyst, corpus luteal cyst, or mature teratoma.[19] Right-sided torsion is more common than the left side. Ultrasound is usually the first imaging modality for suspected ovarian torsion. CT and MR imaging serve as a second-line imaging test after equivocal ultrasound findings but they may be an initial imaging in patients with nonspecific presentation.

MR imaging findings consistent with ovarian torsion (**Fig. 5**) include ovarian enlargement, edematous ovary (increased T2 signal intensity), abnormal location of the torsed ovary, twisted vascular pedicle (so-called whirlpool sign), lack of contrast enhancement,[6,19,20] and restricted diffusion in the wall of the twisted mass.[21] Multiple, small, peripherally located ovarian follicles may be observed, which are a result of pressure effect

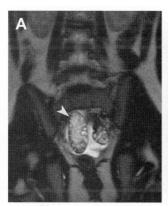
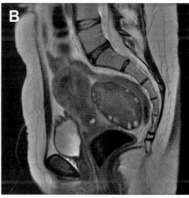

Fig. 5. Ovarian torsion. (*A*) Coronal T2-weighted MR image of the pelvis shows enlargement of the right ovary (*arrowhead*) with increased signal intensity of the ovarian parenchyma. Multiple, small, peripherally located ovarian follicles are also observed. (*B*) Sagittal T2-weighted image in a different patient shows an enlarged ovary with peripheral follicles posterior to the uterus. In both instances a diagnosis of ovarian torsion was made at laparoscopy.

from stromal edema. Other MR imaging findings include abnormal uterine deviation to the side of torsion, adnexal fat infiltration, free fluid, and fallopian tubal thickening. Although MR imaging has been shown to have a good sensitivity of 86% and a positive predictive value of 100% for the diagnosis of ovarian torsion,[8] some pitfalls have been reported. Ovarian lesions containing subacute hemorrhage, such as hemorrhagic corpus luteal cyst (**Fig. 6**) or hypovascular tumor, may mimic torsion. Absence of a twisted vascular pedicle and preserved ovarian enhancement make the diagnosis of torsion unlikely in these cases. Infarction or degeneration of pedunculated or broad ligament leiomyoma may also mimic ovarian torsion. In these cases, identification of a normal ipsilateral ovary is the key to a correct diagnosis.[22]

Testicular Torsion

Testicular torsion refers to abnormal rotation of the testicle around its cord structures, resulting in venous congestion, subsequent arterial compromise, and eventual infarction. Two types of testicular torsion are intravaginal and extravaginal torsion (**Fig. 7**). The former usually occurs in children and is associated with an elongated attachment of the tunica vaginalis.[23] The latter is generally seen in adolescent and young adults, and is commonly associated with a bell-clapper anomaly.[24] The bell-clapper anomaly describes a large tunica vaginalis that completely surrounds the testis, epididymis, and a part of the spermatic cord, increasing the risk for torsion. Accurate, timely diagnosis and surgical intervention of testicular torsion is crucial because testicular salvage rate is nearly 100% if surgery is done within 6 hours after onset. This number drops significantly to 20% after 12 to 24 hours.[24] Color Doppler ultrasound remains the initial imaging modality for evaluation of suspected torsion because of its wide availability and accuracy, reported between 90% to 100%.[23] However, in cases of equivocal or inconclusive ultrasound findings, contrast-enhanced MR imaging can be used as a problem-solving tool.[25,26] Dynamic contrast-

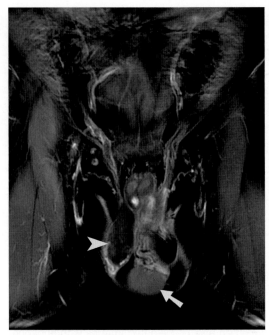

Fig. 7. Testicular torsion. Coronal, contrast-enhanced, fat-suppressed T1-weighted MR image of the scrotum shows an abnormally high position of the right testicle (*arrowhead*). The right testicle has heterogeneous signal intensity with lack of contrast enhancement. The left testicle (*arrow*) is normal.

enhanced MR imaging can show complete torsion with 100% sensitivity. The torsed testicle exhibits no contrast enhancement when compared with the normal side.[2,27,28] Except for an unusual event of spontaneous detorsion, presence of normal testicular enhancement can be used to rule out torsion.[27,28] T2-weighted and T2*-weighted images also can reveal hemorrhagic necrosis by showing low or very low signal intensity with spotty or streaky patterns.[23]

GASTROINTESTINAL EMERGENCIES
Acute Appendicitis

Acute appendicitis is the most common surgical abdominal emergency with a lifetime incidence of 7% to 14%.[29] It is the major differential diagnosis

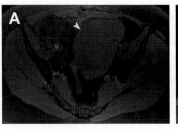
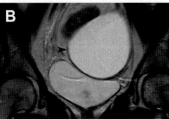

Fig. 6. Corpus luteal cyst. (*A, B*) Axial, fat-suppressed T1-weighted (*A*) and coronal T2-weighted (*B*) MR images demonstrate a large left ovarian cyst (*arrowhead*) with T1 isointensity and T2 near-water hyperintensity.

of acute right lower quadrant pain. The peak incidence is at approximately 10 to 20 years of age with slight male preponderance (male-to-female ratio of 1.4:1.0).[30] The exact cause is probably multifactorial, including luminal obstruction, and dietary and familial factors. A combination of migratory abdominal pain from the periumbilical region to the right iliac fossa, loss of appetite, nausea, and vomiting represent classic clinical presentation. Sensitivity, specificity, and accuracy of MR imaging for acute appendicitis in individuals who are not pregnant are 97% to 100%, 88% to 97%, and 92% to 94%, respectively.[31–35]

On MR imaging, findings of acute appendicitis (**Fig. 8**) include appendiceal dilatation (diameter of >6 mm), fluid distension of the appendix (T2 hyperintense content), appendiceal wall thickness of greater than 2 mm, hyperintense T2 signal change of the periappendiceal tissues, and marked enhancement of the appendix after gadolinium administration.[35–38] The appendicolith may be seen as a round-shaped structure with low signal intensity on all pulse sequences. Air outside the appendiceal lumen (appearing as tiny, round/oval spots of hypointensity on all pulse sequences), T2 hyperintense fluid collection, or abscess formation are MR imaging signs suggestive of perforated appendicitis.[33] For diagnosis of appendiceal perforation, MR imaging demonstrates slightly higher sensitivity (57%) than ultrasound with conditional CT (48% sensitivity).[39]

Acute Diverticulitis

Diverticular disease affects approximately 5% to 10% of people by the age of 45 years and as many as 80% by the age of 80.[40] The most frequently involved colonic segment is the sigmoid colon, but diverticulosis can occur anywhere. *Acute diverticulitis* is diagnosed when there are diverticula with bowel wall thickening and

pericolonic fat stranding[40–42] (**Fig. 9**). The inflamed diverticulum can be identified in 30% of cases[43] and is seen as an outpouching lesion with low signal intensity on both T1-weighted and T2-weighted images with increased T2 signal intensity of the adjacent mesenteric fat.[44,45] A short segment of focal, eccentric, or circumferential colonic wall thickening with intermediate T1 and high T2 signal intensities is present in 70% to 94% of cases.[44] *Complications of acute diverticulitis*, such as perforation, abscess formation, fistulous tract formation, and rectal bleeding, may be depicted on MR imaging. Microperforation is the most common complication reported in approximately 16% of cases, which can lead to phlegmon and abscess formation. Ill-defined soft tissue of intermediate signal intensity suggests phlegmon, whereas an abscess is diagnosed when there is a T1 hypointense, T2 hyperintense fluid collection with rim enhancement. Diverticular abscess most commonly occurs within the inflamed colonic wall (intramural abscess) or adjacent to the wall (paracolic abscess). It can be remote to the site of diverticulitis, such as within the psoas muscle, pelvic floor musculature, uterus, and adnexae. Small foci of extraluminal free air may show low signal intensity on all pulse sequences.[43] Fistulous tract formation mostly connects the inflamed colon to the bladder or vagina. An air-filled or fluid-filled tract extending from the colon to the affected organs can be seen. Focal urinary bladder wall thickening, tethering of the sigmoid colon to the bladder, or gas in the bladder lumen is the imaging clue for colovesical fistula. The major differential diagnosis of acute diverticulitis is colonic cancer. The involved colonic segment in diverticulitis is longer, has circumferential wall thickening with thumbprinting morphology, and shows preserved stratified wall enhancement and a greater degree of pericolonic fat inflammation. Marked wall thickening of greater than 2 cm, eccentric wall

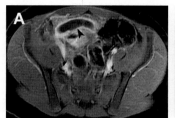 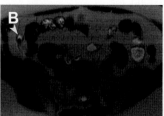 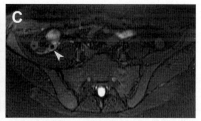

Fig. 8. Acute appendicitis. (*A*) *Patient 1*. Axial, fat-suppressed, contrast-enhanced T1-weighted (*A*) MR image shows an enlarged appendix with thickened and enhancing wall (*arrowhead*). Increased enhancement of the periappendiceal tissue also is observed. (*B*) *Patient 2*. Axial SSFSE T2-weighted MR image shows a T2-hyperintense, fluid-filled appendix (*arrowhead*) with an intraluminal T2 hypointense dot, representing an appendicolith. (*C*) *Patient 3*. Axial SSFSE T2-weighted MR image shows an enlarged appendix with increased T2 signal intensity of its thickened wall. A central T2 hypointense dot represents appendicolith (*arrowhead*).

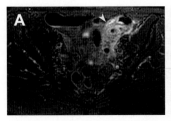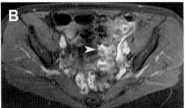

Fig. 9. Sigmoid diverticulitis. (*A, B*) Axial STIR (*A*) and contrast-enhanced, fat-suppressed T1 (*B*) MR images show segmental wall thickening, enhancement, and pericolic fat stranding of the sigmoid colon (*arrowhead*). Multiple colonic diverticula are seen within this inflamed colonic segment.

thickening, homogeneous colonic wall enhancement, pericolic adenopathy, and colonic obstruction are features suggestive of colonic cancer.[43]

Active Crohn Disease

Crohn disease is a chronic granulomatous inflammatory disease of the GI tract, which tends to be relapsing. It commonly affects individuals between 15 and 30 years of age. Clinical signs and symptoms are similar to those of acute appendicitis, including fever, diarrhea, and abdominal pain.[3,46] Inflammatory granulomas start at the submucosal layer, and extend transmurally and then extramurally to the serosa. Strictures, abscesses, fistulae, and sinus tract formation are common. Small bowel is involved in more than 80% of cases and most frequently the terminal ileum.[3] Although an ideal imaging method for the diagnosis and characterization of bowel involvement of Crohn disease is CT or MR enteroclysis, routine MR imaging may be used to assess the extent of disease and complications with a sensitivity more than 95%.[3] Bowel wall thickening (usually greater than 4–5 mm), increased T2 signal intensity of the wall, mural stratification, marked wall enhancement after gadolinium administration, and increased mesenteric vascularity (comb sign) are MR features of active Crohn disease[3,45] (**Fig. 10**). A round area of high T2 signal intensity with rim enhancement is suggestive of abscess formation, whereas a linear high T2 signal-intensity lesion with rim enhancement represents fistulous tract formation. The latter can be between bowel loops or connecting the bowel to other adjacent structures.

Terminal Ileitis

Ileitis refers to an inflammation of the ileum, which is classically caused by Crohn disease. However, a wide variety of diseases are associated with ileitis, including infection (eg, *Campylobacter*, *Yersinia*, *Mycobacterium*), vasculitides, ischemia, neoplasms, drug-induced eosinophilic enteritis, and sarcoidosis. *Typhlitis* or *neutropenic enterocolitis* is an acute inflammatory disease of the cecum and ascending colon. It most often occurs in immunocompromised hosts with profound

neutropenia, therefore impaired host defense immunity. Fever, right lower abdominal pain, and tenderness are the classic signs and symptoms that mimic those of acute appendicitis. Thickened bowel wall at the ileocolic region with increased T2 signal intensity, T2 hyperintense perienteric fluid collection, and edema, fat stranding, or pneumatosis may be seen on MR imaging.[47] *Tuberculous (TB) enteritis* commonly involves ileocecal and jejunoileal areas because of a high density of lymphoid aggregates and physiologic stasis of food bolus causing increased contact time between mycobacteria and the intestinal mucosa.[48] TB ileitis is among common extrapulmonary manifestations of tuberculosis, which accounts for up to 50% in patients positive for human immunodeficiency virus and up to 20% in immunocompetent patients.[47] Asymmetrical ileal wall thickening, enlarged lymph nodes with central high T2 signal intensity of necrosis, ulcerations, luminal narrowing, stricture, and nodularity of the ileocecal valve are suggestive of intestinal TB.[47] However, some MR imaging features overlap between TB ileitis and Crohn disease. High fever in an absence of intra-abdominal abscess, lack of perianal disease, and a shorter duration of signs and symptoms favor TB. *Ischemic ileitis* secondary to splanchnic hypoperfusion and low-flow states (nonocclusive ischemia) also commonly occurs in an ileocecal region. The ileocecal segment is supplied by the most distal branch of superior mesenteric artery (SMA), therefore it is at risk of ischemic change when the patient is in a hypovolemic state. Segmental circumferential ileocecal wall thickening with patent SMA can be seen on MR imaging.[47] Decreased or absent mucosal enhancement may be found after gadolinium administration.

Omental Infarction and Epiploic Appendagitis

Omental infarction is the infarction of the greater omentum, which is usually secondary to omental torsion. Omental torsion leads to venous engorgement and eventually progresses to hemorrhagic infarction and necrosis.[49] Sometimes omental infarction without torsion can occur due to

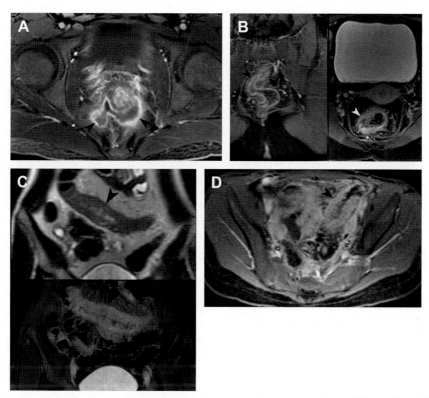

Fig. 10. Crohn disease. (*A*) Perirectal abscess. Axial, fat-suppressed, contrast-enhanced T1-weighted (*A*) MR image shows an irregular-shaped, rim-enhancing perirectal fluid collection (*arrowheads*) with mild perirectal fat stranding. (*B*) Crohn proctitis. Coronal, fat-suppressed, contrast-enhanced T1-weighted (*left*) and axial fat-suppressed T2-weighted (*right*) MR images show segmental thickening, enhancement and T2 hyperintensity of the rectal wall with perirectal fat stranding (*arrowheads*). (*C*) Crohn colitis. Coronal T2 SSFSE (*top*) and fat-suppressed, contrast enhanced T1-weighted (*bottom*) MR images show segmental thickening and enhancement of the transverse colon with pericolic fat stranding (*arrowheads*). (*D*) Crohn enteritis. Axial, fat-suppressed, contrast-enhanced T1-weighted MR image in a patient with active Crohn disease shows marked ileal wall thickening with intense enhancement (*arrowhead*).

hypercoagulable state, vasculitis, or mesenteric venous congestion secondary to congestive heart failure. It commonly affects elderly patients with a slight male preponderance. Anatomic malformation, vascular abnormality, and change in omental consistency serve as primary risk factors, whereas the precipitating factors for torsion include trauma, obesity, overexertion, cough, or sudden change in body positioning.[50] Omental infarction usually occurs on the right side. It can mimic clinical signs and symptoms of acute appendicitis or acute cholecystitis. Acute right-sided abdominal pain, normal or slightly elevated white blood cell count, nausea, vomiting, diarrhea, and fever may be present. On T1-weighted images, omental torsion appears as a fatty mass of larger than 5 cm, which is slightly hypointense to other fatty portions of the omentum.[51] Twisting around a linear hypointensity may be seen and suggests a thrombosed vessel.[50] On T2-weighted images, increased signal intensity of the twisted portion may be seen due to congestion and edema.

Epiploic appendagitis refers to inflammation of appendages epiploicae, which are a small fat-containing peritoneal sac arising from the serosal surface of the colon. Torsion of the vascular stalk or spontaneous venous thrombosis of these appendages is believed to be an etiology that eventually leads to infarction and inflammatory response. This is an uncommon condition with an estimated incidence of 8.8 cases per million population per year.[52] It is commonly found in men between the fourth and fifth decades of life, especially those who are obese. The most frequent sites are sigmoid colon, followed by descending colon and right hemicolon.[53] Epiploic appendagitis is a self-limited disease but its clinical presentation mimics more serious diseases, such as acute diverticulitis and appendicitis.[54]

An oval, inflamed, fatty mass adjacent to the colon can be readily seen on CT or MR imaging, with MR imaging findings closely following those of CT. The inflamed epiploic appendage appears less intense than that of normal adjacent peritoneal fat on T1-weighted images. Surrounding it is a halo of T1 hypointensity and T2 hyperintensity. A central T1 and T2 hypointense dot may be seen, which represents a thrombosed vascular pedicle[55,56] (**Fig. 11**). After gadolinium administration, the inflamed appendage strongly enhances. The degree of fat stranding surrounding the inflamed appendage is disproportionate to the degree of adjacent colonic wall thickening. If there is adjacent colonic wall thickening, this will generally be very short.[54] Abscess, fistula, sinus tract, and bowel obstruction are rarely found in epiploic appendagitis.

Bowel Obstruction

Both small and large bowel obstruction have high morbidity and mortality if left untreated. In small bowel obstruction, the estimated rate of strangulation and necrosis is up to 30% and 15%, respectively.[57] Small bowel obstruction is 4 to 5 times more common than large bowel obstruction[58] and is commonly due to adhesive disease in 60% to 70% of cases. The other causes include volvulus, intussusception, and hernia.[59] Large bowel obstruction, on the other hand, is more likely to be related to obstructive colonic carcinoma in 60% to 80% of cases, followed by volvulus, diverticulitis, and intussusception.[58] Radiography and CT are the mainstay imaging modalities for the evaluation of possible bowel obstruction in patients presenting to the emergency department. MR imaging provides a radiation-free alternative for (1) young patients who had undergone multiple CT scans, (2) children, and (3) pregnant women.[60]

MR imaging diagnosis of small bowel obstruction relies on 2 main findings, which are dilated loops of bowel (greater than 2.5 cm in diameter)

proximal to the collapsed loops and identification of a transition point.[61,62] Fluid within the lumen of dilated loops acts as a natural contrast on T2-weighted images; therefore, these dilated loops can be traced to the transition point. Adhesion is suggested if there is a sharp angulation at the site of transition without an obvious mass. Stricture will be seen as focal narrowing of bowel with abrupt change in caliber without obvious mass. A mass is typically seen as a soft tissue lesion at the transition point, with increased signal intensity on T2-weighted images. The reported sensitivity of MR imaging for diagnosis of small bowel obstruction is as high as 95% and specificity as high as 100%[61,63] and the site of obstruction can be detected correctly in 92.6% by MR imaging.[62] Detection of large bowel obstruction on MR imaging is more difficult because of the intrinsic ability of the colon to absorb the fluid, resulting in less natural contrast and a lesser degree of bowel dilatation.

Intra-abdominal Abscess

There are many potential sources of intra-abdominal abscesses, such as postoperative septic complications, inflammatory or infectious GI tract disease (eg, Crohn disease, appendicitis, diverticulitis), and PID/TOA. Fever and abdominal pain are present in most patients. Although contrast-enhanced CT is the imaging modality of choice in patients with suspected intra-abdominal abscess,[64] MR imaging is helpful in selected patient populations in whom radiation exposure and use of iodinated contrast media are a strong concern.[65] Intra-abdominal abscesses are readily detected as a T1 hypointense and T2 hyperintense fluid collection in the peritoneal cavity. It shows smooth, rim enhancement after gadolinium administration. Layering low signal intensity of debris or fluid-debris level may be seen in the collection. Diffusion-weighed imaging (DWI) sequence can help distinguish abscesses from cystic tumors.[37,65] The abscess generally

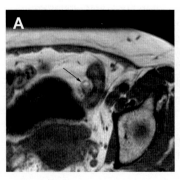 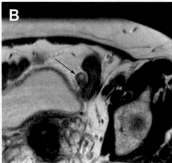

Fig. 11. Acute epiploic appendagitis. Axial T1-weighted (*A*) and T2-weighted (*B*) MR images show a small, oval, fat-containing nodule medial to the sigmoid colon with surrounded hypointense rim, representing an inflamed appendage (*arrows*).

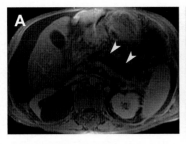
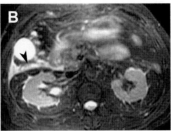

Fig. 12. Necrotizing pancreatitis. (*A*) Axial contrast-enhanced fat-suppressed T1-weighted MR image shows absence of normal pancreatic parenchymal enhancement (*white arrowheads*) and abnormal enhancement of the adjacent peripancreatic fat and ascites. (*B*) Axial fat-suppressed T2-weighted MR image shows enlarged pancreas with increased signal intensity. Hyperintense fluid along the right anterior pararenal space and right lateroconal space is seen (*black arrowhead*).

demonstrates restricted diffusion, and therefore appears markedly hyperintense on DWI and hypointense on apparent diffusion coefficient maps. With combined T2-weighted images and DWI, abscesses can be diagnosed with sensitivity of 96% to 100% and specificity of 100%.[65]

Acute Pancreaticobiliary Diseases

MR imaging and MRCP are considered the most optimal imaging methods to noninvasively evaluate the pancreaticobiliary tract. Although no cross-sectional imaging study is highly recommended by the American College of Radiology in the initial evaluation of acute uncomplicated pancreatitis, MR imaging ranks alongside CT for evaluation of critically ill patients with pancreatitis and systemic inflammatory response syndrome and in patients with ongoing symptoms for longer than 48 hours.[66] The slight advantage in rating given to CT over MR owes largely to its wider availability at most institutions. From a strictly imaging standpoint, MR has the advantage of better characterization of the pancreatic duct, with clear delineation of intraductal stones, strictures, anatomic variations, and duct disruption. In patients who are unable to be evaluated with contrast-enhanced CT due to acute kidney injury, the inherent contrast resolution of T2-weighted images on a noncontrast MR image provide increase sensitivity for the detection of pancreatic necrosis verses noncontrast CT. Last, MR is able to more accurately differentiate between pancreatic and peripancreatic fluid collections and solid necrotic debris. Acute cholecystitis, cholangitis, pancreatitis, and their complications, etiologies, and potentially contributing anatomic variations can usually be depicted on MR. These topics are discussed in detail in the article (See Bates DDB, LeBedis CA, Soto J, et al: Use of MR in Pancreaticobiliary Emergencies, in this issue). Some representative pancreaticobiliary pathologies are demonstrated in **Figs. 12** and **13**.

SUMMARY

MR imaging is a useful method to image emergency patients suspected of having acute pelvic

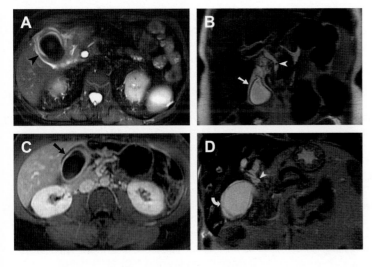

Fig. 13. Acute cholecystitis. (*A*) Axial, fat-suppressed, contrast-enhanced T1-weighted MR image shows thickened gallbladder wall, mural enhancement/stratification, and minimal pericholecystic fluid (*arrowhead*). Coronal T2 SSFSE (*B*) and axial, fat-suppressed, contrast-enhanced T1-weighted (*C*) MR images demonstrate a distended gallbladder (*arrow*) wall thickening with dilatation of the cystic duct to where there is a tiny round filling defect (*arrowhead*), representing an obstructing stone. (*D*) Mirizzi syndrome. Coronal T2 SSFSE MR image reveals a distended gallbladder (*curved arrow*) with T2 hyperintense wall thickening and common duct dilatation (*arrowhead*) secondary to a cystic duct stone.

pathologies and some acute GI disorders, such as appendicitis, diverticulitis, enteritis, and others. MR imaging may be the sole imaging in patients with acute pelvic pain when and where there is a lack of ultrasound expertise, in patients with a strong concern for radiation risk associated with CT, and as a problem solver when ultrasound does not provide definitive answers.

REFERENCES

1. Wasnik AP, Mazza MB, Liu PS. Normal and variant pelvic anatomy on MRI. Magn Reson Imaging Clin N Am 2011;19(3):547–66, viii.

2. Watanabe Y. Instrumentation, technical requirements: MRI. In: Bertolotto M, Trombetta C, editors. Scrotal pathology. Berlin: Springer Berlin Heidelberg; 2012. p. 17–26.

3. Furukawa A, Saotome T, Yamasaki M, et al. Cross-sectional imaging in Crohn disease. Radiographics 2004;24(3):689–702.

4. Gupta S, Manyonda IT. Acute complications of fibroids. Best Pract Res Clin Obstet Gynaecol 2009; 23(5):609–17.

5. Karasick S, Lev-Toaff AS, Toaff ME. Imaging of uterine leiomyomas. AJR Am J Roentgenol 1992;158(4): 799–805.

6. Kamaya A, Shin L, Chen B, et al. Emergency gynecologic imaging. Semin Ultrasound CT MR 2008; 29(5):353–68.

7. Schwartz LB, Zawin M, Carcangiu ML, et al. Does pelvic magnetic resonance imaging differentiate among the histologic subtypes of uterine leiomyomata? Fertil Steril 1998;70(3):580–7.

8. Singh AK, Desai H, Novelline RA. Emergency MRI of acute pelvic pain: MR protocol with no oral contrast. Emerg Radiol 2009;16(2):133–41.

9. Vitiello D, McCarthy S. Diagnostic imaging of myomas. Obstet Gynecol Clin North Am 2006;33(1): 85–95.

10. Shrestha E, Ngangbam HS, Yang Y, et al. Torsion of pedunculated subserous myoma. J Med Cases 2011;2(2):62–3.

11. Roy C, Bierry G, El Ghali S, et al. Acute torsion of uterine leiomyoma: CT features. Abdom Imaging 2005;30(1):120–3.

12. Kim JC, Kim SS, Park JY. "Bridging vascular sign" in the MR diagnosis of exophytic uterine leiomyoma. J Comput Assist Tomogr 2000;24(1):57–60.

13. Sweet RL. Pelvic inflammatory disease: current concepts of diagnosis and management. Curr Infect Dis Rep 2012;14(2):194–203.

14. Lareau SM, Beigi RH. Pelvic inflammatory disease and tubo-ovarian abscess. Infect Dis Clin North Am 2008;22(4):693–708, vii.

15. Workowski KA, Berman S, Centers for Disease Control and Prevention. Sexually transmitted diseases treatment guidelines, 2010. MMWR Recomm Rep 2010;59(RR-12):1–110.

16. Tukeva TA, Aronen HJ, Karjalainen PT, et al. MR imaging in pelvic inflammatory disease: comparison with laparoscopy and US. Radiology 1999;210(1): 209–16.

17. Horrow MM, Rodgers SK, Naqvi S. Ultrasound of pelvic inflammatory disease. Ultrasound Clin 2007; 2(2):297–309.

18. Li W, Zhang Y, Cui Y, et al. Pelvic inflammatory disease: evaluation of diagnostic accuracy with conventional MR with added diffusion-weighted imaging. Abdom Imaging 2013;38(1):193–200.

19. Wilkinson C, Sanderson A. Adnexal torsion–a multimodality imaging review. Clin Radiol 2012;67(5): 476–83.

20. Ghonge NP, Lall C, Aggarwal B, et al. The MRI whirlpool sign in the diagnosis of ovarian torsion. Radiol Case Rep 2012;7(3):1–3.

21. Fujii S, Kaneda S, Kakite S, et al. Diffusion-weighted imaging findings of adnexal torsion: initial results. Eur J Radiol 2011;77(2):330–4.

22. Duigenan S, Oliva E, Lee SI. Ovarian torsion: diagnostic features on CT and MRI with pathologic correlation. AJR Am J Roentgenol 2012;198(2): W122–31.

23. Thompson A, Pearce I. Pain and swelling of the scrotum, epididymitis and torsion. Surgery 2002; 20(12):294–6.

24. Pavlica P, Barozzi L. Imaging of the acute scrotum. Eur Radiol 2001;11(2):220–8.

25. Parenti GC, Feletti F, Brandini F, et al. Imaging of the scrotum: role of MRI. Radiol Med 2009;114(3): 414–24.

26. Muglia V, Tucci S Jr, Elias J Jr, et al. Magnetic resonance imaging of scrotal diseases: when it makes the difference. Urology 2002;59(3):419–23.

27. Watanabe Y, Nagayama M, Okumura A, et al. MR imaging of testicular torsion: features of testicular hemorrhagic necrosis and clinical outcomes. J Magn Reson Imaging 2007;26(1):100–8.

28. Watanabe Y, Dohke M, Ohkubo K, et al. Scrotal disorders: evaluation of testicular enhancement patterns at dynamic contrast-enhanced subtraction MR imaging. Radiology 2000;217(1):219–27.

29. Flum DR. Clinical practice. Acute appendicitis–appendectomy or the "antibiotics first" strategy. N Engl J Med 2015;372(20):1937–43.

30. Humes DJ, Simpson J. Acute appendicitis. BMJ 2006;333(7567):530–4.

31. Barger RL Jr, Nandalur KR. Diagnostic performance of magnetic resonance imaging in the detection of appendicitis in adults: a meta-analysis. Acad Radiol 2010;17(10):1211–6.

32. Nitta N, Takahashi M, Furukawa A, et al. MR imaging of the normal appendix and acute appendicitis. J Magn Reson Imaging 2005;21(2):156–65.

33. Lam M, Singh A, Kaewlai R, et al. Magnetic resonance of acute appendicitis: pearls and pitfalls. Curr Probl Diagn Radiol 2008;37(2):57–66.

34. Incesu L, Coskun A, Selcuk MB, et al. Acute appendicitis: MR imaging and sonographic correlation. AJR Am J Roentgenol 1997;168(3):669–74.

35. Singh A, Danrad R, Hahn PF, et al. MR imaging of the acute abdomen and pelvis: acute appendicitis and beyond. Radiographics 2007;27(5):1419–31.

36. Brown MA. Imaging acute appendicitis. Semin Ultrasound CT MR 2008;29(5):293–307.

37. Loock MT, Fornes P, Soyer P, et al. MRI and pelvic abscesses: a pictorial review. Clin Imaging 2012; 36(5):425–31.

38. Inci E, Hocaoglu E, Aydin S, et al. Efficiency of unenhanced MRI in the diagnosis of acute appendicitis: comparison with Alvarado scoring system and histopathological results. Eur J Radiol 2011; 80(2):253–8.

39. Leeuwenburgh MM, Wiezer MJ, Wiarda BM, et al. Accuracy of MRI compared with ultrasound imaging and selective use of CT to discriminate simple from perforated appendicitis. Br J Surg 2014;101(1): e147–55.

40. Buckley O, Geoghegan T, McAuley G, et al. Pictorial review: magnetic resonance imaging of colonic diverticulitis. Eur Radiol 2007;17(1):221–7.

41. Heverhagen JT, Sitter H, Zielke A, et al. Prospective evaluation of the value of magnetic resonance imaging in suspected acute sigmoid diverticulitis. Dis Colon Rectum 2008;51(12):1810–5.

42. Heverhagen JT, Zielke A, Ishaque N, et al. Acute colonic diverticulitis: visualization in magnetic resonance imaging. Magn Reson Imaging 2001;19(10): 1275–7.

43. Krishnamoorthy S, Israel G. Imaging of acute diverticulitis. J Clin Gastroenterol 2011;45(Suppl 1):S27–35.

44. Cobben LP, Groot I, Blickman JG, et al. Right colonic diverticulitis: MR appearance. Abdom Imaging 2003;28(6):794–8.

45. Hammond NA, Miller FH, Yaghmai V, et al. MR imaging of acute bowel pathology: a pictorial review. Emerg Radiol 2008;15(2):99–104.

46. Ditkofsky NG, Singh A, Avery L, et al. The role of emergency MRI in the setting of acute abdominal pain. Emerg Radiol 2014;21(6):615–24.

47. Dilauro S, Crum-Cianflone NF. Ileitis: when it is not Crohn's disease. Curr Gastroenterol Rep 2010; 12(4):249–58.

48. Leung VK, Law ST, Lam CW, et al. Intestinal tuberculosis in a regional hospital in Hong Kong: a 10-year experience. Hong Kong Med J 2006;12(4): 264–71.

49. Andreuccetti J, Ceribelli C, Manto O, et al. Primary omental torsion (POT): a review of literature and case report. World J Emerg Surg 2011;6:6.

50. Maeda T, Mori H, Cyujo M, et al. CT and MR findings of torsion of greater omentum: a case report. Abdom Imaging 1997;22(1):45–6.

51. Singh AK, Gervais DA, Lee P, et al. Omental infarct: CT imaging features. Abdom Imaging 2006;31(5):549–54.

52. de Brito P, Gomez MA, Besson M, et al. Frequency and epidemiology of primary epiploic appendagitis on computed tomography in adults with abdominal pain. J Radiol 2008;89(2):235–43 [in French].

53. Singh AK, Gervais DA, Hahn PF, et al. Acute epiploic appendagitis and its mimics. Radiographics 2005; 25(6):1521–34.

54. Almeida AT, Melao L, Viamonte B, et al. Epiploic appendagitis: an entity frequently unknown to clinicians–diagnostic imaging, pitfalls, and look-alikes. AJR Am J Roentgenol 2009;193(5):1243–51.

55. Sirvanci M, Balci NC, Karaman K, et al. Primary epiploic appendagitis: MRI findings. Magn Reson Imaging 2002;20(1):137–9.

56. Martinez CAR, Palma RT, Silveira Junior PP, et al. Primary epiploic appendagitis. J Coloproctol 2012; 33(3):161–6.

57. Taylor MR, Lalani N. Adult small bowel obstruction. Acad Emerg Med 2013;20(6):528–44.

58. Jaffe T, Thompson WM. Large-bowel obstruction in the adult: classic radiographic and CT findings, etiology, and mimics. Radiology 2015;275(3):651–63.

59. McKenna DA, Meehan CP, Alhajeri AN, et al. The use of MRI to demonstrate small bowel obstruction during pregnancy. Br J Radiol 2007;80(949):e11–4.

60. Katz DS, Baker ME, Rosen MP, et al. ACR appropriateness criteria® suspected small-bowel obstruction. 2013.

61. Regan F, Beall DP, Bohlman ME, et al. Fast MR imaging and the detection of small-bowel obstruction. AJR Am J Roentgenol 1998;170(6):1465–9.

62. Matsuoka H, Takahara T, Masaki T, et al. Preoperative evaluation by magnetic resonance imaging in patients with bowel obstruction. Am J Surg 2002;183(6):614–7.

63. Beall DP, Fortman BJ, Lawler BC, et al. Imaging bowel obstruction: a comparison between fast magnetic resonance imaging and helical computed tomography. Clin Radiol 2002;57(8):719–24.

64. Yaghmai V, Rosen MP, Lalani N, et al. ACR appropriateness criteria® acute (nonlocalized) abdominal pain and fever or suspected abdominal abscess. American College of Radiology. Available at: https://acsearch. acr.org/docs/69467/Narrative/. Accessed December 15, 2015.

65. Oto A, Schmid-Tannwald C, Agrawal G, et al. Diffusion-weighted MR imaging of abdominopelvic abscesses. Emerg Radiol 2011;18(6):515–24.

66. Baker ME, Nelson RC, Rosen MP, et al. ACR appropriateness criteria® acute pancreatitis. American College of Radiology. Available at: http://www.acr. org/~/media/ACR/Documents/AppCriteria/Diagnostic/ AcutePancreatitis.pdf. Accessed July 30, 2015.

Use of Magnetic Resonance in Pancreaticobiliary Emergencies

CrossMark

David D.B. Bates, MD*, Christina A. LeBedis, MD,
Jorge A. Soto, MD, Avneesh Gupta, MD

KEYWORDS

- Emergency MR imaging • Pancreatitis • Cholecystitis • Biliary obstruction • Cholangitis • Bile leak
- MRCP • Magnetic resonance cholangiopancreatography

KEY POINTS

- Magnetic resonance (MR) plays a role in the evaluation of several acute pancreaticobiliary conditions, including cholecystitis, pancreatitis, biliary obstruction, pancreatic trauma, and bile leak.
- Several MR imaging features may be used to assist in diagnosis and classification of pancreatic and biliary emergencies, including specific complications.
- Several imaging artifacts and pitfalls exist in the MR imaging of pancreaticobiliary emergencies that can mimic pathology.

INTRODUCTION

Acute abdominal symptoms are a common cause of emergency department visits in the United States. According to the results of a 2010 survey, the Department of Health and Human Services reported 7 million emergency department visits for noninjury abdominal pain in 2007 to 2008.[1] Disorders of the biliary system and pancreas constitute a large portion of these conditions, with approximately 250,000 admissions for acute pancreatitis[2] and more than 700,000 emergent cholecystectomies performed annually in the United States.[3] Cross-sectional imaging has become an invaluable tool in the clinicians' armamentarium to aid in the diagnosis and triage of patients presenting with acute abdominal conditions.

Technological advances in multidetector CT (MDCT) over the past several years, particularly involving the increased speed of acquisition and reduced radiation dose, have made it the workhorse of emergency abdominal imaging. The widespread utility of MDCT in abdominal emergencies is well established.

Despite its secondary role to MDCT, certain clinical scenarios may require evaluation with MR imaging. MR cholangiopancreatography (MRCP), first described in 1991 by Wallner and colleagues,[4] has become an essential tool for imaging the pancreas and biliary system. Heavily T2-weighted images enable rapid and noninvasive evaluation of the biliary tree and localization of pathology. In addition, MR may provide relevant information in patients evaluated for pancreatic or biliary trauma, bile leaks, acute cholecystitis, biliary obstruction, or pancreatitis. When compared with MDCT, MR also offers the distinct advantage of avoiding ionizing radiation.

The authors have nothing to disclose.
Department of Radiology, Boston Medical Center, Boston University School of Medicine, 820 Harrison Avenue, FGH Building, 3rd Floor, Boston, MA 02118, USA
* Corresponding author.
E-mail address: david.bates@bmc.org

Magn Reson Imaging Clin N Am 24 (2016) 433–448
http://dx.doi.org/10.1016/j.mric.2015.11.010
1064-9689/16/$ – see front matter © 2016 Elsevier Inc. All rights reserved.

NORMAL ANATOMY AND IMAGING TECHNIQUE

The pancreas is a retroperitoneal organ that arises from the endodermal lining of the duodenum. It is formed by fusion of the dorsal and ventral pancreatic buds.[5] The main pancreatic duct (MPD) (duct of Wirsung) drains the body of the pancreas, whereas in some patients the accessory pancreatic duct of Santorini drains into the minor papilla.[5] Certain congenital anomalies can occur that may be relevant in acute abdominal conditions later in life (discussed later).

The 3 components of the portal triad are the hepatic artery, portal vein, and bile duct. The left and right hepatic ducts join shortly after the porta hepatis to form the common hepatic duct. The common hepatic duct joins the cystic duct to form the common bile duct, which runs in parallel to the pancreatic duct until they merge to form the hepatopancreatic ampulla of Vater.[6] Variant ductal anatomy may have implications in diagnosis and clinical management (discussed later).

Imaging Protocols

At the authors' institution, abdominal MR with MRCP sequences using phased-array surface body or torso coils is standardized (**Table 1**), but certain modifications may be implemented to address a specific clinical question. The contrast agent of choice at the authors' institution is gadobenate dimeglumine. In select cases where detection of a ductal leak is required, gadoxetate disodium may be used, with additional delayed hepatocellular phase images acquired 10 to 20 minutes after the injection of contrast. Currently the use of hepatobiliary contrast agents to detect bile leak is off-label. If a hepatocyte specific agent, such as gadoxetate disodium, is administered, MRCP and other T2-weighted sequences must be acquired prior to contrast administration to prevent T2 shortening in the biliary tree (discussed later).

In addition, MRCP sequences are typically performed when evaluating for pancreaticobiliary pathology. When feasible, patients are administered a negative oral contrast agent immediately prior to imaging to reduce or eliminate the background signal of the proximal gastrointestinal tract. Prior to its discontinuation, an oral suspension of ferumoxsil was routinely administered in the authors' department. Subsequently, the authors have switched to oral administration of pineapple juice. MRCP is typically acquired with both 2-D and 3-D techniques in the authors' department. 2-D MRCP technique is performed using a heavily T2-weighted fat-suppressed single-shot turbo spin-

echo (TSE) with 40-mm slice thickness. Six breath-hold or respiratory-triggered images are acquired in the coronal oblique plane at various angles centered about the head of the pancreas. 2-D MRCP images have the advantage of rapid acquisition. 3-D MRCP images are acquired in the coronal plane using a 3-D TSE technique. Although acquisition time is significantly longer than using a 2-D technique, 3-D MRCP imaging allows high-resolution imaging of the biliary tree and the ability to perform multiplanar reconstructions. Maximum intensity projection reformats are acquired in the coronal oblique plane, and additional multiplanar reconstructions may be performed for additional information, including the distinction between choledocholithiasis and air in the duct (discussed later).

IMAGING FINDINGS AND PATHOLOGY
Pancreatic Trauma

Although MR acquisition times have decreased with advances in technology, MDCT remains the imaging modality of choice in the setting of blunt and penetrating abdominal trauma due to its speed, availability, and high spatial resolution. Select patients with blunt pancreaticobiliary injury on MDCT may benefit, however, from additional MR imaging.[7]

Pancreatic injury in the setting of blunt abdominal trauma is uncommon, with reported incidences ranging from approximately 2% to 12%.[8] The associated mortality is considerable, however, and may be as high as 30% to 50%, largely secondary to concomitant injuries.[7] Factors associated with poor outcomes include a delay in the time to diagnosis, high-grade injury, and disruption of the MPD.[7] Elevated serum amylase may be present, but the clinical presentation of pancreatic injury is variable and nonspecific.[9] Blunt pancreatic injuries occur more commonly in the body of the gland, accounting for two-thirds of cases, and are typically caused by a crushing impact against the vertebral column. Because the main cause for morbidity and mortality is disruption of the MPD, assessment for ductal injuries is critical. Deep lacerations (involving greater than 50% of the thickness of the pancreas) are predictive of ductal disruption and may be detected using T1-weighted postcontrast and T2-weighted sequences. Direct injury to the duct may be visible using T2-weighted sequences, including MRCP images (**Fig. 1**).

Pancreatic lacerations, defined as irregular linear, low-attenuation regions in the pancreatic parenchyma on MDCT,[10] may be either superficial (when involving <50% of the parenchymal

Table 1
Standard magnetic resonance abdomen protocol with intravenous contrast

Parameter	T1-weighted In-phase and Out-of-phase	T2-weighted SPIR	T2-weighted Single-shot Turbo Spin-echo	Diffusion (b = 0, 600 s/mm²)	Magnetic Resonance Cholangiopancreatography	T1-weighted 3-D Gradient-recalled Echo SPIR (THRIVE)
Field of view, mm	400	400	400	400	300	400
Technique	Gradient-recalled echo	Fast spin-echo	Fast spin-echo	Diffusion	Fast spin-echo for 2-D, 3-D TSE for 3-D	Gradient-recalled echo
Scanning mode	Multisection, dual-echo	Multisection	Multisection, 2-D	Multisection, 2-D	Multisection, 2-D or 3-D	3-D
Repetition time (ms)	180	2000	∞	3.6	8000	3.6
Echo time (ms)	2.3 (out of phase)/4.6 (in phase)	80	80	1.8	800	1.7
Section thickness (mm)	5	5	5	7	40 for 2-D, 1.6 for 3-D	4
Flip angle	90	90	90	60	90	15
Sense reduction factor	1.8	2	2	2	2	1.7
Respiration control	Breath holding	Respiratory triggering[a]	Respiratory Triggering[a]	Respiratory triggering[a]	Respiratory triggering[a]	Breath holding

[a] May perform with breath-hold technique as tolerated by patient.
Abbreviations: SPIR, spectral presaturation with inversion recovery; THRIVE, T1 high-res isotropic vol excitation.

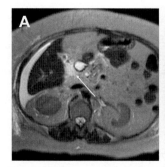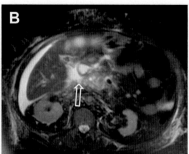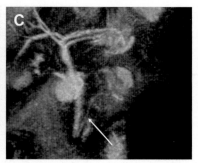

Fig. 1. Pancreatic contusion. A 58-year-old unrestrained driver in an MVC, with stranding around the duodenum and pancreas on MDCT. (*A*) Axial T2-weighted image demonstrating edema in the fat around the neck of the pancreas (*arrow*) and ascites, which becomes more evident on (*B*) T2-weighted fat-suppressed image (*open arrow*). (*C*) 2-D MRCP demonstrates an intact pancreatic duct (*arrow*).

thickness) or deep (>50% of the parenchymal thickness).[11] The sensitivity of MDCT for pancreatic injury is limited, ranging from 47% to 60%.[7] A deep pancreatic laceration is traditionally considered indirect evidence of a MPD injury, and further evaluation with endoscopic retrograde cholangiopancreatography (ERCP) may be warranted if duct integrity is questionable on MR.

Due to the invasive nature of ERCP and its associated complications, particularly in unstable trauma patients, MRCP offers a noninvasive alternative to evaluate the extent of pancreatic injury and MPD involvement. A recent single-center prospective study by Panda and colleagues[7] compared MDCT and MRCP in patients with blunt abdominal trauma using laparotomy as the gold standard. The study found that both MDCT and MRCP performed well in the evaluation of pancreatic injury and suggested that the combination of these modalities increased diagnostic confidence and allowed for more accurate evaluation of MPD involvement.[7] Thus, when pancreatic laceration is suspected, in particular deep lacerations, further evaluation of the MPD with MRCP (if feasible) may be appropriate. Alternatively, an ERCP should be performed.

Bile Leak

Bile leaks may occur after blunt or penetrating hepatic injury or surgical intervention and can present a diagnostic challenge. The lack of specific symptoms may result in a delay in diagnosis. Some of the more common symptoms associated with bile leak include abdominal discomfort, anorexia, and lethargy. Left undiagnosed and untreated, bile leaks can progress to bilomas and bile peritonitis. Eventually, superimposed infection of the intraperitoneal fluid can result in peritonitis and sepsis, often requiring surgical intervention.[12]

Traditionally, hepatobiliary scintigraphy has been used to diagnose bile leaks. Poor anatomic detail and low spatial resolution, however, limit the ability of scintigraphy to precisely localize the source of a bile leak.[12] The addition of single-photon emission CT images may improve the sensitivity and specificity for the detection of leaks but with the disadvantage of increased exposure to ionizing radiation.

With the advent of gadolinium-based hepatobiliary contrast agents, such as gadoxetate disodium, which has 50% renal excretion and 50% hepatic excretion, MRCP may now play a role in the evaluation of patients with suspected bile leaks.[13] Its use for this purpose is currently off-label, but at least 1 recent study has demonstrated improved detection and localization of bile leaks when compared with traditional MRCP[14] (**Fig. 2**).

Gadolinium-based hepatobiliary contrast agents result in T1 shortening of excreted bile, rendering it hyperintense on T1-weighted images. Biliary excretion may begin as early as 10 minutes after intravenous contrast administration, and fat-saturated T1-weighted images to assess for bile leak may be acquired at 20 minutes.[12] Key imaging findings include extraluminal accumulation of contrast in the liver parenchyma or around the liver or free spillage into the peritoneal cavity. Secondary signs of bile leak parallel those seen in other imaging modalities, including a collapsed gallbladder, pericholecystic or perihepatic fluid collections, and ascites.[12]

Acute Cholecystitis

Acute cholecystitis is one of the most common surgical emergencies, with a prevalence of approximately 5%.[15] In approximately 90% to 95% of cases, acute cholecystitis is due to gallstone impaction in the neck of the gallbladder or cystic duct.[16] Cholelithiasis is present in

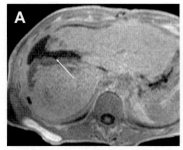 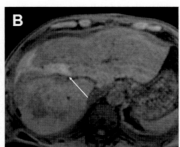 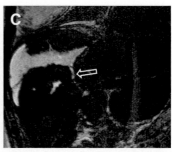

Fig. 2. Hepatic duct laceration. A 63-year-old man after blunt abdominal trauma with grade V liver laceration. (*A*) Precontrast and (*B*) postcontrast T1-weighted fat-suppressed images acquired at 20 minutes after the injection of gadoxetate disodium demonstrate a deep laceration in the right lobe of the liver (*arrows*). Note accumulation of excreted T1 hyperintense bile at the site of laceration (*B*), indicating active biliary leakage. (*C*) 3-D MRCP image demonstrates direct continuity of the fluid collection with the right hepatic duct, indicating the site of ductal injury (*open arrow*).

approximately 10% of the population, with a higher prevalence seen in middle-aged and elderly women.[17] As a result of the obstruction, bile stasis, ischemia, and development of systemic infection can occur.[18] Because cystic duct obstruction leads to increased intraluminal pressure and the gallbladder wall is weakened by ischemia, subsequent gallbladder perforation can result.

Diagnostic imaging plays a central role in the Tokyo Guidelines,[19,20] which seek to improve the diagnostic sensitivity and specificity for acute cholecystitis and acute cholangitis.[21,22] Several imaging modalities are used to assist in the diagnosis of acute cholecystitis, primarily including ultrasound (US), but MDCT and MR imaging may be helpful in select cases. Since its introduction in 1991,[4] MRCP has been an invaluable tool to evaluate the biliary tree.

Imaging features of acute cholecystitis are common to US, MDCT, and MR imaging (**Box 1**) and include cholelithiasis, gallbladder distention to a diameter greater than 40 mm or length greater than 10 cm, gallbladder wall thickening, pericholecystic fluid, and perihepatic fluid (the so-called C sign). CT and MR imaging may also show hyperenhancement of the adjacent liver on postcontrast arterial-phase images.[16] Although not routinely the first modality of choice due to the speed, accuracy, and low cost of abdominal US, MR imaging is more sensitive for the detection of gallstones impacted in the gallbladder neck or cystic duct.[16] The sensitivity and specificity of MR for detection of cholecystitis when any one of these imaging features is present on MR have been reported at 88% and 89%, respectively[23] (**Fig. 3**).

Certain forms of cholecystitis also demonstrate unique imaging features and may be readily classified on MR imaging. Emphysematous cholecystitis is a distinct entity and has a different pathogenesis from typical acute calculous cholecystitis. It is more commonly seen in patients with underlying diabetes mellitus and atherosclerotic disease. Small-vessel ischemia results in gallbladder wall inflammation and necrosis, allowing gas to enter the gallbladder wall. Although US and CT are extremely sensitive for detection of air in the gallbladder wall, this finding may also be detectable by MR. Air in the gallbladder wall appears as signal voids.[16] Air may also be visible as susceptibility artifact on gradient-echo imaging. Other imaging features of emphysematous cholecystitis overlap with gangrenous cholecystitis and include irregular wall thickening or asymmetric heterogeneous hyperintense signal in the gallbladder wall on T2-weighted images[21] (**Fig. 4**).

In addition to demonstrating diagnostic features of acute cholecystitis, MR is an invaluable tool to identify its most common complications, including empyema, perforation, gangrenous cholecystitis, and gallbladder empyema.[16]

Gallbladder empyema refers to filling of the inflamed and distended gallbladder with purulent material. In typical acute cholecystitis, the gallbladder is usually distended with T2-hyperintense bile. In the setting of empyema, the

---

Box 1
Imaging features of acute cholecystitis

- Gallbladder distention >40 mm in diameter (or ≥ 10 cm in length)
- Gallbladder wall thickening >3 mm
- Pericholecystic fluid
- Perihepatic fluid (the C sign)
- Hyperenhancement of the adjacent liver

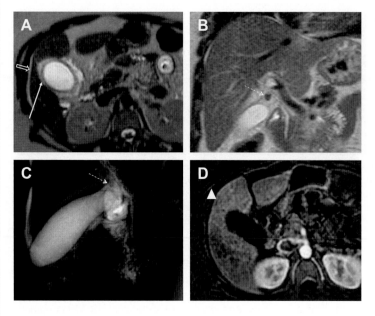

Fig. 3. Acute cholecystitis. A 42-year-old woman with right upper quadrant pain. (*A*) Axial T2-weighted image demonstrates gallbladder wall thickening (*arrow*) and distention, with trace perihepatic ascites (*open arrow*). (*B*) Coronal T2-weighted and (*C*) radial MRCP images demonstrate a T2 hypointense stone (*dashed arrows*) lodged in the cystic duct. (*D*) Arterial-phase postcontrast imaging demonstrates relative hyperenhancement of the adjacent liver parenchyma (*arrowhead*), indicative of inflammation.

inflamed gallbladder fills with pus, which appears as layering-dependent, hypointense, inhomogeneous material on heavily T2-weighted sequences.[16]

Perforation may be diagnosed when there is discontinuity of the gallbladder wall in the setting of acute cholecystitis. MR may aid in the visualization of wall disruption when it is unclear on US or MDCT, particularly on T1-weighted postgadolinium and T2-weighted fat-suppressed images. Although subacute perforation with abscess formation in the gallbladder wall is the most common form, free perforation into the peritoneal cavity and the development of enterocholecystic fistulas may also be seen[16] (**Fig. 5**).

Gangrenous cholecystitis is a complication that occurs when cholecystitis has become advanced.

As with other complications, US and CT findings tend to be specific but insensitive. Ischemia of the gallbladder wall may result in necrosis and sloughing of the mucosa. Key findings suggesting microabscesses or gallbladder wall necrosis include heterogeneous areas of hyperintensity on fat-suppressed T1-weighted and T2-weighted images. Heterogeneous or disrupted wall or mucosal enhancement on postcontrast T1-weighted fat-suppressed images may also be suggestive[16] (**Fig. 6**).

Hemorrhagic cholecystitis may be diagnosed on MDCT by the presence of hyperattenuating blood in the setting of cholecystitis but can be confirmed on MR. When other features of cholecystitis are present on imaging, hemorrhage may be seen in the gallbladder lumen or wall as T1 hyperintense

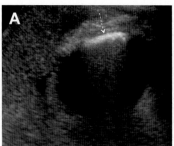
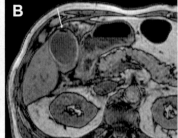
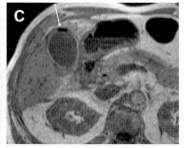

Fig. 4. Emphysematous cholecystitis. A 69-year-old man with abdominal pain. (*A*) Abdominal US demonstrates a linear echogenic area in the anti-dependent aspect of the gallbladder wall (*dashed arrow*), with dirty shadowing posteriorly, consistent with air. (*B*) Out-of-phase and (*C*) in-phase phase T1 gradient-echo images demonstrate patchy decreased T1 signal with prolonged TE (*arrows*, in-phase imaging), consistent with air in the gallbladder wall.

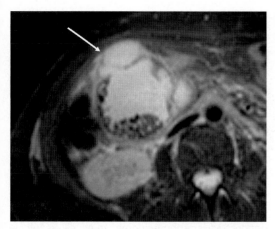

Fig. 5. Cholecystitis with perforation. A 59-year-old man presenting with right upper quadrant pain and cholecystitis. Axial fat-suppressed T2-weighted image demonstrates discontinuity of the anterior gallbladder wall (*arrow*), with loculated fluid collections consistent with gallbladder perforation. This finding was not well seen on US.

signal as a result of the T1-shortening effects of methemoglobin[16] (**Fig. 7**).

Biliary Obstruction

Obstruction of the biliary tree may result in intrahepatic biliary ductal dilation, with associated increase in pressure. In addition to obstructive jaundice, the increased pressure in the biliary tree can result in hepaticovenous reflux of bacteria.[16] The resultant acute cholangitis and biliary sepsis can be life threatening, and emergent intervention may be required with either percutaneous or endoscopic drainage.

Although US and MDCT can demonstrate the presence of biliary obstruction, the exact cause is often most clearly identified by MRCP. Choledocholithiasis, iatrogenic stricture, and malignant obstruction may all contribute to biliary obstruction and can be differentiated on MR.

As discussed previously, choledocholithiasis is common in Western populations. When gallstones migrate through the cystic duct and into the common bile duct, choledocholithiasis occurs and can result in acute biliary obstruction. Identifying gallstones in the common bile duct can help guide therapeutic options. Because choledocholithiasis and cholecystitis may occur together, dilation of the common bile duct greater than 8 mm should raise suspicion for choledocholithiasis when imaging features of cholecystitis are present. Because CT may not detect choledocholithiasis, MRCP may be performed in cases where it is suspected[22] (**Fig. 8**).

In addition to demonstrating a high sensitivity and specificity for detecting choledocholithiasis,[22] excluding the presence of gallstones in the biliary tree may prevent an unnecessary ERCP, an invasive procedure that is associated with complications, such as pancreatitis. On heavily T2-weighted MRCP images, gallstones appear as rounded signal voids within the bile duct, with a meniscus both above and below. Cholesterol stones generally are both T1 and T2 hypointense, but pigmented stones may show variable T1 signal that can be hyperintense. The distinction is significant, because pigmented stones are susceptible to fragmentation via endoscopic lithotripsy, whereas cholesterol stones are not.[17] Rarely, a gallstone may become impacted in the cystic duct and cause extrinsic compression of the common hepatic duct, resulting in intrahepatic biliary duct obstruction (Mirizzi syndrome). This unique condition is named after Pablo Luis Mirizzi, the Argentinian surgeon who first described it (**Fig. 9**).

Several congenital anomalies of the biliary tree have been described that may have an impact on diagnosis and treatment of patients with

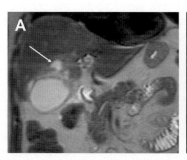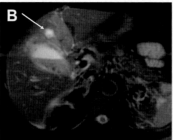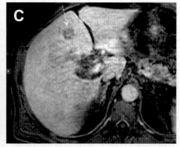

Fig. 6. Cholecystitis with perforation and liver abscess formation. A 70-year-old man with cholelithiasis and abdominal pain. (*A*) Coronal T2-weighted and (*B*) axial fat-suppressed T2-weighted images show a hyperintense fluid collection in the hepatic parenchyma adjacent to an inflamed gallbladder (*arrows*). (*C*) Axial T1-weighted postcontrast imaging during equilibrium phase demonstrates mild peripheral enhancement around the collection, consistent with intrahepatic abscess (*dashed arrow*).

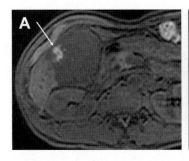 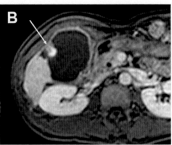

Fig. 7. Hemorrhagic cholecystitis. Axial fat-suppressed T1-weighted precontrast (A) and postcontrast (B) images show an area of focal T1 hyperintensity in the gallbladder fundus (arrows). Pathology showed cholecystitis with an area of focal hemorrhage corresponding to the imaging findings.

choledocholithiasis.[24] Low medial insertion of the cystic duct is one such anomaly and may be diagnosed when the cystic duct inserts at or near the hepatopancreatic ampulla. In this setting, superimposition of the cystic duct on the distal bile duct may appear to represent a stone in the distal bile duct on ERCP. Mirizzi syndrome may also occur due to a low cystic duct insertion. In addition, ERCP may be more technically difficult in patients with this anomaly, and the gastroenterologist should be alerted to its presence prior to endoscopy.[24]

A second but rare cause of acute biliary obstruction worth noting is inadvertent occlusion of the cystic duct during surgery. This may occur during liver transplant, hepatic resection, or cholecystectomy. The rate of iatrogenic bile duct injury remains low, with reported rates of 1.0% for laparoscopic and 0.5% for open cholecystectomy.[25] Given the large volume of cholecystectomies performed each year, however, as high as 700,000 per year in the United States, even a low rate of 0.5% to 1.0% can result in a substantial incidence of iatrogenic bile duct injuries.[17] It is associated with significant need for reintervention, increased hospital costs, and decreased quality of life for the patients.[26]

Malignant biliary obstruction does not occur acutely in the same manner as choledocholithiasis or iatrogenic biliary stricture, but patients may present emergently with obstructive jaundice and complicating cholangitis as the growing tumor

occludes the biliary tree. Cholangiocarcinoma, gallbladder carcinoma, ampullary tumors, and pancreatic adenocarcinoma may all result in obstruction of the biliary tree once they have progressed. Identifying the level of obstruction helps guide therapeutic options, whether via percutaneous biliary decompression, endoscopic stent placement, or surgical resection.[27]

Lastly, acute (ascending) cholangitis represents a feared complication of biliary obstruction and is diagnosed clinically by the presence of right upper quadrant pain, jaundice, and fever[23] (Box 2). In 1 study, the most common imaging finding in patients with cholangitis was cholestasis, characterized by dilation of the intrahepatic bile ducts. Biliary sludge, periductal edema (increased T2 signal), and ascites/retroperitoneal fluid are additional findings associated with acute cholangitis. Pus within the biliary tree may be identified as intraductal hypointense signal on heavily T2-weighted images[16] (Fig. 10).

Care must be taken to avoid mistaking certain imaging findings for biliary obstruction. Potential pitfalls that may cause apparent filling defects in the bile ducts and mimic stones include impression from the right hepatic artery, intraductal air, signal voids from flow of bile through the bile ducts, and metal artifact from surgical clips or stents. Impression from the right hepatic artery appears as an extrinsic signal void in the common hepatic duct on MRCP images, but this pitfall may be avoided by recognizing the characteristic

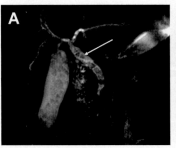 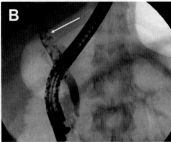

Fig. 8. Choledocholithiasis. A 25-year-old woman with right upper quadrant pain and cholelithiasis on US. (A) MRCP demonstrates choledocholithiasis and dilation of the common bile duct to 11 mm (arrow). (B) ERCP was performed with stone retrieval (arrow).

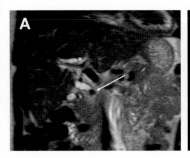
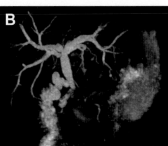

Fig. 9. Mirizzi syndrome. A 59-year-old man with prior cholecystectomy, abdominal pain and intrahepatic biliary ductal dilation seen on US. (A) Coronal T2-weighted image demonstrates a retained hypointense stone (arrow) in the remnant cystic duct, causing mass effect on the common hepatic duct. (B) Maximum intensity projection of 3-D MRCP demonstrates intrahepatic and extrahepatic biliary ductal dilation.

location of this artifact and by identifying the right hepatic artery on T2-weighted and T1-weighted postgadolinium sequences. Intraductal air appears as rounded signal voids within the bile ducts, but, unlike gallstones, air is antidependent on axial images. Axial reformatted images of 3-D MRCP data may be particularly valuable to determine if such rounded filling defects are dependent or antidependent. Flowing bile can create a central signal void in the bile duct. This pitfall may be avoided by noting the characteristic central location of the signal void, which usually is not reproducible on repeat sequences. Susceptibility artifact from metal clips or stents may create artificial signal voids, particularly on gradient-echo sequences (**Figs. 11–15**).

Pancreatitis

Acute pancreatitis is a common cause of acute abdominal pain in the Western hemisphere, and the incidence has increased in recent decades.[28] Acute pancreatitis accounts for one-quarter of a million hospital admissions each year in the United States. Choledocholithiasis and alcohol are the leading causes of acute pancreatitis, but no inciting factor is identified in as many as one-third of cases.[29] The clinical course of acute pancreatitis is variable. Mild pancreatitis typically follows a self-limited course and requires only

---

Box 2
Imaging features of acute cholangitis

- Cholestasis (dilated intrahepatic ducts)
- Biliary sludge
- Periductal increased T2 signal (edema)
- Ascites and/or retroperitoneal fluid
- Intraductal T2 hypointense signal (purulent material)

^a Note that acute cholangitis is a clinical diagnosis, and imaging features are merely supportive.

[a] Note that acute cholangitis is a clinical diagnosis, and imaging features are merely supportive.

---

supportive care with low associated morbidity and mortality. In its severe acute form, necrotizing pancreatitis can be life threatening, with morbidity and mortality as high as 36% to 50%.[30]

In response to considerable variability and confusion regarding the classification and terminology of acute pancreatitis in the medical literature, the Atlanta classification was developed[31] and most recently updated in 2012.[30]

The revised Atlanta classification states that acute pancreatitis may be diagnosed when 2 of the following 3 criteria are met: elevated lipase 3 times the upper limit of normal, characteristic abdominal pain, and radiologic findings suggestive of pancreatic inflammation. The report suggests that when acute pancreatitis is suspected based on characteristic abdominal pain but serum lipase is less than 3 times the upper limit of normal, cross-sectional imaging is indicated to establish the diagnosis.

Acute pancreatitis is divided into early and late phases, and the severity is classified as mild, moderate, or severe. The early phase of acute pancreatitis typically lasts up to 1 week and is the result of systemic response to local pancreatic inflammation. During the early phase, the presence and duration of organ failure determine the severity. In mild acute pancreatitis, there is no associated organ failure or systemic complication. Moderate pancreatitis occurs when transient organ failure (<48 hours) is present and may be associated with local or systemic complications, such as exacerbation of preexisting cardiac or pulmonary disease. Severe acute pancreatitis is diagnosed when organ failure, either single or multiple, persists beyond 48 hours.[30]

The late phase of acute pancreatitis occurs after the first week of presentation and only in moderate and severe cases. Local complications include the development of pancreatic or peripancreatic fluid collections, vascular complications (thrombosis or pseudoaneurysm), or gastric outlet obstruction.[30] Cross-sectional imaging, with either MDCT or MR, plays an essential role in the

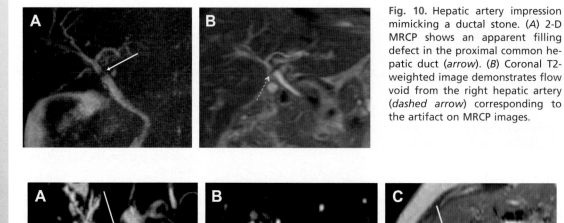

Fig. 10. Hepatic artery impression mimicking a ductal stone. (*A*) 2-D MRCP shows an apparent filling defect in the proximal common hepatic duct (*arrow*). (*B*) Coronal T2-weighted image demonstrates flow void from the right hepatic artery (*dashed arrow*) corresponding to the artifact on MRCP images.

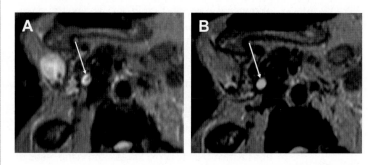

Fig. 11. Air in the cystic duct mimicking a stone. (*A*) 3-D and (*B*) 2-D MRCP show antidependent signal void consistent with air (*arrows*). (*C*) Axial T2-weighted image shows antidependent signal void in the bile ducts, consistent with pneumobilia.

Fig. 12. (*A*) Axial T2-weighted image shows a central signal void in the CBD due to flow of bile (*arrow*), which does not persist on (*B*) repeat imaging (*arrow*).

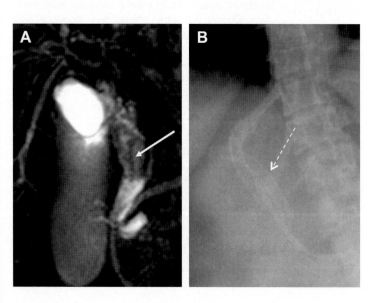

Fig. 13. (*A*) Apparent filling defect in the bile duct on 2-D MRCP (*arrow*) is due to (*B*) metallic artifact from a biliary stent (*dashed arrow*).

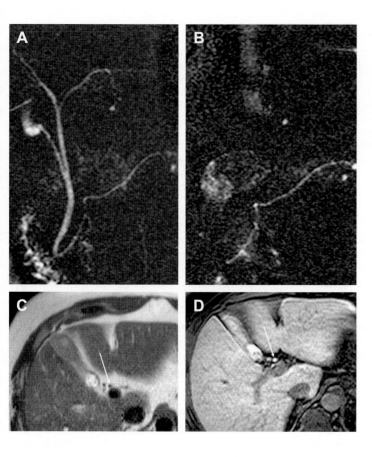

Fig. 14. MRCP acquired (*A*) before and (*B*) several minutes after the administration of hepatobiliary contrast. Signal in the biliary tree is obscured on delayed postcontrast images due to the T2-shortening effect of excreted contrast in the bile ducts. (*C*) Axial T2-weighted image acquired several minutes after the administration of gadoxetate disodium shows corresponding hypointense signal in the bile duct (*arrow*). (*D*) T1-weighted fat-suppressed image acquired 10 minutes postcontrast demonstrates hyperintense signal in the duct (*arrow*), indicating biliary excretion of contrast.

characterization of local complications in acute pancreatitis and has significant implications in management.

Although MDCT is generally the preferred modality due to widespread availability and rapid acquisition, MR may be desirable for a variety of reasons. Detection of cholelithiasis or choledocholithiasis, characterization of nonliquefied collections, or a contraindication to iodinated CT contrast may make MR the modality of choice in certain clinical situations. Familiarity with the MR imaging appearance of acute pancreatitis and its causes and complications is essential.

When first evaluating a patient with acute pancreatitis, the distinction must first be made between interstitial edematous pancreatitis (IEP) and necrotizing pancreatitis. IEP appears as diffuse or local pancreatic enlargement with homogenous or slightly heterogeneous enhancement (**Fig. 16**). T2 hyperintense signal may also be seen in the surrounding fat, indicating inflammation and edema. Pancreatic necrosis is present when an area of

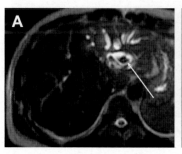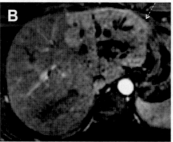

Fig. 15. Acute pyogenic cholangitis. A 26-year-old man with severe epigastric pain, leukocytosis and intrahepatic biliary ductal dilation on abdominal US. (*A*) Axial T2-weighted image demonstrates intrahepatic biliary ductal dilation isolated to the left lobe of the liver, with rounded hypointense filling defects in the bile ducts consistent with stones (*arrow*). The liver parenchyma in the left lobe is asymmetrically T2 hyperintense. (*B*) T1-weighted postcontrast imaging demonstrates early enhancement of the left lobe of the liver (*dashed arrow*).

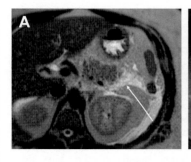
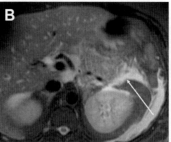

Fig. 16. IEP. A 25-year-old man with abdominal pain. (*A*) Axial T2-weighted image through the upper abdomen demonstrates an enlarged pancreas with edema and fluid in the surrounding fat (*arrow*). (*B*) The degree of inflammation is more readily apparent on axial fat-suppressed T2-weighted image through the same location, with adjacent APFC (*arrow*).

the pancreas does not enhance on postcontrast imaging. In addition, the presence of nonliquefied components in the collection (hemorrhage, fat, or necrotic fat) should be classified as necrotizing pancreatitis and not IEP.[32] If the presence or absence of necrosis is indeterminate, repeat imaging may be performed 5 to 7 days later (**Figs. 17–19**).

Four types of fluid collections are described in the new classification, stratified by the presence or absence of necrosis and duration (**Table 2**). A peripancreatic fluid collection that is present during the first 4 weeks of IEP that does not contain a solid component is described as an *acute peripancreatic fluid collection (APFC)*. A fluid collection present within the parenchyma of the pancreas should not be described as an APFC and should be considered necrosis.[32] When the fluid collection persists beyond 4 weeks in IEP, it is termed, *pancreatic pseudocyst*. To qualify as a pancreatic pseudocyst, the collection must be entirely fluid and must have a well-defined wall.[30] Pancreatic pseudocysts may communicate with the pancreatic duct via a side branch or the MPD. MRCP may demonstrate the communication, indicating a pseudocyst may be amenable to transpapillary drainage[32,33] (**Fig. 20**).

Within the category of necrotizing pancreatitis, 3 subtypes are described: pancreatic parenchymal necrosis alone, peripancreatic necrosis alone, and combined pancreatic parenchymal necrosis with peripancreatic necrosis. The combined form is most common (75%–80%), with peripancreatic necrosis typically seen in the retroperitoneum and lesser sac.[32] Once necrotizing pancreatitis has been diagnosed, a peripancreatic fluid collection should be termed, *acute necrotic collection (ANC)*, in the first 4 weeks and may contain variable amounts of solid components. After 4 weeks, once a capsule has developed, the collection should be termed, *walled-off necrosis (WON)*, not a pseudocyst[32] (**Fig. 21**).

Treatment of the collections associated with acute pancreatitis is variable. Any of the 4 types of collection may be either sterile or infected. An APFC does not generally require intervention and often resolves spontaneously on its own. Likewise, pseudocysts generally do not require intervention unless the patient is symptomatic from local mass effect or superimposed infection is suspected. If infection is suspected, percutaneous drainage of the pseudocyst is often sufficient. In contrast, patients with WON require débridement via percutaneous catheter drainage

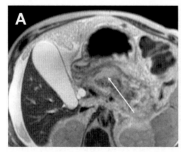
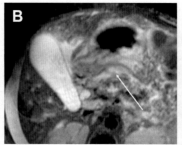
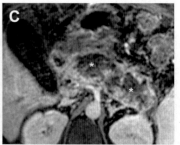

Fig. 17. Necrotizing pancreatitis. A 51-year-old man with pancreatitis. (*A*) Axial T2-weighted and (*B*) fat-suppressed T2-weighted images through the upper abdomen demonstrate ascites and significant edema in the region of the pancreas and an adjacent ANC (*arrow*). (*C*) Postcontrast fat-suppressed T1-weighted image acquired during the portal venous phase shows hypoenhancement of nearly the entire pancreatic body and tail (*asterisks*), consistent with necrotizing pancreatitis.

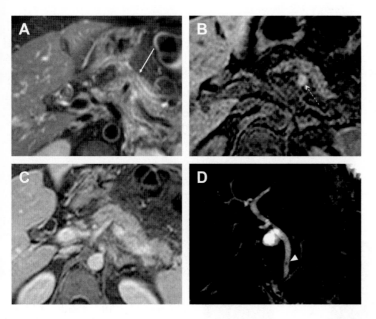

Fig. 18. Pancreatitis with hemorrhage. A 52-year-old man with pancreatitis. (*A*) Axial fat-suppressed T2-weighted image shows an edematous pancreas with surrounding inflammation (*arrow*). (*B*) Precontrast fat-suppressed T1-weighted shows a hyperintense focus along the superior, posterior aspect of the pancreas consistent with hemorrhage (*dashed arrow*). (*C*) Postcontrast fat-suppressed T1-weighted image demonstrates homogenous enhancement without evidence of necrosis. (*D*) 2-D MRCP images show a small stone in the distal CBD (*arrowhead*).

or surgery to remove all of the nonliquid components.[32]

In addition to collections, potential vascular complications should be identified in patients with acute pancreatitis. Venous complications are common and typically involve thrombosis of the splenic or portal vein. Venous thrombosis is more common in necrotizing pancreatitis, with some investigators reporting an incidence as high as 45%.[34] Arterial complications in acute pancreatitis are far less common, with the main complications pseudoaneurysm formation and acute hemorrhage. The left gastric, splenic, gastroduodenal, superior mesenteric, and hepatic arteries are most commonly involved.[34] Identification of pseudoaneurysm formation is crucial, and

timely intervention must be performed to prevent life-threatening hemorrhage (**Fig. 22**).

The identification of hemorrhagic pancreatitis is another distinct advantage of MR imaging. The presence of T1 hyperintense methemoglobin is easily recognized to aid in this diagnosis. Hemorrhage in the pancreatic bed is typically thought the result of erosion of a vessel, and prompt surgical intervention may be required to prevent potentially fatal consequences.[22]

A final complication of acute necrotizing pancreatitis is disrupted duct syndrome, a condition in which the MPD is interrupted along its course. Due to its noninvasive nature, MRCP is preferred over ERCP to evaluate for pancreatic duct disruption. On imaging, the presence of an

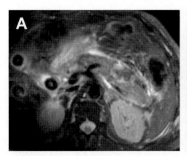
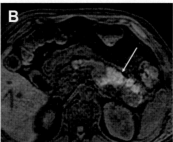
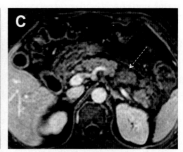

Fig. 19. Pancreatitis with necrosis and hemorrhage. A 43-year-old man admitted with abdominal pain and pancreatitis on CT. (*A*) Axial fat-suppressed T2-weighted demonstrates extensive inflammation in the pancreatic bed and enlargement of the gland. (*B*) Precontrast fat-suppressed T1-weighted image shows a large area of T1 hyperintensity in the body and tail of the pancreas consistent with hemorrhage (*arrow*). (*C*) Postcontrast fat-suppressed T1-weighted image shows hypoenhancement in the area of hemorrhage (*dashed arrow*), indicating concurrent necrosis.

Table 2
Fluid collections in pancreatitis

Interstitial Edematous Pancreatitis	Necrotizing Pancreatitis
APFC • <4 wk • No discernible wall • No solid component	ANC • <4 wk • Variable amounts of solid component • Any fluid collection *within* the pancreatic parenchyma
Pancreatic pseudocyst • >4 wk • Well-defined wall • No solid component	Walled-off necrosis • >4 wk • Variable amounts of solid component • Any fluid collection *within* the pancreatic parenchyma

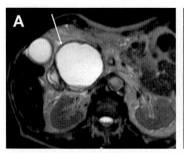 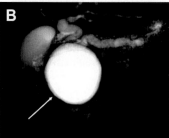

Fig. 20. Pancreatic pseudocyst. A 67-year-old man with acute on chronic pancreatitis. (*A*) Axial T2-weighted image demonstrates a T2 hyperintense fluid collection adjacent to the head of the pancreas (*arrow*). (*B*) 2-D MRCP image demonstrates the pseudocyst (*arrow*).

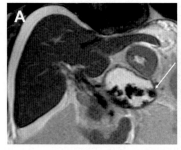 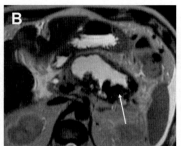 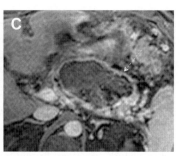

Fig. 21. WON. A 45-year-old man with history of pancreatitis and abdominal pain. (*A*) Coronal and (*B*) axial T2-weighted images demonstrate a T2 hyperintense fluid collection in the body of the pancreas with hypointense internal debris (*arrows*). (*C*) Postcontrast fat-suppressed T1-weighted image acquired during equilibrium demonstrates peripheral enhancement and a clearly defined capsule (*dashed arrow*).

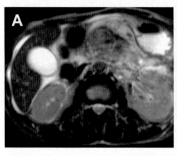 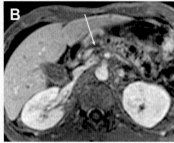

Fig. 22. Pancreatitis with splenic vein and SMV thrombosis. A 58-year-old man with pancreatitis. (*A*) Axial T2-weighted image demonstrates ascites, pancreatic edema, and surrounding fluid. (*B*) Axial fat-suppressed T1-weighted postcontrast image acquired in the equilibrium phase shows abrupt tapering of the portal vein (*arrow*) at the expected confluence of the splenic and superior mesenteric veins, which were not visualized. The splenic vein and SMV were patent on abdominal CT performed 3 months prior, suggesting thrombosis.

intrapancreatic fluid collection along the expected course of the duct is suggestive of ductal disruption,[35] a finding that increases the risk of pancreatic fistula formation and often requires surgical treatment.[36]

SUMMARY

Evaluation of patients with acute abdominal conditions is common in diagnostic radiology, and a multimodality approach to imaging is often required. Although MDCT is the main workhorse of emergency abdominal imaging, additional information gathered from modalities, such as US, MR, and nuclear medicine, can be of the utmost value. In the evaluation of patients with pancreaticobiliary trauma, suspected bile leak, cholecystitis, biliary obstruction, and pancreatitis, MR is invaluable. Familiarity with the optimal imaging protocols, imaging appearance of pathology and mimics, established guidelines, and therapeutic implications is key to the accurate diagnosis and management of these patients.

REFERENCES

1. Bhuiya FA, Pitts SR, McCaig LF. Emergency department visits for chest pain and abdominal pain: United States, 1999–2008. Hyattsville (MD): Centers for Disease Control; 2010.
2. Lowenfels AB, Maisonneuve P, Sullivan T. The changing character of acute pancreatitis: epidemiology, etiology, and prognosis. Curr Gastroenterol Rep 2009;11(2):97–103.
3. Knab LM, Boller A, Mahvi DM. Cholecystitis. Surg Clin North Am 2014;94:455–70.
4. Wallner BK, Schumacher KA, Weidenmaier W, et al. Dilated billary tract: evaluation with MR cholanglography with a T2-weighted contrast-enhanced fast sequence. Radiology 1991;181:805–8.
5. Sadler TW. Langman's medical embryology. 12th edition. Baltimore (MD): Lippincott Williams & Wilkins; 2012.
6. Moore KL, Dalley AF II, Agur AMR. Clinically oriented anatomy. 7th edition. Baltimore (MD): Williams & Wilkins; 2014.
7. Panda A, Kumar A, Gamanagatti S, et al. Evaluation of diagnostic utility of multidetector computed tomography and magnetic resonance imaging in blunt pancreatic trauma: a prospective study. Acta Radiol 2015;56(4):387–96.
8. Gupta A, Stuhlfaut J, Fleming K, et al. Blunt trauma of the pancreas and biliary tract: a multimodality imaging approach to diagnosis. Radiographics 2004; 24(5):1381–95.
9. Bradley EL, Young PR, Chang MC, et al. Diagnosis and initial management of blunt pancreatic trauma: guidelines from a multi-institutional review. Ann Surg 1998;227(6):861–9.
10. Rekhi S, Anderson SW, Rhea JT, et al. Imaging of blunt pancreatic trauma. Emerg Radiol 2010;17: 13–9.
11. Wong Y, Wang L, Lin B. CT grading of blunt pancreatic injuries: prediction of ductal disruption and surgical correlation. J Comput Assist Tomogr 1997; 21(1):246–50.
12. Melamud K, LeBedis CA, Anderson SW, et al. Biliary imaging: multimodality approach to imaging of biliary injuries and their complications. Radiographics 2014;34:613–23.
13. LeBedis CA, Luna A, Soto J. Use of magnetic resonance imaging contrast agents in the liver and biliarys tract. Magn Reson Imaging Clin N Am 2012; 20:715–37.
14. Kantarcı M, Pirimoglu B, Karabulut N, et al. Noninvasive detection of biliary leaks using Gd-EOB-DTPA-enhanced MR cholangiography: comparison with T2-weighted MR cholangiography. Eur Radiol 2013;23:2713–22.
15. Kiewiet JJ, Leeuwenburgh MM, Bipat S, et al. A systematic review and meta-analysis of diagnostic performance of imaging in acute cholecystitis. Radiology 2012;264(3):708–20.
16. Watanabe Y, Nagayama M, Okumura A, et al. MR Imaging of acute biliary disorders. Radiographics 2007;27:477–95.
17. Yam BL, Siegelman ES. MR imaging of the biliary system. Radiol Clin North Am 2014;52:725–55.
18. O'Connor OJ, Maher MM. Imaging of cholecystitis. AJR Am J Roentgenol 2011;196:W367–74.
19. Takada T, Kawarada Y, Nimura Y, et al. Background: Tokyo Guidelines for the management of acute cholangitis and cholecystitis. J Hepatobiliary Pancreat Surg 2007;14:1–10.
20. Takada T, Strasberg SM, Solomkin JS, et al. TG13: Updated Tokyo Guidelines for the management of acute cholangitis and cholecystitis. J Hepatobiliary Pancreat Sci 2013;20:1–7.
21. Adusumilli S, Siegelman E. MR imaging of the gallbladder. Magn Reson Imaging Clin N Am 2002;10: 165–84.
22. Tkacz JN, Anderson SA, Soto J. MR imaging in gastrointestinal emergencies. Radiographics 2009; 29:1767–80.
23. Hakansson K, Leander P, Ekberg O, et al. MR imaging in clinically suspected acute cholecystitis: a comparison with ultrasonography. Acta Radiol 2000;41:322–8.
24. Turner MA, Fulcher AS. The cystic duct normal anatomy and disease processes. Radiographics 2001; 21:3–22.
25. Mungai F, Berti V, Colagrande S. Bile leak after elective laparoscopic cholecystectomy: role of MR imaging. J Radiol Case Rep 2013;7:25–32.

26. Buddingh KT, Nieuwenhuijs B, van Buuren L, et al. Intraoperative assessment of biliary anatomy for prevention of bile duct injury: a review of current and future patient safety interventions. Surg Endosc 2011;25:2449–61.

27. Soto JA, Alvarez O, Lopera JE, et al. Biliary obstruction: findings at MR cholangiography and cross-sectional MR imaging. Radiographics 2000;20:353–66.

28. Goldacre MJ, Roberts SE. Hospital admission for acute pancreatitis in an English population, 1963-98: database study of incidence and mortality. BMJ 2004;328:1466–9.

29. Murphy KP, O'Connor KJ, Maher MM. Updated imaging nomenclature for acute pancreatitis. AJR Am J Roentgenol 2014;203:W464–9.

30. Banks P, Bollen T, Dervenis C, et al. Classification of acute pancreatitis—2012: revision of the Atlanta classification and definitions by international consensus. Gut 2013;62:102–11.

31. Bradley EL III. A clinically based classification system for acute pancreatitis. Arch Surg 1993;128:586–90.

32. Thoeni RF. The revised Atlanta classification of acute pancreatitis: its importance for the radiologist and its effect on treatment. Radiology 2012; 262(3):751–64.

33. Aghdassi A, Mayerle J, Kraft M, et al. Pancreatic pseudocysts–when and how to treat? HPB (Oxford) 2006;8(6):432–41.

34. Mendelson R, Anderson J, MarshallL M, et al. Vascular complications of acute pancreatitis. ANZ J Surg 2005;75:1073–9.

35. Manikkavasakar S, AlObaidy M, Busireddy KK, et al. Magnetic resonance imaging of pancreatitis: an update. World J Gastroenterol 2014;20(40):14760–77.

36. Sandrasegaran K, Tann M, Jennings SG, et al. Disconnection of the pancreatic duct: an important but overlooked complication of severe acute pancreatitis. Radiographics 2007;27(5):1389–400.

Pediatric Emergency Magnetic Resonance Imaging
Current Indications, Techniques, and Clinical Applications

Patricia T. Chang, MD[a], Edward Yang, MD, PhD[a],
David W. Swenson, MD[a], Edward Y. Lee, MD, MPH[b],*

KEYWORDS

- Children • Pediatric emergency • Trauma • Appendicitis • Stroke • Sinus thrombosis • Meningitis
- Abscess

KEY POINTS

- MR imaging is valuable in the confirmation and characterization of emergent pediatric disorders because of its ease of performance, superior soft tissue contrast, multiplanar capabilities, lack of ionizing radiation, and ability to detect multiple lesions with minimal patient manipulation.
- Emergent MR imaging can be critical when clinical, laboratory, and ultrasound or computed tomography findings are nonspecific.
- Recognition of some of the characteristic imaging features of emergent pediatric disorders is important because it can allow rapid institution of therapy, which reduces morbidity and mortality.
- MR imaging can be an effective and efficient method for the timely and appropriate management of pediatric disease entities that can occur in the emergent setting.

INTRODUCTION

MR imaging in the pediatric population can be difficult to obtain because of noise, fear, claustrophobia, and inability to remain motionless. Sedation or general anesthesia is often required to obtain quality images. Despite these limitations, the uses of pediatric MR imaging have expanded over time to include a growing number of emergency indications. This shift is a reflection of the intrinsic advantages of MR imaging in depicting soft tissue disease processes and bone marrow edema as well as the heightened awareness of radiation exposure associated with alternative work-up strategies that use computed tomography (CT). Additionally, rapid MR imaging protocols have reduced the length of MR imaging examinations while still obtaining clinically usable information.[1] The use of single-shot fast spin-echo (SSFSE) MR imaging, for example, has been shown to be useful in the evaluation of ventriculostomy shunt malfunction in children treated for hydrocephalus. Similarly, rapid protocols can also be used to diagnose appendicitis without the need for CT imaging. In this article, the authors discuss a variety of pediatric emergencies that can be diagnosed with MR imaging and review the clinical features that are specific for each disease entity.

The authors have nothing to disclose.
a Department of Radiology, Boston Children's Hospital, Harvard Medical School, 300 Longwood Avenue, Boston, MA 02115, USA; b Division of Thoracic Imaging, Department of Radiology, Boston Children's Hospital, Harvard Medical School, 300 Longwood Avenue, Boston, MA 02115, USA
* Corresponding author.
E-mail address: Edward.Lee@childrens.harvard.edu

1064-9689/16/$ – see front matter © 2016 Elsevier Inc. All rights reserved.

IMAGING TECHNIQUE

Pediatric magnetic resonance (MR) evaluation in the emergent setting is typically performed on a 1.5T or 3T MR scanner with patients supine, using a phased array receiver coil. Higher field strength imaging on a 3T MR scanner offers several benefits for pediatric imaging, including improved signal-to-noise ratio (SNR) and contrast-to-noise ratio, with potential for improved spatial and temporal resolution.[2,3] However, 3T MR imaging also has disadvantages that can be particularly challenging for abdominal imaging, including increased susceptibility artifacts from air within bowel loops as well as increased energy deposition, which can approach patients' specific absorbed ratio limits in children. Nevertheless, the current trend in academic centers in the United States is toward higher-field-strength pediatric MR imaging.

The receiver coil used for pediatric MR depends on the body part being imaged. For brain imaging, a 32-channel head coil is typically used at the authors' institution. For spine imaging, whole-body coils that include coil elements embedded in the scan table are used. The receiver coil used in pediatric musculoskeletal imaging also depends on the body part being imaged, with either a flex coil or a whole-body coil in combination with a body matrix coil used. The receiver coil for pediatric abdominal imaging should fit snugly around patients to maximize spatial resolution and SNR. This fit can be difficult, as various adult MR coils need to be fitted to pediatric patients ranging from infants to adolescents. A head coil is often used for infants and small children, whereas a body coil is typically used for larger children and adolescents.[4] Whole-body coils have also been used with success.

Compared with adult imaging, patient motion is a more substantial problem with pediatric MR imaging. Sources of motion include voluntary motion from patients' muscular movements in the scanner as well as involuntary motion predominantly due to respiratory motion in children unable to suspend respiration on command. In order to minimize scan times, parallel and fast imaging techniques can be used.[5] An additional consideration unique to children is the prevalence of orthodontic hardware, the presence of which can render susceptibility-weighted imaging (SWI) and diffusion-weighted imaging (DWI) nondiagnostic. Therefore, removal of braces should be considered in cases whereby these sequences are vital (eg, acute stroke).

PATIENT PREPARATION

Patients older than 6 years are usually able to cooperate with MR imaging after an explanation of the procedure and reassurance. Distraction techniques including the use of MR imaging–compatible music and video players as well as scanning during off hours to minimize ambient noise and activity can also be helpful. Similarly, newborns and young infants may tolerate MR imaging without the need for sedation, if they are well fed and comfortably swaddled. For young children less than 6 years of age, conscious or deep sedation may be required to relieve patient anxiety and minimize patient motion during imaging.

Sedation

Several sedation medications are currently used for pediatric MR imaging, including chloral hydrate, pentobarbital, propofol, and midazolam.[6,7] Advantages of sedation in children who cannot tolerate MR imaging while awake include reduction in scan time and improvement in image quality. Generally, the least amount of sedation necessary for patients to tolerate MR imaging is administered, both to minimize post-MR imaging side effects and to facilitate patient induction and emergence from sedation. As always, the proper balance should be maintained between adequate sedation for patient comfort and scan performance and minimization of potential neurologic and cognitive effects associated with prolonged anesthesia.[8]

Intravenous Contrast Administration

Contrast agents used for clinical pediatric MR imaging are gadolinium chelated, extracellular contrast agents that cause T1 shortening within blood vessels and perfused tissues. The typical dose for intravenous administration is 0.1 mmol/kg.[9]

IMAGING SEQUENCES
Brain

A minimal MR imaging examination of the brain (termed *brain screen* at the authors' institution) includes sagittal T1, axial T2 fluid-attenuated inversion recovery (FLAIR), axial T2 fast spin echo, coronal T2, and axial DWI. Additional sequences are obtained based on the clinical indication (**Table 1**). When the clinical question is limited to change in ventricle size for chronically shunted patients, SSFSE imaging is adequate for this evaluation, requires only a few minutes of scanner time, and can typically be performed without sedation in the authors' experience (**Fig. 1**).

Spine

The MR imaging sequences for the evaluation of pediatric spine emergencies also depend on the

Table 1
3T brain MR imaging techniques based on clinical indication

Indication	Sequences
Hydrocephalus	Axial SSFSE
Stroke	• Brain screen • Axial SWI • MRA 3D time-of-flight circle of Willis, neck • Option: axial T1 fat-saturated and high-resolution T2 imaging of the neck for dissection
Sinus thrombosis	• Brain screen • Axial SWI • Coronal time-of-flight MRV • Postcontrast, isotropic T1 MPRAGE/SPGR
Encephalitis and meningitis Cerebral abscess/ empyema	• Brain screen • Postcontrast axial T1 TSE (optional fat saturation) • Postcontrast sagittal T1 3D TSE (replace with SPGR/ MPRAGE if sinus venous thrombosis suspected)
New intracranial neoplasm	• Brain screen • 3D spectroscopy • Arterial spin labeled perfusion imaging • Postcontrast axial T1 TSE • Postcontrast sagittal T1 3D TSE • Postcontrast sagittal T1 entire spine • Optional: axial SWI, balanced steady-state gradient-echo sequences

Abbreviations: 3D, 3 dimensional; MPRAGE, magnetization prepared rapid gradient echo; MRA, MR angiography; MRV, MR venography; SPGR, spoiled gradient echo; TSE, turbo spin-echo.

disease process, whether it is infectious/inflammatory, neoplastic, or traumatic in cause (**Table 2**).

Body

Septic arthritis, osteomyelitis, and appendicitis are the 3 most common clinical indications for emergent body MR imaging in pediatric patients. In the case of acute hip pain, the following sequences are obtained for evaluation of septic arthritis and/or osteomyelitis: coronal T1, coronal fast spin-echo inversion recovery (FSEIR), sagittal oblique proton density with fat saturation, axial T2 with fat saturation, and postcontrast axial and coronal T1 with fat saturation. The main MR imaging sequences for the evaluation of osteomyelitis in other regions of the body include coronal T1, axial T2 with fat saturation, sagittal FSEIR, postcontrast axial T1 with fat saturation, and postcontrast coronal/sagittal T1 with fat saturation (**Table 3**).

Appendix MR imaging sequences are acquired from the level of the kidneys through the urinary bladder without sedation or contrast media. Although there is variability in the published literature about the necessary sequences, most institutions include multiplanar T2-weighted single-shot turbo spin-echo (ie, half-Fourier acquisition single-shot turbo spin-echo) without fat saturation and at least a single-plane short-tau inversion recovery (STIR) sequence.[10–13] At the authors' institution, additional sequences that have been considered useful include a coronal T2-weighted 3-dimensional (3D) turbo spin-echo (TSE) sequence with multiplanar reconstructions and/or axial true fast imaging with steady-state precession. All sequences except 3D TSE are obtained with breath holding, whereas 3D TSE is acquired during shallow free breathing (see **Table 3**).

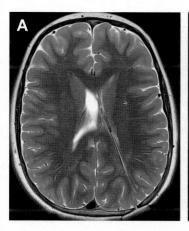 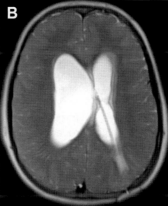

Fig. 1. Shunt malfunction. A chronically shunted 12-year-old girl presented with headache and vomiting. Compared with baseline axial fast spin-echo T2 imaging (*A*), the SSFSE T2 imaging (*B*) demonstrates marked ventricular enlargement and periventricular signal increase diagnostic of hydrocephalus with transependymal CSF resorption. Note the poorer soft tissue detail of the SSFSE technique relative to normal fast spin-echo T2-weighted imaging.

Table 2 3T spine MR imaging techniques based on clinical indication	
Indication	**Sequences**
Discitis/osteomyelitis	• Sagittal T1 • Sagittal T2 fat saturated • Axial T1 and T2 • Postcontrast axial and sagittal T1 fat saturated
Transverse myelitis/ acute neurologic abnormality	• Sagittal T1 and T2 whole spine • Axial T2 entire spine • Axial T1 lumbar spine • Sagittal DWI • Postcontrast sagittal and T1 entire spine
New primary tumor	• Sagittal T1 and T2 of entire spine • Axial T1 FLAIR and T2 through lesion • Axial T1 and T2 through lumbar spine • Postcontrast sagittal T1 fat saturated through lesion • Postcontrast axial T1 through lesion • Postcontrast sagittal T1 to cover rest of spine • Sagittal DWI
Metastatic disease	• Postcontrast sagittal T1 entire spine • Postcontrast axial T1 imaging targeted to any region of interest
Trauma	• Sagittal T1 and T2 • Sagittal short-tau inversion recovery • Axial T1 and T2 • Axial T2* GRE • Optional: sagittal DWI, CISS/FIESTA

Table 3 3T body MR imaging techniques based on clinical indication	
Indication	**Sequences**
Septic arthritis (hip)	• Coronal T1 • Coronal FSEIR/STIR • Sagittal oblique proton density with fat saturation • Axial T2 with fat saturation • Postcontrast multiplanar T1 with fat saturation
Osteomyelitis	• Coronal T1 • Axial T2 with fat saturation • Sagittal FSEIR/STIR • Postcontrast multiplanar T1 with fat saturation
Appendicitis	• Axial and coronal T2 HASTE, kidneys through bladder • Axial STIR • Coronal SPACE with multiplanar reconstruction • Axial and/or coronal true fast imaging with steady-state precession

Abbreviation: STIR, short-tau inversion recovery.

estimates,[14] the immediate care of these patients often revolves around managing mass effect from the hematoma or hydrocephalus from decompression into the ventricular system, something usually done adequately and with maximal efficiency with head CT. Therefore, it is not further discussed in detail here.

Arterial ischemic stroke
The incidence of AIS in children has been estimated in the range of 0.2 to 7.8 cases per 100,000 children per year, with neonates having roughly 10-fold higher incidence.[14] Well-known risk factors include underlying congenital heart disease and sickle cell anemia, the latter increasing the risk of an ischemic event by roughly a factor of 100 times.[15] Most children presenting with AIS are previously well, and up to 30% to 50% of AIS cases have been historically thought to lack an identifiable risk factor.[14] However, the increasing recognition of children with some kind of risk factor, such as an arteriopathy (eg, moyamoya, spontaneous intracranial dissection), prothrombotic state (eg, hyperhomocysteinemia), or recent infection, have reduced the number of cases with no known cause.[16]

Unlike adults, significant numbers of pediatric patients with AIS present with seizure. This feature is particularly striking in neonates whereby seizures may affect up to 40% of newborns with territorial

SPECTRUM OF DISORDERS
Vasculopathic Disorders

A stroke is a syndrome of spontaneous, prolonged neurologic dysfunction secondary to brain injury. Like adults, childhood strokes can be divided into those due to insufficient arterial inflow (arterial ischemic stroke [AIS]) and those due to thrombosis of the venous outflow (cerebral venous thrombosis [CVT]). Although hemorrhagic strokes are more common in children than adults, composing up to 30% to 50% by some

infarcts.[17] These newborns may also have vague findings, such as generalized encephalopathy or abnormalities of tone. In older children, focal neurologic symptoms are more common; but the clinical picture may be obfuscated by nonspecific symptoms, such as headache or altered mental status.[18,19] These atypical presentations may be a contributor to considerable delays in diagnosis of pediatric AIS and also represent an impediment to investigation of stroke interventions.[20]

In the authors' institution, emergent evaluation of a potential AIS is generally sought using brain MR imaging, MR angiography (MRA) (brain and neck), and in many cases MR venography (MRV) because this combined MR work-up provides the quickest means of unambiguously differentiating AIS from alternative diagnoses, such as CVT, posterior reversible encephalopathy syndrome, or acute disseminated encephalomyelitis (ADEM).[21] Imaging typically begins with diffusion imaging early in the examination to detect sites of infarction should patients prove too unstable or uncooperative to continue imaging. As is the case for adults, diffusion restriction is visible within minutes of thromboembolic compromise of inflow, and T2 signal abnormality develops after the first 6 to 8 hours with peak mass effect anticipated a few days after the onset of infarction. The vascular imaging typically allows for definition of the level of inflow compromise (Fig. 2); special sequences,

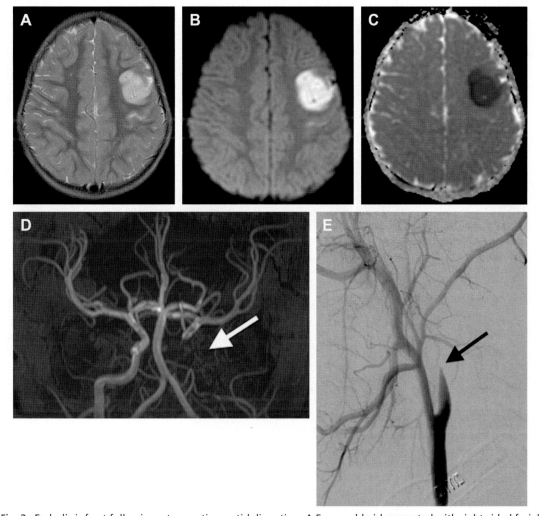

Fig. 2. Embolic infarct following a traumatic carotid dissection. A 5-year-old girl presented with right-sided facial droop and seizures after blunt trauma to the left neck. Axial T2 (A), diffusion trace (B), and apparent diffusion coefficient (C) images demonstrate an acute infarct within the left frontal lobe. Time-of-flight MRA frontal projection (D) demonstrates absence of flow-related enhancement within the left internal carotid artery (*white arrow*). Left common carotid artery catheter angiogram in the lateral projection (E) demonstrates flamelike tapering of the proximal internal carotid artery consistent with dissection and vessel occlusion (*black arrow*).

such as fat-saturated or vessel wall imaging, may be used in certain circumstances, such as suspected dissection. SWI is a useful adjunct to diffusion imaging as it can detect areas of petechial hemorrhage, intraluminal clot, and areas of increased oxygen extraction from decreased blood flow (**Fig. 3**). In the dictation, special comment should be made on the general geographic extent of the infarction and involvement of critical structures, such as the corticospinal tract, because these imaging markers correlate with long-term disability.[22,23]

Therapy for AIS begins with correction of any exacerbating conditions, such as decompensated cardiac function or prothrombotic states.

Investigation for predisposing risk factors, such as prothrombotic conditions, is usually undertaken unless a known risk factor accounts for the stroke. Additional therapies then depend on underlying causes of the stroke. For arterial dissection, therapeutic anticoagulation with heparin/warfarin is generally begun in patients with infarction, though anticoagulation for intracranial dissections is more controversial. For patients with sickle cell, transfusions are usually performed to optimize oxygen carrying capacity. At this time, thrombolytic agents are considered experimental in children, though clinical trials are currently evaluating their use. Aspirin is often used as a medication for secondary prevention, but special considerations are

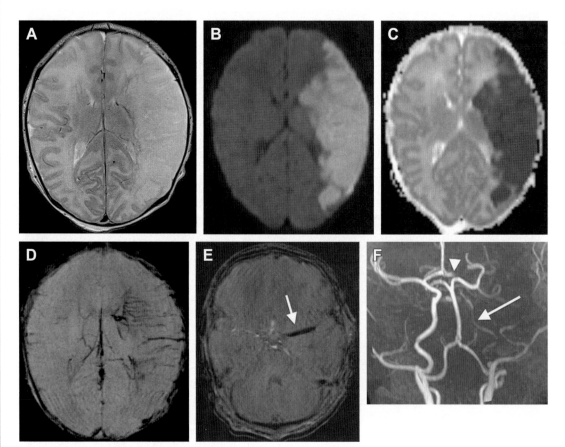

Fig. 3. Focal infarct of infancy (idiopathic). A full-term newborn presented with apneic episodes and a subsequent electroencephalogram demonstrating seizures originating in the left temporal lobe. Axial T2 (*A*), diffusion trace (*B*), and apparent diffusion coefficient (*C*) images of the brain demonstrate an acute infarct involving the entirety of the left middle cerebral artery territory, including the left basal ganglia. SWI (*D*, *E*) is notable for prominent susceptibility within the left hemisphere venous drainage consistent with increased oxygen extraction and thrombus within the proximal left middle cerebral artery (*white arrow* in *E*). Frontal maximum intensity projection of time-of-flight MRA (*F*) demonstrates absence of flow-related enhancement in the left middle cerebral artery and poor flow-related enhancement of the upstream left internal carotid artery from nonocclusive thrombus (*white arrow*). There is retrograde flow within the left anterior cerebral artery A1 segment via the anterior communicating artery (*white arrowhead*). Coagulopathy and infectious work-ups were negative, and the ultimate cause of the thromboembolic stroke could not be determined.

required for minimizing the risk of Reye syndrome. The therapies available for AIS as well as expected outcomes for specific causes of AIS are comprehensively reviewed in the American Heart Association's (AHA) scientific statement on pediatric stroke.[14]

Cerebral venous thrombosis
CVT is abnormal clot formation within the cortical veins, deep cerebral veins, or the dural sinuses. When of hemodynamically significant size or occlusive, these clots cause venous hypertension, which can result in congestion of the drained brain parenchyma, in some cases manifesting as venous ischemia or hemorrhage (up to 40%).[24] CVT is estimated to be twice as common in children as in adults, with an estimated incidence of slightly less than 1 case per 100,000 children per year; neonates represent the most susceptible population accounting for more than 25% of all affected children ascertained in the largest study of childhood CVT.[25] Myriad causes may trigger CVT episodes, including prothrombotic states (eg, malignancy; nephrotic syndrome; lupus anticoagulant; medications, such as L-asparaginase or oral contraceptives), dehydration, and underlying infection/inflammation (eg, inflammatory bowel disease or complicated otomastoiditis).[26,27] Although focal neurologic deficits or headaches often accompany CVT, the clinical picture may be confusing in very young patients whereby altered sensorium or seizure may be the primary manifestation.[26,28] Additionally, more insidious symptoms, such as elevated intracranial pressure, communicating hydrocephalus, or papilledema (ie, vision loss), can be the primary symptom in some patients.

Therefore, imaging is often pivotal in correctly identifying the cause of nonspecific symptoms, such as headache, seizure, or altered mental status; the appropriateness of MRV in infants should always be considered as part of the evaluation for unexplained seizure, and scrutiny of the venous flow voids is required when MR imaging for headache has no other positive findings. In the authors' institution, MR imaging and MRV are the preferred means of evaluating and following CVT because of the absence of radiation and the ability to characterize parenchymal complications in detail as well as evaluate the cerebral venous system. Clot within the cerebral sinuses evolves in a manner paralleling parenchymal hematomas, being initially T1 isointense and T2 hypointense followed by evolution to more T1/T2 hyperintense signal over a course of a few weeks.[29] Deoxygenated hemoglobin from clot is most conspicuous on SWI or T2* gradient echo (GRE) sequences (**Fig. 4**). MRV can

be performed using the time-of-flight technique (T1 hyperintense clot can spuriously appear as flow due to the T1 weighting of this sequence, and in-plane flow can falsely simulate clot) or phase contrast technique (artifacts related to aliasing or flow below the velocity encoding can occur). Postcontrast 3D gradient echo sequences, such as MPRAGE or SPGR, circumvent many of the technical limitations of noncontrast MRV sequences and offer isotropic resolution, often enabling more confident determination of the extent/occlusiveness of a thrombus. It should be noted that isolated cortical vein thrombosis is frequently best seen on susceptibility and conventional noncontrast 3D gradient echo sequences. These technical details have been recently reviewed elsewhere.[30]

Treatment of CVT in children begins with management of systemic contributors to the thrombosis, including cessation of offending medications, rehydration, and treatment of inciting infections (eg, mastoidectomy and antibiotics for complicated sinusitis).[26] However, the use of anticoagulation is more controversial because of the frequent co-occurrence of intracranial hemorrhage with CVT and lack of age-specific randomized controlled trials. Based on a large case series, however, the AHA's Stroke Council endorses the use of therapeutic anticoagulation for CVT experienced in children outside the neonatal age group.[14] For neonates, the AHA does not recommend use of heparin/warfarin unless there is radiographic evidence of thrombus propagation or multiple thrombosed dural sinuses. However, there is considerable heterogeneity in actual practice patterns regarding neonatal CVT treatment.[31]

Posterior reversible encephalopathy syndrome
Posterior reversible encephalopathy syndrome (PRES) merits consideration in a discussion of pediatric stroke because it is also a disorder that may present with headaches, altered mental status, and seizure. Although studies of children with PRES are scarce, the risk factors seem similar to those for adult PRES and include use of immunosuppressive medication (eg, tacrolimus, cyclosporine), some chemotherapeutic agents, and hypertensive crisis.[32] However, there is some evidence that these children may lack the severity of hypertension common to adults presenting with this diagnosis.[33,34] Regardless of cause, the treatment of PRES is generally to remove the inciting cause.

Although frequently subtle on CT examinations, the MR imaging manifestations of PRES are usually quite obvious. Typical features are areas of subcortical and cortical signal abnormality within the perfusion watershed (**Fig. 5**) with occasional

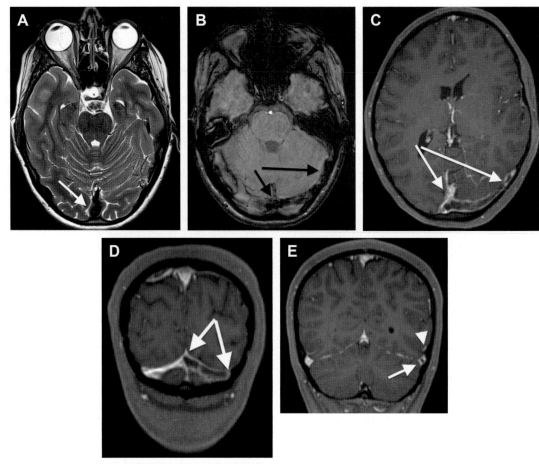

Fig. 4. Thrombosis of the dural sinuses. A 17-year-old girl with recent initiation of oral contraception was evaluated for acute onset of unremitting headache. Axial T2 imaging (*A*) suggests faint heterogeneous material within the torcula (*white arrow*). Axial SWI (*B*) indicates clot within the left transverse sinus (*black arrows* denote susceptibility from clot). Axial oblique (*C*) and coronal (*D, E*) postcontrast T1-weighted spoiled gradient echo images reveal the filling defect from the clot (*white arrows*). Of note, the clot is nonobstructive distally and there is normal opacification of the only superficial vein draining into the left transverse sinus, the left vein of Labbé (*white arrowhead*).

involvement of deeper structures, such as the deep white matter, deep gray matter, brainstem, and cerebellum.[35] Small areas of diffusion restriction or hemorrhage occur in a minority of cases[36] and probably account for the rare cases where imaging findings are not truly reversible.[37] It has been suggested that pediatric PRES may present in a more florid manner than typical adult PRES,[38] but many adult cases of PRES have been reported with similarly extensive findings.

INFECTIOUS AND INFLAMMATORY DISORDERS
Brain

Meningitis
Meningitis is inflammation of the leptomeninges by a virus (most commonly enteroviruses), bacterium,

autoimmunity, or drug/chemical exposure.[39] In an emergency setting, bacterial meningitis is the most feared type of meningitis because of mortality rates approaching 30% to 50% in some studies and significant morbidity in those who survive.[40,41] It is also frequently a difficult diagnosis for the referring physician, reportedly representing the most common cause of malpractice litigation among pediatric emergency department physicians: symptoms are neither sensitive nor specific, featuring headache, fever, seizure, and mental status changes seen with many of the other infectious disorders discussed in this section.[42] The incidence of bacterial meningitis among children of all ages is reported as 1 to 3 per 100,000 individuals per year, but this frequency can be 2 orders of magnitude higher among newborns and in some developing countries.[41] The most common

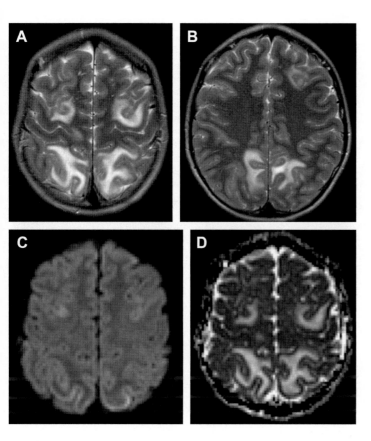

Fig. 5. PRES. A chronically ill 11-year-old boy presented with hypertension and seizures. Axial T2-weighted images of the brain (*A, B*) demonstrate symmetric subcortical white matter and cortical signal increase within the parieto-occipital and frontal lobes. There is no corresponding restricted diffusion on the DWI trace (*C*) and apparent diffusion coefficient (*D*) maps.

neonatal causes of meningitis are group B streptococcus (*Streptococcus agalactiae*), gram-negative rods, such as *Escherichia coli*, and *Listeria monocytogenes*. The most common causes of bacterial meningitis among older children are bacteria known to colonize the upper respiratory tract, including *Haemophilus influenza* type b, *Streptococcus pneumonia*, and *Neisseria meningitidis*, though the epidemiology is evolving because of vaccination campaigns against these organisms.[43,44] Complicated sinusitis/otomastoiditis are also important though infrequent causes of meningitis in older children.[45,46]

Cerebrospinal fluid (CSF) sampling is critical in confirming an acute infection, suggesting a bacterial cause, and eventually identifying a specific organism by CSF culture.[47] Such an analysis is recommended in febrile seizure patients with additional features, such as encephalopathy or without immunization against the major meningitic bacteria, *H influenza* type b and *S pneumonia*.[48] Although antibiotic therapy before lumbar puncture can diminish the yield from CSF culture, the typical bacterial meningitis CSF pattern can still be observed: high protein, low glucose, and polymorphonuclear cell-predominant white blood cells.[49] Once the diagnosis of bacterial meningitis is secured, broad-spectrum antibiotics are continued until culture identifies a specific agent and its sensitivities; steroids are occasionally also used.[41]

Imaging is performed to exclude parenchymal complications (ie, infarction, abscess), empyema, ventriculitis, or hydrocephalus from bacterial meningitis rather than to confirm the diagnosis itself. Although some articles have suggested remarkable sensitivity for diagnosing meningitis by imaging alone, expert opinion is that imaging remains much less sensitive in detecting meningeal inflammation than CSF sampling.[50,51] MR imaging with diffusion imaging provides the most sensitive evaluation for parenchymal changes, allowing early detection of areas of microinfarction from meningitis; DWI/FLAIR allows differentiation of proteinaceous exudates from purulent material (**Fig. 6**).[52] MR imaging can also be used to follow disturbances of CSF resorption (ie, hydrocephalus) that ensue in many cases of bacterial meningitis. In cases of tuberculous meningitis, areas of leptomeningeal nodularity, thick basilar exudates, and parenchymal tuberculomas may suggest this specific diagnosis.[53] As detailed later, MR imaging has

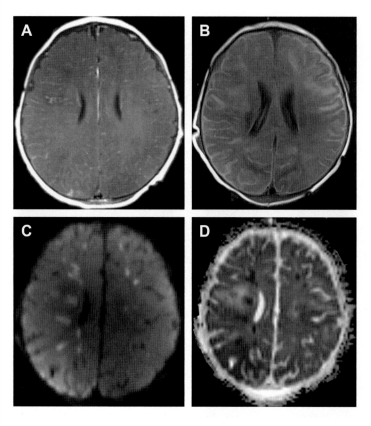

Fig. 6. Bacterial meningitis with parenchymal complications. A 5-month-old girl presents with fever, sleepiness, vomiting, and a bulging fontanelle. CSF sampling recovered streptococcus pneumonia. Axial T1-weighted postcontrast image of the brain (*A*) demonstrates diffuse leptomeningeal enhancement with an area of cerebritis versus venous congestion in the right frontal lobe. Axial FLAIR image (*B*) demonstrates sulcal signal increase consistent with exudate from the meningitis as well as parenchymal edema suggesting cerebritis and/or vascular complications from the meningitis. Diffusion trace (*C*) and apparent diffusion coefficient (*D*) maps confirm the presence of small complicating infarctions from the meningitis. The patient also had complicating dural sinus thrombosis and petechial hemorrhage within some of the sites of infarction (not shown).

additional advantages in definitively characterizing parenchymal abscess versus cerebritis and effusions from empyema. Should there be concern regarding arterial or venous occlusion in the setting of meningitis, MRA and MRV can be added on during the examination with minimal prolongation in total examination time.

Encephalitis and acute disseminated encephalomyelitis

Encephalitis is a condition of parenchymal inflammation due to an infectious agent other than pyogenic bacteria or due to autoimmune inflammation. Although relatively uncommon in the population as a whole, encephalitis is relatively common in children, particularly young children, with quoted incidences of 10.5 and 27.7 cases per 100,000 children yearly for all children and infants, respectively.[54] The list of potential causes is lengthy and includes viruses (respiratory, such as influenza A; enteroviruses; arboviruses, such as West Nile; and herpes viruses, such as herpes simplex virus type 1 [HSV-1], varicella zoster, and Epstein-Barr viruses) and nonpyogenic bacteria, such as *Mycoplasma*, *Bartonella*, and *Borrelia* species.[55] Depending on the case series, a significant minority or most cases will ultimately remain

without a defined infectious agent as the cause. Of interest, the California Encephalitis Project suggests that *Mycoplasma pneumoniae*–associated encephalitis may represent the single most common infectious cause of childhood encephalitis and autoimmune (ie, anti–N-methyl-d-aspartate receptor) encephalitis may represent the single most common noninfectious cause excluding ADEM.[56,57] ADEM is a monophasic demyelinating event associated with recent vaccination or infection, most commonly seen in children whereby the incidence is up to 0.8 cases per 100,000 individuals per year.[58]

The encephalitides and ADEM present with fever, headache, other symptoms of elevated intracranial pressure (nausea, vomiting), changes in mental status, and seizure[55] making it difficult to distinguish the different encephalitides among each other and from other possibilities, such as meningitis. However, neuropsychiatric manifestations and movement disorders are a much more pronounced feature of autoimmune encephalitis, with elevations in temperature usually occurring in the setting of autonomic instability.[59] Also, ADEM symptoms are reported to have more subacute onset than infectious encephalitis, over a couple of days.[60] Laboratory analysis (serum and

CSF) is a critical component of an encephalitis work-up and typically reveals CSF pleocytosis with a mononuclear/lymphocyte predominance. ADEM CSF studies usually show normal or more modest levels of CSF pleocytosis and may have transient oligoclonal immunoglobulin G detected.[60]

MR imaging is the most sensitive imaging modality for detecting encephalitis, in the case of HSV-1 being positive in more than 90% of cases.[61] The advantages of MR imaging are particularly striking with the use of diffusion imaging, which can detect areas of nascent cytotoxic injury before the onset of florid parenchymal edema.[62] In most cases, a specific viral agent cannot be suggested based on the imaging pattern alone.[63] One exception is reactivation pattern HSV-1 infection, which classically involves one or both temporal lobes with associated diffusion restriction and hemorrhage (**Fig. 7**). In this regard, the radiologist may play an important role in diagnosis because

polymerase chain reaction (PCR) of CSF from early HSV-1 encephalitis may occasionally be falsely negative.[64] This pattern stands in contrast to the neonatal, HSV-2 encephalitis pattern, which is less spatially restricted and frequently involves areas outside the limbic system (eg, deep gray matter, brainstem, cerebellum).[65] There is a propensity for deep gray matter structures by the respiratory viruses and some arboviruses, such as West Nile.[66] The pattern of involvement may also suggest a noninfectious cause because ADEM typically has less mass effect, smaller lesions, and a propensity for subcortical/deep white matter. MR imaging of the spine also commonly reveals additional lesions in up to 28% of ADEM cases.[58] However, ADEM also commonly involves the deep gray matter as well as the deep white matter; hyperacute lesions may restrict diffusion, raising uncertainty about the diagnosis.[67]

When encephalitis is clinically suspected, it is standard to administer acyclovir until HSV PCR

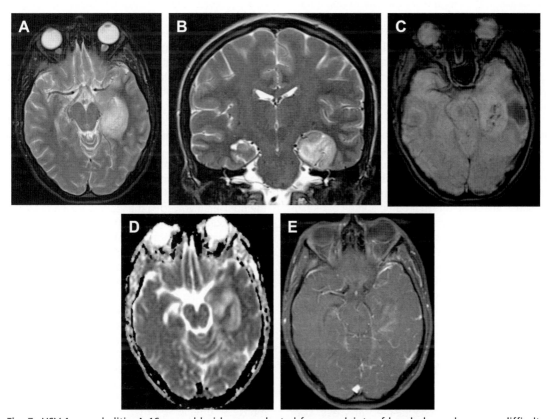

Fig. 7. HSV-1 encephalitis. A 16-year-old girl was evaluated for complaints of headache and memory difficulty after a recent episode of left-sided perioral vesicle eruptions. The axial (A) and coronal (B) T2-weighted images of the brain demonstrate diffuse edema throughout the medial left temporal lobe, including the hippocampus. SWI (C) demonstrate areas of punctate susceptibility artifact consistent with petechial hemorrhage within the edema. There is mild cortically based diffusion restriction visible on the apparent diffusion coefficient maps (D) and faint gyral enhancement on postcontrast T1-weighted imaging (E). Findings are consistent with reactivation pattern HSV infection. Subsequent PCR of CSF was positive for HSV-1.

has returned negative with administration of antibiotics for indeterminate CSF cell count (ie, possible bacterial meningitis) or suspected exposure to atypical bacteria (eg, doxycycline for suspected tick exposure).[54] This practice reflects the fact that therapy for most encephalitides besides herpes viridae (mainly HSV-1 and HSV-2) are only supportive at the present time.[68] Should the clinical history, CSF analysis, and imaging support a diagnosis of ADEM instead, steroids are commonly given because there is evidence of reduced duration of symptoms and possibly better outcomes with immunosuppression.[67]

Cerebritis and cerebral abscess

Cerebritis is an infection of the brain parenchyma by pyogenic bacteria and, left untreated, will result in progressive liquefaction/necrosis of the involved brain tissue until surrounded by a capsule that indicates an organized abscess. The incidence of cerebral abscess is difficult to estimate. However, it is clearly quite rare with case series suggesting incidence in the range of 1 case per million inhabitants per year.[69,70] Risk factors for cerebritis and cerebral abscess include cyanotic congenital heart disease, meningitis, trauma, and intracranial complications from otomastoiditis or sinusitis; making allowances for roughly one-third of cases with polymicrobial or nongrowing cultures, grampositive cocci seem to be the most common single infectious agents.[69,71] Demographic risk factors include male sex and age in the early first or second decade.[71,72] It should be noted that intracranial complications from bacterial sinusitis are estimated to be 4%, and abscess is less common than empyema (see later discussion).[73] Although abscess is also an unusual complication of meningitis, certain organisms are known to have a high propensity for this complication; neonatal *Citrobacter* meningitis can be complicated by abscess in greater than 70% of cases.[74] Symptoms of abscess include headache (particularly older children), irritability (particularly young children or infants), altered mental status, and seizure.[75] However, fever is present in only half of cases, and the white blood cell count may be normal.[69,75]

Cerebritis and abscess have been studied experimentally and with radiologic-pathologic correlation, demonstrating evolution through 4 discrete stages (beginning with early cerebritis and ending with an encapsulated abscess) over a period of 2 weeks.[76] The imaging abnormalities recapitulate these stages with ill-defined T2 signal abnormality and absence of enhancement in early cerebritis, followed by incomplete peripheral enhancement in late cerebritis.[77] By the time an organized abscess has formed, a well-defined rim of T2 hypointensity and enhancement (usually thinner on the ventricular side of the abscess) can be defined with a center of restricted diffusion (**Fig. 8**). As expected, extensive edema surrounds the abscess and manifests as facilitated diffusion.

Although usually fatal in the era before antibiotics and imaging-guided neurosurgical care, the outcomes from modern series suggest fairly good outcomes: 6% and 33% mortality has been reported for immunocompetent and immunosuppressed populations, respectively.[71] Although most published literature suggests open craniotomy or stereotactic aspiration of abscesses for diagnosis and treatment,[69,78] a trial of antibiotics with serial imaging may be considered for some neurologically stable patients without generalized mass effect or ventriculitis.[76]

Empyema

Epidural empyema (EE) and subdural empyema (SE) represent extra-axial accumulations of pus superficial to the dura or deep to the dura, respectively. Precise location and risk factors for empyema depend on age. For infants, isolated SE are usually encountered after meningitis; although the precise rate of meningitis complicated by empyema is somewhat uncertain in children, the best available adult data suggest 3% of meningitis cases are complicated by subdural empyema.[79,80] On the other hand, older children more typically experience some combination of epidural and subdural empyemas from local extension through the skull secondary to trauma, a small percentage from complicated otomastoiditis, and a small percentage from complicated sinusitis.[45,46,73,80,81] The bacteria found within the empyemas reflect the species involved in the inciting cause of infection (eg, gram-positive organisms for trauma, upper respiratory flora for sinusitis).[82,83] Clinical symptoms associated with EE and SE depend on several factors, including mass effect (ie, quantity of pus), proximity to the subarachnoid space, brain parenchyma (ie, risk of meningitis and cerebritis), and complications, such as dural sinus thrombosis. Because the epidural space is partly obliterated by fusion to the periosteum, accumulation of pus in EE is slower and the symptoms are often less severe than those seen in SE. Although fever is common in both SE and EE, seizures, altered mental status, and focal neurologic deficits are more common in SE.[84]

Although CT plays an important role in detecting the presence of complicated otomastoiditis or sinusitis, MR imaging allows more accurate determination of the nature of any fluid collections, their extent, and cerebral venous complications.[51,85] Diffusion-weighted MR imaging is particularly

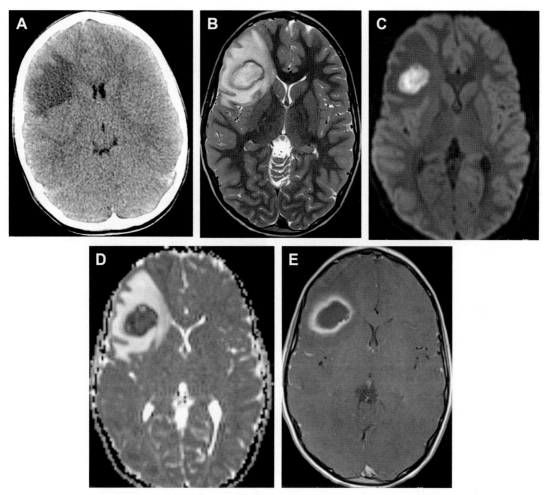

Fig. 8. Intracranial abscess. An 8-year-old boy presented to the emergency department with 1 week of headache. Axial noncontrast CT (*A*) demonstrates right frontal edema suggestive of an underlying mass lesion or abscess. Axial T2 imaging (*B*) confirms the presence of a circumscribed lesion with T2 hypointense walls and marked surrounding edema. The diffusion trace (*C*) and apparent diffusion coefficient (*D*) images demonstrate homogeneous diffusion restriction corresponding to the T2 hyperintense material within the center of lesion, diagnostic of abscess. There is a thick rim of surrounding enhancement of axial T1 postcontrast images (*E*).

useful in discriminating subdural effusions that can be seen with meningitis from true accumulations of pus (ie, diffusion restriction) because the former does not require emergent evacuation.[86] The extent of the collection is also very sensitively depicted using diffusion imaging and can inform the extent of the craniotomy chosen at surgery. As mentioned earlier, MR imaging is the preferred means of definitively evaluating for cerebritis/abscess, signs of meningeal irritation, and dural sinus thrombosis, which frequently accompanies empyema. All these advantages are depicted in **Fig. 9**.

In the early days of CT, there was some enthusiasm for medically treating subdural empyemas rather than evacuating these collections emergently.[87] However, most neurosurgeons advocate

emergent drainage of SE because of the potential for rapid evolution and irreversible brain injury (eg, venous infarction) from inadequately treated SE.[82,88] On the other hand, epidural abscesses can be safely observed while treated with medical therapy and/or decompression of any infected extracranial cavities that contribute to EE (eg, mastoidectomy).[83]

Spine

Epidural abscess

Spinal epidural abscesses represent organized purulent infections within the spinal epidural space. Although data specific to children are scarce, case series suggest that the incidence is

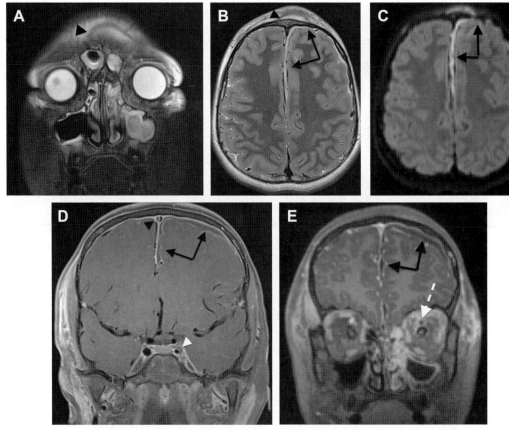

Fig. 9. Acute sinusitis complicated by subdural empyema, venous thrombosis, and orbital thrombophlebitis. An 8-year-old boy presented with headaches and facial swelling. After CT demonstrated orbital cellulitis and subperiosteal abscess, MR imaging was obtained for further evaluation of intracranial complications. Coronal (*A*) and axial (*B*) T2-weighted images demonstrate a frontal subperiosteal abscess (*black arrowhead*) known as a Pott puffy tumor as well as subdural collections over the left frontal lobe (*black arrows*). Note paranasal sinus opacification. Diffusion imaging (*C*) demonstrates restricted diffusion consistent with pus in the subdural collections (ie, subdural empyema). The coronal T1 fat-saturated postcontrast image (*D*) additionally shows filling defects within the left cavernous sinus (*white arrowhead*) and the superior sagittal sinus (*black arrowhead*) consistent with cavernous and sagittal sinus thrombus, respectively. Postcontrast T1 spoiled gradient echo coronal images (*E*) demonstrate clot within the left superior ophthalmic vein (*dashed white arrow*) and surrounding fat stranding, consistent with thrombophlebitis.

similar to adults, approximately 1 per 10,000 hospital admissions.[89] These data also suggests that although the most common causative organisms in children remain *Staphylococcus spp*, children frequently lack a typical risk factor unlike in adults, such as a condition predisposing to bacteremia (eg, intravenous drug use, endocarditis), immunosuppression, diabetes, or localized infections of the spine (eg, spontaneous, traumatic, or postoperative diskitis/osteomyelitis).[83] For both children and adults, the clinical presentation seems to be similarly nonspecific, featuring pain and (as the collection enlarges over a variable period of days to weeks) neurologic deficit.[90] Accompanying signs of fever, leukocytosis, and increased

inflammatory markers are usually present, but not invariably.

MR imaging is the study of choice for suspected spinal epidural abscess because of the ability to simultaneously characterize the full extent of the collection and to determine any signs of cord compression. As with abscesses elsewhere, spinal epidural abscesses demonstrate rim enhancement and restricted diffusion,[91,92] the contrast-enhanced study being preferably performed with fat saturation to suppress signal from adjacent marrow and epidural fat (**Fig. 10**). Adult and pediatric data both suggest a preference for posterior epidural space collections in the thoracolumbar spine with a variable

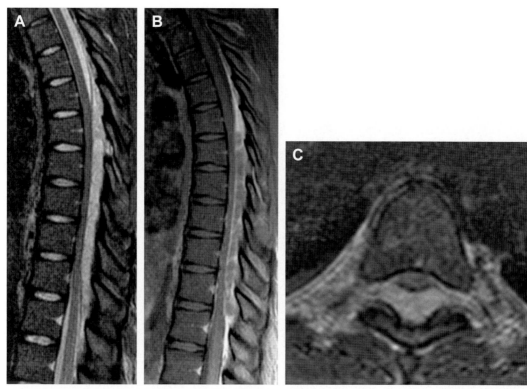

Fig. 10. Epidural abscess. An 18-year-old boy with lupus and chronic immunosuppression presents with back pain and fever. Sagittal T2 (*A*), sagittal T1 postcontrast with fat saturation (*B*), and axial T2 (*C*) images demonstrate a large dorsal epidural collection in the thoracic spine with peripheral enhancement. Note absence of associated discitis/osteomyelitis implying hematogenous seeding. There is exclusion of CSF from the thecal sac and mild cord compression but no visible cord signal abnormality. Although initially the patient had a benign neurologic examination, he developed lower extremity clonus by the time of neurosurgical consultation for abscess evacuation.

degree of extension (1 to more than 5 vertebral body lengths).[89,93]

Epidural abscess is generally treated as a neurosurgical emergency because there is evidence to suggest that patients managed conservatively with antibiotics have a tendency to deteriorate even if initially asymptomatic.[93] This practice is also supported by the intuitive observation that patients who go on to develop symptoms often have greater neurologic deficit despite decompression given the size of epidural abscess required to cause symptoms in the first place.[94]

Discitis with or without osteomyelitis
Discitis represents an infectious process of the disk space, whereas vertebral body osteomyelitis represents infection of the bone itself, either from extension of discitis or direct hematogenous dissemination to the end vessels in the end plates. Isolated discitis is mostly a disease of infants and very young children due to the end vessels present in the intervertebral disks at this age, whereas

vertebral body osteomyelitis is more commonly a disease of older children.[95] In children with either discitis or osteomyelitis, back pain and refusal to walk are the most common symptoms with nonspecific mild leukocytosis and increase in inflammatory markers. However, children with osteomyelitis more frequently have fever and toxic clinical appearance.[95] The incidence of discitis and osteomyelitis in children is difficult to estimate, but it has been suggested that it is lower than in the adult population for whom cited incidence is in the range of 1 per 100,000 individuals.[96,97]

Discitis can often be suggested on plain radiography as narrowed disk spaces. However, MR imaging provides details regarding potential complications (eg, paraspinal or epidural abscess), subtle indications of osteomyelitis, and exclusion of alternative diagnoses, such as epidural abscess.[96,98] Fluid signal or rim enhancement within the disk space suggests discitis, and marrow edema with end plate destruction suggests accompanying osteomyelitis (**Fig. 11**).[99] It should

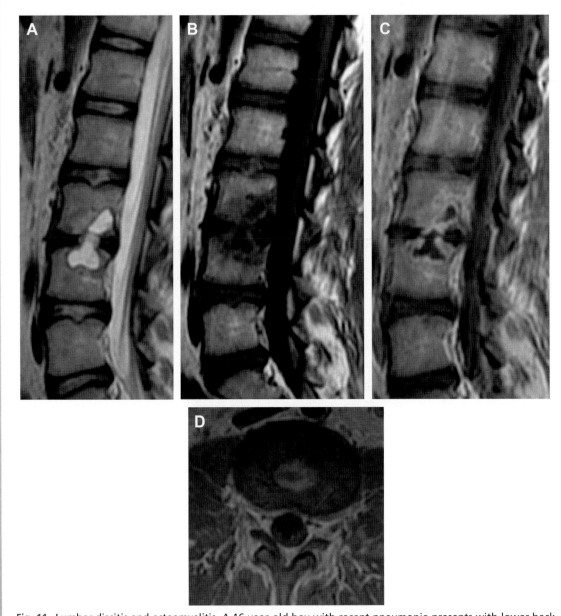

Fig. 11. Lumbar discitis and osteomyelitis. A 16-year-old boy with recent pneumonia presents with lower back pain and elevated C-reactive protein. Sagittal T2 (*A*), sagittal T1 precontrast (*B*), and sagittal T1 postcontrast (*C*) images demonstrate a rim enhancing abscess crossing the L2-3 disk space (ie, discitis) with surrounding edema/enhancement consistent with osteomyelitis. Axial T1 postcontrast imaging (*D*) confirms absence of associated paraspinal or epidural abscess. Biopsy of the disk space confirmed coagulase-negative staphylococcus.

be noted that a special variant of disk pathology may sometimes be confused with discitis. In intervertebral disk calcification of childhood, there may also be disk space narrowing as well as calcification; but this entity typically resolves without treatment and is usually encountered in the cervical spine unlike discitis/osteomyelitis, which preferentially affects thoracolumbar spine.[100]

Both discitis and osteomyelitis are treated with antibiotics. Osteomyelitis is often evaluated with biopsy should blood cultures fail to identify an organism.[96] However, it should be noted that although patients treated with antibiotics for discitis have been shown to have better outcomes, biopsy of isolated discitis in infancy is almost always culture negative.[101,102]

Transverse myelitis and other fulminant demyelinating disease; Guillain-Barré syndrome

Transverse myelitis (TM) is a syndrome of myelopathy secondary to acute spinal cord inflammation, which can be seen in the setting of ADEM, neuromyelitis optica, multiple sclerosis (MS), some collagen vascular disorders, cord infarct, infections, as well as idiopathic cases for which an associated disorder cannot be established in approximately half of cases.[103] Even in cases whereby ADEM has been excluded on clinical and radiologic grounds (no seizures, headaches, or cerebral lesions), idiopathic TM seems to be associated with antecedent infection/immunization or a family history of autoimmune disease in up to a half of childhood cases.[103,104] Overall incidence is estimated in the range of 1400 cases per year, of which only 20% are children.[103] However, the fulminant symptoms of motor (virtually all have paraparesis within a few days of presentation), sensory (including sensory level and dysesthesia), and autonomic (bladder dysfunction) usually result in urgent imaging evaluation due to the need to exclude a compressive lesion and to improve outcomes through early use of steroids if TM is confirmed and an infectious cause of myelitis is excluded.[104–106] The outcome for children treated with steroids is variable, with reports of residual sensorimotor or bladder dysfunction anywhere from 20% to 80% depending on the series.[103,106]

MR imaging defines the presence and level of an acute inflammatory cord lesion while excluding alternative explanations for patients' symptoms (eg, cord compression). The adult literature demonstrates that TM lesions typically manifest as central expansile T2 signal abnormality and enhancement that can appear nodular or diffuse; enhancement may not manifest until the subacute period, after the first few weeks (**Fig. 12**).[107] Child-specific imaging studies suggest a similar appearance, though there is evidence that the lesions are more commonly expansile and have greater longitudinal extent (greater than 3 vertebral bodies), with cervical or cervicothoracic lesions being most common.[103,104,106] One potential pitfall to imaging in the hyperacute stage of TM is the paucity or even absence of cord signal abnormality, something that can take a few days to fully manifest.[104,108] Compared with TM, ADEM and MS are usually associated with multiple cord/brain lesions, which in the case of MS lesions are less extensive, more peripheral in the cord, and associated with asymmetric neurologic findings.[104,109,110] However, neuromyelitis optica cannot be readily distinguished from idiopathic TM at presentation unless there is presence of neuromyelitis optica (NMO) autoantibodies or optic neuritis.[111]

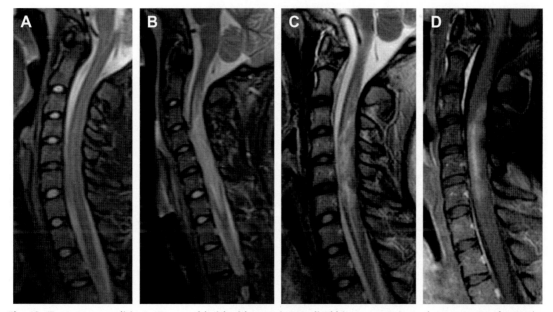

Fig. 12. Transverse myelitis. A 17-year-old girl with no prior medical history experienced acute onset of paresthesias followed within hours by quadriparesis. Sagittal T2-weighted images on the day of presentation (*A*) and 5 days later (*B*) demonstrate progressive cervical cord edema spanning multiple vertebral body levels. Although there was no initial enhancement, a follow-up examination during the subacute period 2 weeks later demonstrates subsidence of edema on sagittal T2-weighted imaging (*C*) and patchy cord enhancement on sagittal T1 postcontrast imaging with fat saturation (*D*).

Another disease entity worth mentioning in terms of inflammatory causes of paralysis is Guillain-Barré syndrome (GBS), a demyelinating polyneuropathy that is, the most common cause of flaccid paralysis in children with cited incidence of 1 case per 100,000 children per year.[112] Most cases are associated with respiratory illness, gastroenteritis, or vaccinations in the couple of weeks before symptoms.[113] In addition to the classic ascending paralysis, patients may complain of pain, paresthesia, and ataxia.[113] Unlike TM, there is usually no pleocytosis seen on lumbar puncture, though increased CSF protein may be present.[114] In contrast to TM, there is no cord lesion visible in GBS. Rather, there is enhancement of the cauda equina nerve roots with a ventral predominance (**Fig. 13**); at least in children, there is some evidence of frequent enhancement involving cranial nerves even in children without clinical diagnosis of the so-called Miller-Fisher variant of GBS.[115–117]

Body

Osteomyelitis and septic arthritis

Hematogenous osteomyelitis is an inflammation of bone and bone marrow that is seen predominantly

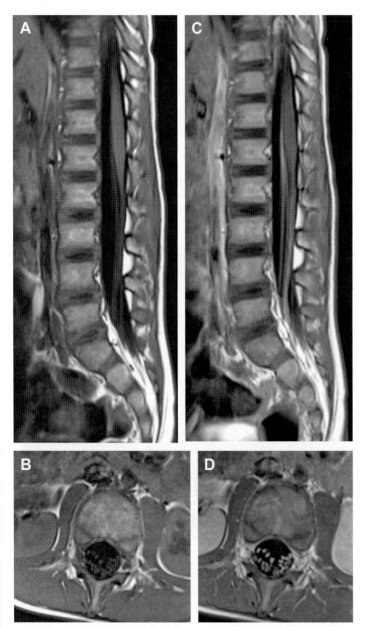

Fig. 13. GBS (acute inflammatory demyelinating polyradiculoneuropathy). A 4-year-old boy with recent diarrheal illness presented with a limp. Within 24 hours, he was unable to walk and had episodes of urinary incontinence. Comparison of sagittal (*A*) and axial (*B*) precontrast images with postcontrast sagittal T1 (*C*) and axial T1 (*D*) images demonstrates profound enhancement of the cauda equina nerve roots, most conspicuous in the ventral nerve roots.

in patients in the first 2 decades of life, with more than half of pediatric patients younger than 5 years of age. Boys are affected about twice as often as girls.[118,119] In contrast, septic arthritis is an infection of a synovial joint that can occur in all age groups in children. Both septic arthritis and acute osteomyelitis typically have an acute onset, and septic arthritis can result from contiguous spread of osteomyelitis. The organism most commonly responsible for osteoarticular infections is *Staphylococcus aureus*. *Neisseria gonorrhoeae* is the most common cause of septic arthritis in the United States but more commonly affects older adolescents and adults.[120] Risk factors for hematogenous osteomyelitis in children include sickle cell disease, immunodeficiency disorders, sepsis, and indwelling vascular catheters.[121]

Clinical manifestations of acute osteomyelitis and septic arthritis are similar. Children typically initially present with focal bone tenderness, high fever, and oftentimes unwillingness to move the affected extremity. If the infection is located in the lower limb, patients may limp or refuse to walk.

MR findings of osteomyelitis include confluent bone marrow edema that is T1 hypointense and T2 hyperintense (**Fig. 14**). Edema is typically present within the surrounding deep soft tissues. Osteomyelitis frequently copresents with associated intraosseous, subperiosteal, and/or soft tissue abscesses (**Fig. 15**). For septic arthritis, MR is more sensitive (100%) and specific (77%) than other imaging modalities; suspicious imaging findings can be seen within 24 hours of onset.[122] On T1-weighted sequences, low signal can be seen within subchondral bone on both sides of the

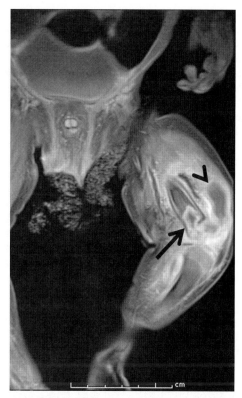

Fig. 15. Osteomyelitis with intraosseous abscess and synovitis. A 36-day-old boy with left thigh and knee swelling and low-grade fever. Coronal postcontrast T1 imaging with fat saturation shows a rim-enhancing collection (*black arrow*) involving the distal femoral metaphysis, compatible with an intraosseous abscess. There is also a large associated septic joint effusion with robustly enhancing reactive synovitis (*black arrowhead*).

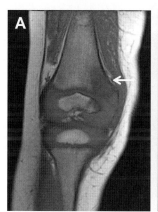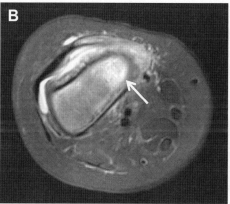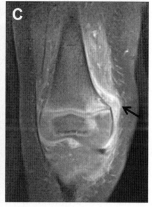

Fig. 14. Osteomyelitis. A 17-month-old girl with failure to bear weight and swollen right knee. On coronal precontrast T1 imaging (*A*), there is abnormal low T1 signal (*white arrow*) in the distal medial femoral metaphysis that corresponds on axial T2 fat-saturated imaging (*B*) to high T2 signal (*white arrow*). Coronal postcontrast T1 imaging with fat-saturation (*C*) shows abnormal enhancement in the same region, crossing the physis and involving the medial aspect of the femoral epiphysis. There is also enhancement within the adjacent distal vastus medialis (*black arrow*), consistent with myositis.

affected joint. Hyperintense effusion, hyperintense subchondral bone, and hyperintense perisynovial soft tissue can be seen on fluid-sensitive sequences. Postcontrast T1 fat-saturated imaging may show synovial thickening surrounding an effusion, subchondral bone enhancement, or an occasional adjacent soft tissue abscess (see **Fig. 15**; **Fig. 16**).

The basic treatment is antibiotics. However, if an abscess is present, drainage is mandatory. Untreated osteomyelitis and septic arthritis have a dismal prognosis with a mortality rate close to 50% and with the remaining patients with protracted disability for the rest of their lives.[123] Both diseases are curable if recognized early and adequately treated. As joint infection destroys the articular cartilage and may cause permanent joint destruction, septic arthritis is a more serious disease than osteomyelitis and a real emergency.

Appendicitis

Appendicitis is the most common surgical cause of atraumatic abdominal pain among children presenting to the emergency department and is ultimately diagnosed in 1% to 8% of such children.[124,125] It results from acute obstruction of the appendiceal lumen, which leads to progressive luminal dilatation, followed sequentially by mural ischemia, superimposed infection, and eventually perforation with abscess formation. Optimal outcomes require early diagnosis followed by appendectomy before gangrene or perforation develops.

Affected pediatric patients classically present with periumbilical pain, which ultimately migrates to the right lower quadrant as visceral irritation is overshadowed by inflammation of the peritoneal lining of the abdomen. Patients generally experience nausea, vomiting, and fever. Very young children may also present with diarrhea. Unfortunately, this classic scenario is present in less than one-third of all pediatric patients and is rare in children younger than 5 years of age.[126] Therefore, diagnostic imaging plays a crucial role in the accurate and timely diagnosis of this common pediatric surgical emergency.

Because of its low cost, lack of ionizing radiation, and ability to delineate gynecologic disease, graded-compression ultrasonography is considered the most appropriate first test for the

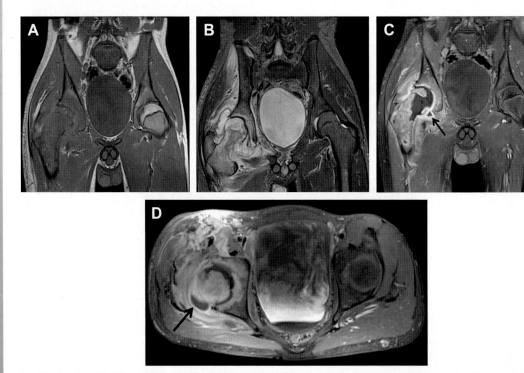

Fig. 16. Septic arthritis and osteomyelitis. A 13-year-old boy after right hip septic washout with ongoing fever and hemodynamic instability. Coronal precontrast T1 (*A*) and T2 fat-saturated (*B*) images show abnormal low T1 and corresponding high T2 bone marrow signal in the right femoral head and neck as well as within the right anterosuperior acetabulum. On coronal (*C*) and axial (*D*) postcontrast T1 images with fat saturation, there is intense enhancement of the synovium (*black arrows*). There is also high T2 signal abnormality and marked enhancement within the obturator, adductor, gluteal, and iliacus muscles as well as within the surrounding fascia, compatible with adjacent myositis and fasciitis.

work-up of children with suspected appendicitis. At many institutions, an equivocal ultrasound is typically followed by abdominal CT scan if clinical suspicion remains high for acute appendicitis. However, given concerns over exposing children to the ionizing radiation of CT, some institutions have begun using MR imaging in place of CT. Multiple single-institution studies have demonstrated that MR imaging has high sensitivity (98%–100%) and specificity (96%–99%) for appendicitis in pediatric patients and that MR imaging can be performed in children in the emergent setting.[10–12,127] Although no study has yet compared CT and MR imaging directly for the diagnosis of appendicitis, these available studies suggest that MR imaging can replace CT after inconclusive ultrasound in the work-up of acute lower abdominal pain in pediatric patients.[10–12,127]

A normal appendix on MR should meet classic size criteria for CT, measuring less than 6 mm in width and without associated inflammatory changes in the wall or adjacent tissues (**Fig. 17**). Previously published MR criteria for acute appendicitis include an enlarged appendix measuring at least 7 mm in width, with T2 hyperintense intraluminal fluid, occasional mural thickening with T2 hyperintense edema, and T2 hyperintense periappendiceal inflammatory edema and free fluid (**Figs. 18 and 19**).[10–13,127]

Treatment is surgical appendectomy. If there are clinical or radiological signs of perforation, antibiotics with gram-negative and anaerobic coverage should be started. Percutaneous drainage of loculated peritoneal fluid collections can also be performed. Acute appendicitis has a benign course in most cases, especially if there are classic symptoms; prompt surgery is performed. Morbidity and mortality increase with perforation, and complications include hepatic abscess and pylephlebitis.

NEOPLASTIC DISORDERS
Brain

Intracranial neoplasms
Primary brain tumors are uncommon, with a reported incidence of up to 4 per 100,000 children per year; they typically manifest with nonspecific symptoms (ie, headache, nausea/vomiting) that have numerous alternative explanations.[128,129] However, primary brain tumors are obviously much feared because of their potentially grave implications for patients; it has long been appreciated that there can be long delays before diagnosis of a brain tumor is made.[130] Therefore, early imaging evaluation is recommended when headaches are accompanied by atypical features, such as early morning vomiting, focal neurologic deficits, or seizures, particularly when the symptoms are of relatively short duration (less than 6 months).[128,131]

As a result, it is not uncommon for patients with atypical headaches or signs of elevated intracranial pressure to present for urgent or emergent imaging. The specific appearances of particular tumor histologies is beyond the scope of this article and has been recently reviewed elsewhere.[132,133] However, MR imaging has the advantage of providing, in addition to an assessment of mass effect or herniation, an indication of tumor aggressiveness or CSF dissemination. This information is necessary before surgery to allow a rationale assessment of risk-benefit in terms of how aggressive a resection to perform. In attempting to judge tumor histology, diffusion MR imaging is particularly helpful in distinguishing a cellular tumor, such as medulloblastoma (diffusion restriction), from a benign tumor, such as a pilocytic astrocytoma (**Figs. 20 and 21**).[134] MR imaging can also allow for definitive characterization of intracranial masses, which are not true

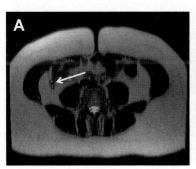
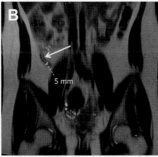

Fig. 17. Normal appendix. A 14-year-old girl discharged from the emergency department with diagnosis of abdominal pain, not otherwise specified. Axial T2 HASTE imaging (*A*) shows that the appendix loops in the right mid abdomen, arising from a high riding cecum. The appendix has a thin, low signal wall and high signal intraluminal fluid (*white arrow*). Small mesenteric lymph nodes are partially demonstrated medially, adjacent to nondilated small bowel loops. On coronal T2 HASTE imaging (*B*), the distal appendix (*white arrow*) is seen in plane, measuring up to 5 mm in cross section.

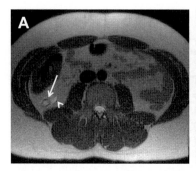

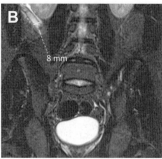

Fig. 18. Acute nonperforated appendicitis. A 16-year-old boy with acute appendicitis, not perforated at time of surgery. On axial T2 HASTE imaging (*A*), the appendix is retrocecal in location (*white arrow*). The lumen is distended; there is high signal within the wall, and there is periappendiceal fluid and stranding of the adjacent fat (*white arrowhead*). Coronal STIR imaging (*B*) shows the appendix in plane, measuring up to 8 mm in cross section.

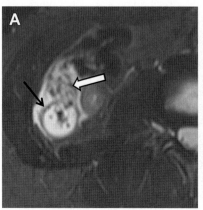

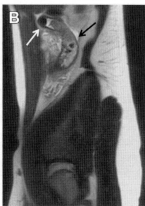

Fig. 19. Acute perforated appendicitis. A 13-year-old boy with gangrenous appendicitis, perforated at time of surgery. The appendix can be seen retrocecal in location on axial STIR imaging (*A*) and markedly dilated (*black arrow*) with heterogeneous internal contents, periappendiceal fluid, and stranding of the adjacent fat (*open white arrow*). Sagittal T2 HASTE imaging (*B*) demonstrates the appendix in plane, measuring up to 20 mm in cross section. An appendicolith is seen at its tip (*white arrow*); there are heterogeneous luminal contents, corresponding to mixed hemorrhage, pus, and smaller appendicoliths (*black arrow*).

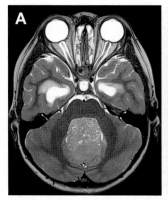

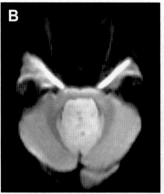

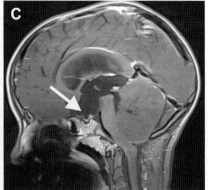

Fig. 20. Classic medulloblastoma. An 8-year-old girl was referred to the emergency department after an ophthalmology office visit for left-sided vision loss revealed bilateral papilledema. Parents also noted recent deterioration of motor coordination. Axial T2 imaging (*A*) demonstrates an intraventricular mass arising from the vermis and having T2 intermediate signal intensity suggestive of hypercellularity. This series also demonstrates hydrocephalus with transependymal CSF resorption. Axial diffusion imaging confirms hypercellularity with marked hyperintensity on the trace maps (*B*). Sagittal T1 SPACE imaging (*C*) characterizes the mass as nonenhancing. Note ballooning of the infundibular recess of the third ventricle (*white arrow, C*) from resultant noncommunicating hydrocephalus. Although medulloblastomas can have variable enhancement, the absence of enhancement, the diffusion restriction, and the location of this mass are typical of a medulloblastoma.

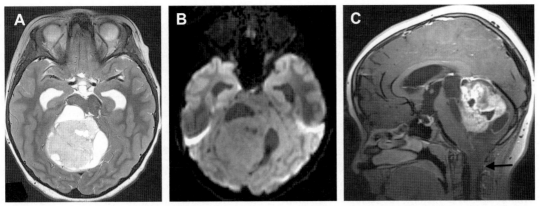

Fig. 21. Juvenile pilocytic astrocytoma. An 8-year-old girl presented to the emergency department with a few weeks of escalating headaches and vomiting. Axial T2-weighted imaging (*A*) demonstrates a cystic and solid mass, the solid portions having T2 hyperintensity relative to normal brain parenchyma. The mass causes noncommunicating hydrocephalus visible as temporal horn enlargement in (*A*). The diffusion trace map covering this region (*B*) confirms absence of restricted diffusion. Sagittal T1 SPACE postcontrast imaging (*C*) demonstrates avid enhancement of the solid portions of the mass and tonsillar herniation (*black arrow*).

neoplasms, for example, a cavernous malformation (**Fig. 22**).

Spine

Oncologic spinal cord compression

Of children with an underlying cancer in the United States, approximately 5% develop signs of metastatic spinal cord compression during their disease course.[135] These metastases are overwhelmingly in the epidural space with responsible tumors varying by age: neuroblastoma more commonly for younger children and sarcomas (eg, Ewing sarcoma) more common for older children.[136] In children, epidural compression is frequently due to a paraspinal malignancy insinuating into the epidural space through the neural

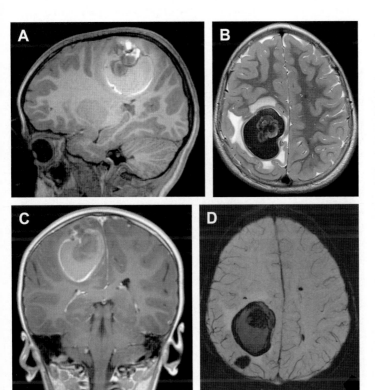

Fig. 22. Symptomatic hemorrhage from cavernous malformations. A previously healthy 6-year-old girl presented with 1 week of headache and left-hand weakness. Sagittal T1 MPRAGE (*A*) and axial T2 (*B*) images demonstrate the presence within the right frontal lobe of a large hemorrhagic mass containing blood products of differing ages. There is surrounding edema suggesting acuity. The coronal T1 MPRAGE images (*C*) characterize the lesion as nonenhancing, In the setting of multiple other similar lesions elsewhere in the brain on SWI (*D*), findings are consistent with multiple cavernous malformations, the right frontal one having recently bled.

foramina (ie, local extension), whereas in adults hematogenous metastases to vertebrae are the more common inciting cause of compression.[137] Although back pain is a prevalent symptom in cord compression in both children and adults (for whom it is the far most common presenting symptom),[138,139] there is some evidence that children more commonly present with neurologic deficit initially (dysesthesia, paraparesis/paraplegia).[136,140,141] Although intramedullary lesions usually present with back pain as the initial symptom,[142] these patients can present with deficits that are indistinguishable from extrinsic cord compression in a minority of cases.[136,140] Most of these intramedullary tumors are astrocytomas, ependymomas, or gangliogliomas.[143] The thoracic spine is the most common level affected by epidural metastatic disease,[136] and the cervicothoracic/thoracic levels are the most common to be affected by intramedullary tumor.[143] Although resection of intramedullary tumors is usually attempted,[143] the specific combination of laminectomy, radiotherapy, and chemotherapy for epidural metastasis depends on tumor histology.[135]

MR imaging is the study of choice for the evaluation of suspected cord compromise with cited sensitivity and specificity greater than 90%.[137] MR imaging serves to delineate the degree of thecal sac or cord compression and detect cord signal abnormality that can confirm acuity (**Fig. 23**). Unlike CT, MR imaging can also definitively characterize intrinsic cord lesions, which may clinically mimic cord compression from an extradural metastasis, such as TM or an intramedullary tumor. In the case of intramedullary tumors, the lesions are typically more circumscribed and may have surrounding syringohydromyelia that allows for differentiation from an inflammatory process, such as TM (**Fig. 24**).[144]

Traumatic Disorders

Spinal compression, contusion, and transection

Traumatic injury to the spinal column and the spinal cord is infrequent, with a yearly incidence in children generally quoted in the range of 1 case per 1,000,000 children or approximately a tenth that of adults.[145] However, the morbidity associated with these relatively rare injuries can be significant: of the 2% of trauma patients with spinal trauma ascertained by a level I pediatric trauma center, 20% had cord injuries and 50% associated injuries, such as intracranial trauma.[146]

Spinal injuries in children more frequently involve the cervical spine than in adults, the cervico-cranial junction for children less than 9 (with the exception of birth injuries, usually due to pedestrian vs motor collisions or falls), and the lower cervical spine for older children (usually due to motor vehicle accidents and sports-related accidents).[147] This epidemiology is a reflection of the disproportionately larger head and higher flexion point in younger children as

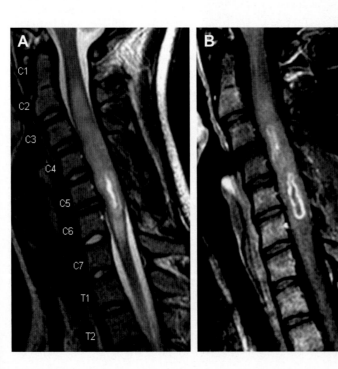

Fig. 23. Cord glioblastoma. A 12-year-old girl presented for evaluation of worsening left upper extremity paresthesias and neck pain. Sagittal T2-weighted (*A*) and postcontrast T1 (*B*) images demonstrate expansile, T2 intermediate signal abnormality within the cervical cord, and patchy areas of enhancement. There is an area of cavitation within the inferior aspect of the lesion. The T2 intermediate signal is lower than edema seen in transverse myelitis, and the cavitation would also be unusual for an inflammatory process. Biopsy confirmed glioblastoma.

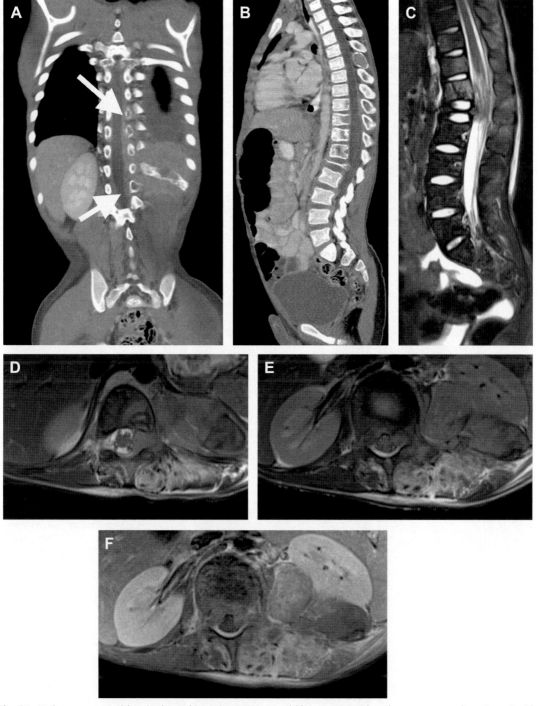

Fig. 24. Ewing sarcoma with spinal canal invasion. A 6-year-old boy presented to the emergency department with abdominal pain and question of a left upper quadrant mass on plain radiographs. Coronal reformat of contrast-enhanced chest/abdomen/pelvis CT (*A*) demonstrates a soft tissue mass arising from the partially destroyed left T11 rib and entering the epidural space of the thoracic spine (*white arrows*). Sagittal reformats (*B*) of the same study also demonstrate collapse of the L1 vertebra and scattered lucencies throughout the remainder of the spinal column (eg, T6 spinous process) suggesting local invasion and metastatic disease. Sagittal T2 (*C*) and axial T2 (*D, E*) MR imaging of the spine demonstrates minimal conus and cauda equina compression from a combination of osseous retropulsion from the pathologic L1 compression fracture and epidural infiltration by the tumor. The axial T2 images (*D, E*) and T1 postcontrast images (*F*) failed to demonstrate any violation of the thecal sac or CSF dissemination. The MR images also nicely depict infiltration of the paraspinal musculature and elevation of the left kidney by the mass.

well as the laxity of ligamentous structures, undeveloped musculature, and open vertebral synchondroses.[148] As a result, there is an approximately 35% incidence of soft tissue, synchondrosis, disk, or cord injury among childhood trauma patients with pain or transient/ongoing neurologic deficit but with negative CT or plain radiographs, a phenomenon termed *spinal cord injury without radiographic abnormality* (SCIWORA).[149]

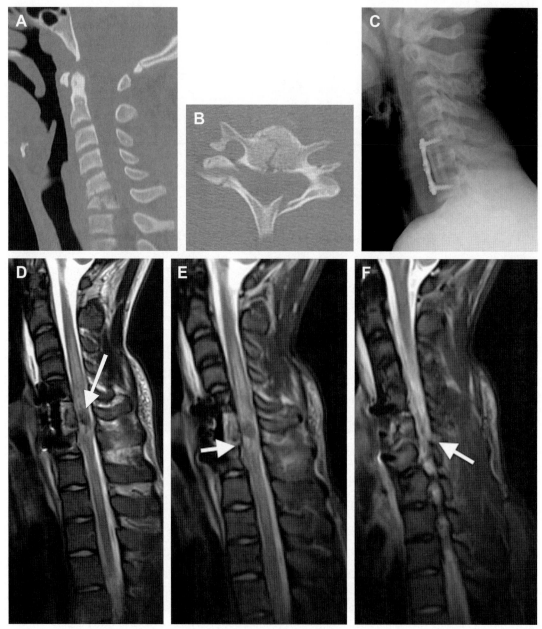

Fig. 25. Traumatic spinal cord compression. A 17-year-old boy was referred for hyperflexion injury after a sports collision with resultant thoracic sensory level and lower extremity plegia. The patient was hypotensive consistent with spinal shock. Sagittal reformatted (*A*) and axial source (*B*) CT of the cervical spine reveals burst fracture of the C6 vertebra with fracture extending into the posterior elements. Because of retropulsed bone and neurologic deficit, MR imaging was omitted and the patient was emergently brought to surgery for anterior fusion and corpectomy, documented by a lateral postoperative radiograph (*C*). Sagittal T2 imaging (*D*) demonstrates extensive cord edema with a focal T2 hypointensity (*white arrow*) at the level of the burst fracture indicating hemorrhagic cord contusion. STIR imaging better depicts disruption of the posterior longitudinal ligament (*white arrow, E*) and the ligamentum flavum (*white arrow, F*) as well as interspinous edema suggestive of interspinous ligament sprain/disruption.

All of these radiographically occult injuries can be detected by MR imaging, which is, therefore, recommended in evaluating this population of patients because of the frequency with which clinically significant findings are identified.[150,151] MR imaging is also used to clear the cervical spine in patients who are obtunded or otherwise unable to participate in clinical evaluation.[152] The actual imaging manifestations of these injuries are similar to those encountered in adults and may include edema/disruption of the major spinal stabilizing ligaments and edema/hemorrhage within the cord (**Fig. 25**). The degree of cord signal abnormality or hemorrhage is critical as it is highly predictive of patients' neurologic outcomes in SCIWORA.[149]

SUMMARY

MR imaging is valuable in the confirmation and characterization of emergent pediatric disorders because of its ease of performance, superior soft tissue contrast, multiplanar capabilities, lack of ionizing radiation, and ability to detect multiple lesions with minimal patient manipulation. In addition, emergent MR imaging can be critical when clinical, laboratory, and ultrasound or CT findings are nonspecific. Recognition of some of the characteristic imaging features of emergent pediatric disorders is important because it can allow rapid institution of therapy, which reduces morbidity and mortality. MR imaging can be both an effective and efficient method for the timely and appropriate management of pediatric disease entities that can occur in the emergent setting. Furthermore, MR imaging in combination with pertinent clinical facts can often help narrow the differential diagnosis and lead to the correct diagnosis, thus ultimately optimizing management for patients.

REFERENCES

1. Baker N, Woolridge D. Emerging concepts in pediatric emergency radiology. Pediatr Clin North Am 2013;60(5):1139–51.
2. Chavhan GB, Babyn PS, Singh M, et al. MR imaging at 3.0 T in children: technical differences, safety issues, and initial experience. Radiographics 2009; 29(5):1451–66.
3. Chang KJ, Kamel IR, Macura KJ, et al. 3.0-T MR imaging of the abdomen: comparison with 1.5 T. Radiographics 2008;28(7):1983–98.
4. Anupindi S, Jaramillo D. Pediatric magnetic resonance imaging techniques. Magn Reson Imaging Clin N Am 2002;10(2):189–207.
5. Pruessmann KP. Parallel imaging at high field strength: synergies and joint potential. Top Magn Reson Imaging 2004;15(4):237–44.
6. Slovis TL. Sedation and anesthesia issues in pediatric imaging. Pediatr Radiol 2011;41(Suppl 2): 514–6.
7. Cravero JP, Blike GT. Pediatric sedation. Curr Opin Anaesthesiology 2004;17(3):247–51.
8. Rappaport B, Mellon RD, Simone A, et al. Defining safe use of anesthesia in children. N Engl J Med 2011;364(15):1387–90.
9. Haliloglu M, Hoffer FA, Gronemeyer SA, et al. Applications of 3D contrast-enhanced MR angiography in pediatric oncology. Pediatr Radiol 1999; 29(11):863–8.
10. Cobben L, Groot I, Kingma L, et al. A simple MRI protocol in patients with clinically suspected appendicitis: results in 138 patients and effect on outcome of appendectomy. Eur Radiol 2009; 19(5):1175–83.
11. Johnson AK, Filippi CG, Andrews T, et al. Ultrafast 3-T MRI in the evaluation of children with acute lower abdominal pain for the detection of appendicitis. AJR Am J Roentgenol 2012;198(6):1424–30.
12. Moore MM, Gustas CN, Choudhary AK, et al. MRI for clinically suspected pediatric appendicitis: an implemented program. Pediatr Radiol 2012;42(9): 1056–63.
13. Herliczek TW, Swenson DW, Mayo-Smith WW. Utility of MRI after inconclusive ultrasound in pediatric patients with suspected appendicitis: retrospective review of 60 consecutive patients. AJR Am J Roentgenol 2013;200(5):969–73.
14. Roach ES, Golomb MR, Adams R, et al. Management of stroke in infants and children: a scientific statement from a Special Writing Group of the American Heart Association Stroke Council and the Council on Cardiovascular Disease in the Young. Stroke 2008;39(9):2644–91.
15. Earley CJ, Kittner SJ, Feeser BR, et al. Stroke in children and sickle-cell disease: Baltimore-Washington Cooperative Young Stroke Study. Neurology 1998;51(1):169–76.
16. Ganesan V, Prengler M, McShane MA, et al. Investigation of risk factors in children with arterial ischemic stroke. Ann Neurol 2003;53(2):167–73.
17. Nelson KB, Lynch JK. Stroke in newborn infants. Lancet Neurol 2004;3(3):150–8.
18. Mackay MT, Wiznitzer M, Benedict SL, et al. Arterial ischemic stroke risk factors: the International Pediatric Stroke Study. Ann Neurol 2011;69(1):130–40.
19. Singhal AB, Biller J, Elkind MS, et al. Recognition and management of stroke in young adults and adolescents. Neurology 2013;81(12):1089–97.
20. Gabis LV, Yangala R, Lenn NJ. Time lag to diagnosis of stroke in children. Pediatrics 2002;110(5): 924–8.

21. Hunter JV. Magnetic resonance imaging in pediatric stroke. Top Magn Reson Imaging 2002;13(1):23–38.

22. Zecavati N, Singh R, Farias-Moeller R, et al. The utility of infarct volume measurement in pediatric ischemic stroke. J Child Neurol 2014;29(6):811–7.

23. Domi T, deVeber G, Shroff M, et al. Corticospinal tract pre-wallerian degeneration: a novel outcome predictor for pediatric stroke on acute MRI. Stroke 2009;40(3):780–7.

24. Stam J. Thrombosis of the cerebral veins and sinuses. N Engl J Med 2005;352(17):1791–8.

25. deVeber G, Andrew M, Adams C, et al. Cerebral sinovenous thrombosis in children. N Engl J Med 2001;345(6):417–23.

26. Jackson BF, Porcher FK, Zapton DT, et al. Cerebral sinovenous thrombosis in children: diagnosis and treatment. Pediatr Emerg Care 2011;27(9):874–80 [quiz: 881–3].

27. Kenet G, Lutkhoff LK, Albisetti M, et al. Impact of thrombophilia on risk of arterial ischemic stroke or cerebral sinovenous thrombosis in neonates and children: a systematic review and meta-analysis of observational studies. Circulation 2010;121(16): 1838–47.

28. Sebire G, Tabarki B, Saunders DE, et al. Cerebral venous sinus thrombosis in children: risk factors, presentation, diagnosis and outcome. Brain 2005; 128(Pt 3):477–89.

29. Isensee C, Reul J, Thron A. Magnetic resonance imaging of thrombosed dural sinuses. Stroke 1994;25(1):29–34.

30. Hedlund GL. Cerebral sinovenous thrombosis in pediatric practice. Pediatr Radiol 2013;43(2): 173–88.

31. Jordan LC, Rafay MF, Smith SE, et al. Antithrombotic treatment in neonatal cerebral sinovenous thrombosis: results of the International Pediatric Stroke Study. J Pediatr 2010;156(5):704–10, 710. e1–2.

32. Bartynski WS. Posterior reversible encephalopathy syndrome, part 1: fundamental imaging and clinical features. AJNR Am J Neuroradiol 2008;29(6): 1036–42.

33. Onder AM, Lopez R, Teomete U, et al. Posterior reversible encephalopathy syndrome in the pediatric renal population. Pediatr Nephrol 2007;22(11): 1921–9.

34. Morris EB, Laningham FH, Sandlund JT, et al. Posterior reversible encephalopathy syndrome in children with cancer. Pediatr Blood Cancer 2007; 48(2):152–9.

35. Bartynski WS, Boardman JF. Distinct imaging patterns and lesion distribution in posterior reversible encephalopathy syndrome. AJNR Am J Neuroradiol 2007;28(7):1320–7.

36. McKinney AM, Short J, Truwit CL, et al. Posterior reversible encephalopathy syndrome: incidence of atypical regions of involvement and imaging findings. AJR Am J Roentgenol 2007;189(4): 904–12.

37. Pande AR, Ando K, Ishikura R, et al. Clinicoradiological factors influencing the reversibility of posterior reversible encephalopathy syndrome: a multicenter study. Radiat Med 2006;24(10): 659–68.

38. Ishikura K, Ikeda M, Hamasaki Y, et al. Posterior reversible encephalopathy syndrome in children: its high prevalence and more extensive imaging findings. Am J Kidney Dis 2006;48(2):231–8.

39. Lee BE, Davies HD. Aseptic meningitis. Curr Opin Infect Dis 2007;20(3):272–7.

40. Saezllorens X, McCrackenjr G. Bacterial meningitis in children. Lancet 2003;361(9375):2139–48.

41. Agrawal S, Nadel S. Acute bacterial meningitis in infants and children: epidemiology and management. Paediatr Drugs 2011;13(6):385–400.

42. Curtis S, Stobart K, Vandermeer B, et al. Clinical features suggestive of meningitis in children: a systematic review of prospective data. Pediatrics 2010;126(5):952–60.

43. Schuchat A, Robinson K, Wenger JD, et al. Bacterial meningitis in the United States in 1995. Active Surveillance Team. N Engl J Med 1997;337(14): 970–6.

44. Stockmann C, Ampofo K, Byington CL, et al. Pneumococcal meningitis in children: epidemiology, serotypes, and outcomes from 1997-2010 in Utah. Pediatrics 2013;132(3):421–8.

45. Gallagher RM, Gross CW, Phillips CD. Suppurative intracranial complications of sinusitis. Laryngoscope 1998;108(11 Pt 1):1635–42.

46. Luntz M, Brodsky A, Nusem S, et al. Acute mastoiditis–the antibiotic era: a multicenter study. Int J Pediatr Otorhinolaryngol 2001;57(1):1–9.

47. Bonsu BK, Harper MB. Differentiating acute bacterial meningitis from acute viral meningitis among children with cerebrospinal fluid pleocytosis. Pediatr Infect Dis J 2004;23(6):511–7.

48. Neurodiagnostic evaluation of the child with a simple febrile seizure. Pediatrics 2011;127(2):389–94.

49. Nigrovic LE, Malley R, Macias CG, et al. Effect of antibiotic pretreatment on cerebrospinal fluid profiles of children with bacterial meningitis. Pediatrics 2008;122(4):726–30.

50. Upadhyayula S. Question 2 is there a role for MRI as an adjunct for diagnosing bacterial meningitis? Arch Dis Child 2013;98(5):388–90.

51. Nickerson JP, Richner B, Santy K, et al. Neuroimaging of pediatric intracranial infection–part 1: techniques and bacterial infections. J Neuroimaging 2012;22(2):e42–51.

52. Parmar H, Ibrahim M. Pediatric intracranial infections. Neuroimaging Clin N Am 2012;22(4): 707–25.

53. Pienaar M, Andronikou S, van Toorn R. MRI to demonstrate diagnostic features and complications of TBM not seen with CT. Childs Nerv Syst 2009;25(8):941–7.

54. Weingarten L, Enarson P, Klassen T. Encephalitis. Pediatr Emerg Care 2013;29(2):235–41 [quiz: 242–4].

55. Simon DW, Da Silva YS, Zuccoli G, et al. Acute encephalitis. Crit Care Clin 2013;29(2):259–77.

56. Gable MS, Sheriff H, Dalmau J, et al. The frequency of autoimmune N-methyl-D-aspartate receptor encephalitis surpasses that of individual viral etiologies in young individuals enrolled in the California Encephalitis Project. Clin Infect Dis 2012;54(7):899–904.

57. Christie LJ, Honarmand S, Talkington DF, et al. Pediatric encephalitis: what is the role of Mycoplasma pneumoniae? Pediatrics 2007;120(2):305–13.

58. Tenembaum S, Chitnis T, Ness J, et al. Acute disseminated encephalomyelitis. Neurology 2007; 68(16 Suppl 2):S23–36.

59. Florance NR, Davis RL, Lam C, et al. Anti-N-methyl-D-aspartate receptor (NMDAR) encephalitis in children and adolescents. Ann Neurol 2009; 66(1):11–8.

60. Menge T, Hemmer B, Nessler S, et al. Acute disseminated encephalomyelitis: an update. Arch Neurol 2005;62(11):1673–80.

61. Koelfen W, Freund M, Guckel F, et al. MRI of encephalitis in children: comparison of CT and MRI in the acute stage with long-term follow-up. Neuroradiology 1996;38(1):73–9.

62. McCabe K, Tyler K, Tanabe J. Diffusion-weighted MRI abnormalities as a clue to the diagnosis of herpes simplex encephalitis. Neurology 2003;61(7):1015–6.

63. Crawford JR. Advances in pediatric neurovirology. Curr Neurol Neurosci Rep 2010;10(2):147–54.

64. Weil AA, Glaser CA, Amad Z, et al. Patients with suspected herpes simplex encephalitis: rethinking an initial negative polymerase chain reaction result. Clin Infect Dis 2002;34(8):1154–7.

65. Vossough A, Zimmerman RA, Bilaniuk LT, et al. Imaging findings of neonatal herpes simplex virus type 2 encephalitis. Neuroradiology 2008;50(4): 355–66.

66. Beattie GC, Glaser CA, Sheriff H, et al. Encephalitis with thalamic and basal ganglia abnormalities: etiologies, neuroimaging, and potential role of respiratory viruses. Clin Infect Dis 2013;56(6): 825–32.

67. Marin SE, Callen DJ. The magnetic resonance imaging appearance of monophasic acute disseminated encephalomyelitis: an update post application of the 2007 consensus criteria. Neuroimaging Clin N Am 2013;23(2):245–66.

68. Tunkel AR, Glaser CA, Bloch KC, et al. The management of encephalitis: clinical practice guidelines by the Infectious Diseases Society of America. Clin Infect Dis 2008;47(3):303–27.

69. Shachor-Meyouhas Y, Bar-Joseph G, Guilburd JN, et al. Brain abscess in children - epidemiology, predisposing factors and management in the modern medicine era. Acta Paediatr 2010;99(8):1163–7.

70. Sharma R, Mohandas K, Cooke RP. Intracranial abscesses: changes in epidemiology and management over five decades in Merseyside. Infection 2009;37(1):39–43.

71. Felsenstein S, Williams B, Shingadia D, et al. Clinical and microbiologic features guiding treatment recommendations for brain abscesses in children. Pediatr Infect Dis J 2013;32(2):129–35.

72. Menon S, Bharadwaj R, Chowdhary A, et al. Current epidemiology of intracranial abscesses: a prospective 5 year study. J Med Microbiol 2008;57(Pt 10):1259–68.

73. Clayman GL, Adams GL, Paugh DR, et al. Intracranial complications of paranasal sinusitis: a combined institutional review. Laryngoscope 1991; 101(3):234–9.

74. Chowdhry SA, Cohen AR. Citrobacter brain abscesses in neonates: early surgical intervention and review of the literature. Childs Nerv Syst 2012;28(10):1715–22.

75. Saez-Llorens X. Brain abscess in children. Semin Pediatr Infect Dis 2003;14(2):108–14.

76. Gaskill SJaM, Marlin AE. Brain abscesses and encephalitis. In: Albright AL, Pollack IF, Adelson PD, editors. Principles and practice of pediatric neurosurgery. New York: Thieme; 2008. p. 1162–81.

77. Osborn AG. Abscess. Osborn's brain: imaging, pathology, and anatomy. Manitoba (Canada): Amirsys; 2013. p. 311–7.

78. Moorthy RK, Rajshekhar V. Management of brain abscess: an overview. Neurosurg Focus 2008; 24(6):E3.

79. Jim KK, Brouwer MC, van der Ende A, et al. Subdural empyema in bacterial meningitis. Neurology 2012;79(21):2133–9.

80. Legrand M, Roujeau T, Meyer P, et al. Paediatric intracranial empyema: differences according to age. Eur J Pediatr 2009;168(10):1235–41.

81. Germiller JA, Monin DL, Sparano AM, et al. Intracranial complications of sinusitis in children and adolescents and their outcomes. Arch Otolaryngol Head Neck Surg 2006;132(9):969–76.

82. Osborn MK, Steinberg JP. Subdural empyema and other suppurative complications of paranasal sinusitis. Lancet Infect Dis 2007;7(1):62–7.

83. Pradilla G, Ardila GP, Hsu W, et al. Epidural abscesses of the CNS. Lancet Neurol 2009;8(3): 292–300.

84. Cochrane DD, Price A, Dobson S. Intracranial epidural and subdural infections. In: Albright AL, Pollack IF, Adelson PD, editors. Principles and

practice of pediatric neurosurgery. New York: Thieme; 2008. p. 1148–61.

85. Younis RT, Anand VK, Davidson B. The role of computed tomography and magnetic resonance imaging in patients with sinusitis with complications. Laryngoscope 2002;112(2):224–9.

86. Wong AM, Zimmerman RA, Simon EM, et al. Diffusion-weighted MR imaging of subdural empyemas in children. AJNR Am J Neuroradiol 2004;25(6): 1016–21.

87. Leys D, Destee A, Petit H, et al. Management of subdural intracranial empyemas should not always require surgery. J Neurol Neurosurg Psychiatry 1986;49(6):635–9.

88. Nathoo N, Nadvi SS, van Dellen JR, et al. Intracranial subdural empyemas in the era of computed tomography: a review of 699 cases. Neurosurgery 1999;44(3):529–35 [discussion: 535–6].

89. Auletta JJ, John CC. Spinal epidural abscesses in children: a 15-year experience and review of the literature. Clin Infect Dis 2001;32(1):9–16.

90. Darouiche RO, Hamill RJ, Greenberg SB, et al. Bacterial spinal epidural abscess. Review of 43 cases and literature survey. Medicine 1992;71(6):369–85.

91. Sadato N, Numaguchi Y, Rigamonti D, et al. Spinal epidural abscess with gadolinium-enhanced MRI: serial follow-up studies and clinical correlations. Neuroradiology 1994;36(1):44–8.

92. Eastwood JD, Vollmer RT, Provenzale JM. Diffusion-weighted imaging in a patient with vertebral and epidural abscesses. AJNR Am J Neuroradiol 2002;23(3):496–8.

93. Curry WT Jr, Hoh BL, Amin-Hanjani S, et al. Spinal epidural abscess: clinical presentation, management, and outcome. Surg Neurol 2005;63(4): 364–71 [discussion: 371].

94. Soehle M, Wallenfang T. Spinal epidural abscesses: clinical manifestations, prognostic factors, and outcomes. Neurosurgery 2002;51(1): 79–85 [discussion: 86–7].

95. Fernandez M, Carrol CL, Baker CJ. Discitis and vertebral osteomyelitis in children: an 18-year review. Pediatrics 2000;105(6):1299–304.

96. Fucs PM, Meves R, Yamada HH. Spinal infections in children: a review. Int Orthop 2012; 36(2):387–95.

97. Zimmerli W. Vertebral osteomyelitis. N Engl J Med 2010;362(11):1022–9.

98. Offiah AC. Acute osteomyelitis, septic arthritis and discitis: differences between neonates and older children. Eur J Radiol 2006;60(2):221–32.

99. Hedlund G, Bale JF, Barkovich AJ. Infections of the developing and mature nervous system. Pediatric neuroimaging. 5th edition. Philadelphia: Lippincott; 2012.

100. Lernout C, Haas H, Rubio A, et al. Pediatric intervertebral disk calcification in childhood: three case reports and review of literature. Childs Nerv Syst 2009;25(8):1019–23.

101. Ring D, Johnston CE 2nd, Wenger DR. Pyogenic infectious spondylitis in children: the convergence of discitis and vertebral osteomyelitis. J Pediatr Orthop 1995;15(5):652–60.

102. Brown R, Hussain M, McHugh K, et al. Discitis in young children. J Bone Joint Surg Am 2001;83(1): 106–11.

103. Pidcock FS, Krishnan C, Crawford TO, et al. Acute transverse myelitis in childhood: center-based analysis of 47 cases. Neurology 2007;68(18): 1474–80.

104. Alper G, Petropoulou KA, Fitz CR, et al. Idiopathic acute transverse myelitis in children: an analysis and discussion of MRI findings. Mult Scler 2011; 17(1):74–80.

105. Lahat E, Pillar G, Ravid S, et al. Rapid recovery from transverse myelopathy in children treated with methylprednisolone. Pediatr Neurol 1998; 19(4):279–82.

106. Yiu EM, Kornberg AJ, Ryan MM, et al. Acute transverse myelitis and acute disseminated encephalomyelitis in childhood: spectrum or separate entities? J Child Neurol 2009;24(3):287–96.

107. Choi KH, Lee KS, Chung SO, et al. Idiopathic transverse myelitis: MR characteristics. AJNR Am J Neuroradiol 1996;17(6):1151–60.

108. Thomas T, Branson HM. Childhood transverse myelitis and its mimics. Neuroimaging Clin N Am 2013;23(2):267–78.

109. Jeffery DR, Mandler RN, Davis LE. Transverse myelitis. Retrospective analysis of 33 cases, with differentiation of cases associated with multiple sclerosis and parainfectious events. Arch Neurol 1993;50(5):532–5.

110. Scott TF, Bhagavatula K, Snyder PJ, et al. Transverse myelitis. Comparison with spinal cord presentations of multiple sclerosis. Neurology 1998; 50(2):429–33.

111. Pittock SJ, Lucchinetti CF. Inflammatory transverse myelitis: evolving concepts. Curr Opin Neurol 2006;19(4):362–8.

112. Devos D, Magot A, Perrier-Boeswillwald J, et al. Guillain-Barre syndrome during childhood: particular clinical and electrophysiological features. Muscle Nerve 2013;48(2):247–51.

113. Ryan MM. Pediatric Guillain-Barré syndrome. Curr Opin Pediatr 2013;25(6):689–93.

114. Rantala H, Uhari M, Niemela M. Occurrence, clinical manifestations, and prognosis of Guillain-Barre syndrome. Arch Dis Child 1991;66(6):706–8 [discussion: 708–9].

115. Zuccoli G, Panigrahy A, Bailey A, et al. Redefining the Guillain-Barre spectrum in children: neuroimaging findings of cranial nerve involvement. AJNR Am J Neuroradiol 2011;32(4):639–42.

116. Gorson KC, Ropper AH, Muriello MA, et al. Prospective evaluation of MRI lumbosacral nerve root enhancement in acute Guillain-Barre syndrome. Neurology 1996;47(3):813–7.

117. Mulkey SB, Glasier CM, El-Nabbout B, et al. Nerve root enhancement on spinal MRI in pediatric Guillain-Barre syndrome. Pediatr Neurol 2010; 43(4):263–9.

118. Nelson JD. Acute osteomyelitis in children. Infect Dis Clin North Am 1990;4(3):513–22.

119. Goergens ED, McEvoy A, Watson M, et al. Acute osteomyelitis and septic arthritis in children. J Paediatr Child Health 2005;41(1–2):59–62.

120. Gutierrez K. Bone and joint infections in children. Pediatr Clin North Am 2005;52(3):779–94, vi.

121. Schuppen J, Doorn MAC, Rijn R. Childhood osteomyelitis: imaging characteristics. Insights Imaging 2012;3(5):519–33.

122. Pineda C, Espinosa R, Pena A. Radiographic imaging in osteomyelitis: the role of plain radiography, computed tomography, ultrasonography, magnetic resonance imaging, and scintigraphy. Semin Plast Surg 2009;23(2):80–9.

123. De Boeck H. Osteomyelitis and septic arthritis in children. Acta Orthop Belg 2005;71(5):505–15.

124. Andersson RE, Hugander A, Ravn H, et al. Repeated clinical and laboratory examinations in patients with an equivocal diagnosis of appendicitis. World J Surg 2000;24(4):479–85 [discussion: 485].

125. Callahan MJ, Rodriguez DP, Taylor GA. CT of appendicitis in children. Radiology 2002;224(2): 325–32.

126. Lessin MS, Chan M, Catallozzi M, et al. Selective use of ultrasonography for acute appendicitis in children. Am J Surg 1999;177(3):193–6.

127. Hormann M, Paya K, Eibenberger K, et al. MR imaging in children with nonperforated acute appendicitis: value of unenhanced MR imaging in sonographically selected cases. AJR Am J Roentgenol 1998;171(2):467–70.

128. Reulecke BC, Erker CG, Fiedler BJ, et al. Brain tumors in children: initial symptoms and their influence on the time span between symptom onset and diagnosis. J Child Neurol 2008;23(2):178–83.

129. Mehta V, Chapman A, McNeely PD, et al. Latency between symptom onset and diagnosis of pediatric brain tumors: an Eastern Canadian geographic study. Neurosurgery 2002;51(2):365–72 [discussion: 372–3].

130. Flores LE, Williams DL, Bell BA, et al. Delay in the diagnosis of pediatric brain tumors. Am J Dis Child 1986;140(7):684–6.

131. Medina LS, Kuntz KM, Pomeroy S. Children with headache suspected of having a brain tumor: a cost-effectiveness analysis of diagnostic strategies. Pediatrics 2001;108(2):255–63.

132. Borja MJ, Plaza MJ, Altman N, et al. Conventional and advanced MRI features of pediatric intracranial tumors: supratentorial tumors. AJR Am J Roentgenol 2013;200(5):W483–503.

133. Plaza MJ, Borja MJ, Altman N, et al. Conventional and advanced MRI features of pediatric intracranial tumors: posterior fossa and suprasellar tumors. AJR Am J Roentgenol 2013;200(5):1115–24.

134. Koral K, Zhang S, Gargan L, et al. Diffusion MRI improves the accuracy of preoperative diagnosis of common pediatric cerebellar tumors among reviewers with different experience levels. AJNR Am J Neuroradiol 2013;34(12):2360–5.

135. Klein SL, Sanford RA, Muhlbauer MS. Pediatric spinal epidural metastases. J Neurosurg 1991;74(1): 70–5.

136. Conrad EU 3rd, Olszewski AD, Berger M, et al. Pediatric spine tumors with spinal cord compromise. J Pediatr Orthop 1992;12(4):454–60.

137. Cole JS, Patchell RA. Metastatic epidural spinal cord compression. Lancet Neurol 2008;7(5): 459–66.

138. Byrne TN. Spinal cord compression from epidural metastases. N Engl J Med 1992;327(9):614–9.

139. Lewis DW, Packer RJ, Raney B, et al. Incidence, presentation, and outcome of spinal cord disease in children with systemic cancer. Pediatrics 1986; 78(3):438–43.

140. Pollono D, Tomarchia S, Drut R, et al. Spinal cord compression: a review of 70 pediatric patients. Pediatr Hematol Oncol 2003;20(6):457–66.

141. De Bernardi B, Pianca C, Pistamiglio P, et al. Neuroblastoma with symptomatic spinal cord compression at diagnosis: treatment and results with 76 cases. J Clin Oncol 2001;19(1):183–90.

142. Hsu W, Jallo GI. Pediatric spinal tumors. Handb Clin Neurol 2013;112:959–65.

143. Constantini S, Miller DC, Allen JC, et al. Radical excision of intramedullary spinal cord tumors: surgical morbidity and long-term follow-up evaluation in 164 children and young adults. J Neurosurg 2000;93(2 Suppl):183–93.

144. Smith AB, Soderlund KA, Rushing EJ, et al. Radiologic-pathologic correlation of pediatric and adolescent spinal neoplasms: Part 1, intramedullary spinal neoplasms. AJR Am J Roentgenol 2012;198(1):34–43.

145. Reilly CW. Pediatric spine trauma. J Bone Joint Surg Am 2007;89(Suppl 1):98–107.

146. Carreon LY, Glassman SD, Campbell MJ. Pediatric spine fractures: a review of 137 hospital admissions. J Spinal Disord Tech 2004;17(6):477–82.

147. Li Y, Glotzbecker MP, Hedequist D, et al. Pediatric spinal trauma. Trauma 2011;14(1):82–96.

148. McCall T, Fassett D, Brockmeyer D. Cervical spine trauma in children: a review. Neurosurg Focus 2006;20(2):E5.

149. Pang D. Spinal cord injury without radiographic abnormality in children, 2 decades later. Neurosurgery 2004;55(6):1325–43.
150. Flynn JM, Closkey RF, Mahboubi S, et al. Role of magnetic resonance imaging in the assessment of pediatric cervical spine injuries. J Pediatr Orthop 2002;22(5):573–7.
151. Rozzelle CJ, Aarabi B, Dhall SS, et al. Spinal cord injury without radiographic abnormality (SCIWORA). Neurosurgery 2013;72(Suppl 2): 227–33.
152. Frank JB, Lim CK, Flynn JM, et al. The efficacy of magnetic resonance imaging in pediatric cervical spine clearance. Spine 2002;27(11):1176–9.

Index

Note: Page numbers of article titles are in **boldface** type.

Magn Reson Imaging Clin N Am 24 (2016) 481–484
http://dx.doi.org/10.1016/S1064-9689(16)30010-1
1064-9689/16/$ – see front matter © 2016 Elsevier Inc. All rights reserved.